Exposure

Also by Wim Hof

The Wim Hof Method

The Way of the Iceman

Becoming the Iceman

Exposure
The Life of the Iceman in Photos

How an Outlier's Journey Illuminates the
Extremes of Power, Vitality, and Possibility

Wim Hof

Photography by Henny Boogert

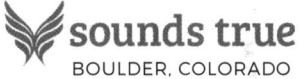

sounds true
BOULDER, COLORADO

Sounds True
Boulder, CO

Text © 2024 Wim Hof

Cover and interior photographs
© 2024 Henny Boogert

This book is not intended as a substitute for the medical recommendations of physicians, mental health professionals, or other health-care providers. Rather, it is intended to offer information to help the reader cooperate with physicians, mental health professionals, and health-care providers in a mutual quest for optimal well-being.

Do not practice the method during pregnancy or if you are epileptic. People with cardiovascular, respiratory, or any other health conditions should always consult a medical professional before starting the Wim Hof Method®.

The cold is a powerful force, and extreme cold can be a shock to your body. We strongly advise to start slowly and gradually build up exposure. If not practiced responsibly, there is risk of hypothermia. The breathing exercises in this book can likewise have strong physiological effects and must be practiced as instructed. Always perform them in a safe environment, sitting or lying down. Never practice the Wim Hof Method breathing exercises before or during diving, driving, swimming, taking a bath, or in any other circumstance where loss of consciousness could result in bodily harm. Wim Hof Method breathing may cause tingling sensations, a ringing in the ears, and/or lightheadedness. These are normal responses and are no cause for alarm. If you faint, however, you have gone too far, and should take it more slowly next time. It is not necessary to take the method to extremes to receive its benefits. Listen to the signals from your body and never force any of the practices of the Wim Hof Method.

Neither the author nor Sounds True make any representations, warranties, or covenants as to fitness or suitability of the Wim Hof Cold Therapy Method for any particular purpose or personal situation.

Published 2024

Cover and jacket design by Rachael Murray
Book design by Meredith Jarrett

Printed in China

BK06773

Library of Congress Cataloging-in-
   Publication Data
Names: Hof, Wim, 1959- author. | Boogert,
   Henny, 1962- photographer.
Title: Exposure: how an outlier's journey
   illuminates the extremes of power,
   vitality, and possibility / Wim Hof ;
   photography by Henny Boogert.
Description: Boulder, CO : Sounds True,
   2024.
Identifiers: LCCN 2023056226 (print)
   | LCCN 2023056227 (ebook) | ISBN
   9781649631688 (hardcover) | ISBN
   9781649631695 (ebook)
Subjects: LCSH: Hof, Wim,
   1959---Philosophy. | Daredevils--
   Netherlands--Psychology. | Cold--
   Physiological effect. | Mind and body. |
   Portrait photography.
Classification: LCC GV1839.H64 A3 2024
   (print) | LCC GV1839.H64 (ebook) |
DDC 612/.014465--dc23/eng/20240415
LC record available at https://lccn.loc.
   gov/2023056226
LC ebook record available at https://lccn.
   loc.gov/2023056227

The feats included in the following pages are not related to the Wim Hof Method protocol. These are extreme acts performed by a highly trained individual. Please speak with a professional whenever investigating and engaging in new modalities.

If you wish to learn more about the Wim Hof Method, please refer to the website and strictly follow the safety guidelines.

The Wim Hof Method breathing can affect motor control and, in rare cases, lead to loss of consciousness. Always sit or lie down when practicing the techniques. **Never practice the Wim Hof Method breathing exercises in or near bodies of water—that includes before or during diving, swimming, or taking a bath—piloting a vehicle**, or in any other situation where loss of consciousness could result in bodily harm.

Additionally, the cold is a powerful force, and extreme cold can be a shock to your body. We strongly advise to start slowly and gradually build up exposure. Be sure to follow the proper cold exposure protocol.

Introduction

WITHIN THESE PAGES ARE SOME of the moments, now frozen in time, that have made up my life.

Always a bit of an outcast, I sought to understand the Soul. To live life unconditionally, uninhibited, open to whatever came my way. It can be unforgiving terrain but glorious all the same. Looking back through these images, I would never have thought I would be where I am now. I had no reference point. I always just followed my feeling. In turn, life has taken me on an unforeseen journey, wandering like a river, with unexpected twists and turns, through valleys and mountaintops.

I'm very fortunate to have a visual record of some of these pivotal seasons and moments in my life, thanks to my friend Henny. We met in a squat in Amsterdam when he was a budding photographer who needed a subject for his portfolio, and I was the guy always doing crazy stuff! Two completely different personalities united by a common goal . . . freedom. It was an instant friendship. Henny challenged me to be my best, and having him with me made me challenge myself to get the best out of myself. It was a specific dynamic. Unique. Henny has been there through many of the challenges I put my mind and body through, photographing and documenting a life lived on the outskirts of society—the early years of fatherhood, the adventures in the mountains, the world records, the scientific triumphs.

My life, as you will see in this photo book, has not been straightforward. I wasn't able to see around corners in life. I am no wizard. I'm just an ordinary guy following his feeling, but I always had faith and belief in myself, in living every moment fully no matter what was in front of me. It is as simple as that. That's always been the heart of my method. Following your gut and feelings isn't a magic bullet that makes everything easy, but it takes you on a path that unfurls you like a beautiful piece of nature.

You become one with it. Whatever form it takes. My wish is for you to live life fully, no matter what is in front of you. To live life with heart and soul and a good laugh. You see, we are all unique and have the ability to live huge. I didn't come from much, but my enduring belief in life got me here. Living life every day with playfulness, attention, and soul, while holding true to my belief that we are so much more than we think. If it has shown me anything, it is that life happens in a wondrous moment, beyond thoughts. Spontaneous being, that is where your ultimate potential resides.

This is a book for the dreamer. For the person who wants to discover new frontiers. Who knows there is something more not only out there but in here, in their own body and mind. It is for the many, many people who have found joy and strength in practicing my method for years. It is for first-timers who still shiver at the idea of jumping into a frozen lake or even just taking a cold shower. It is for every curious person in between. You're capable of so much more than you know. Than what you give yourself credit for.

That doesn't mean you should go free solo a mountain or run a half marathon barefoot in the arctic circle. I've done a lot of crazy things that no one else should do. Reaching your full potential isn't about pushing the extreme to your breaking point. It's more than just cold plunges. It's about going inward. About tapping into the part of you that's been buried. The part where you allow feeling and intuition to guide you. Where you trust yourself and your connection to the earth.

May you be inspired by the photos, poetry, and stories in this book. I took life on as something to be discovered. I had to go out there and experience it all. No thinking, just being. I went into the extremes, pushing past many perceived boundaries to bring you the simplest of truths. We can do more than we think! Life can be experienced by anyone, simply and without having to complicate it. It is all as nature provided, right there waiting.

Know that you are incredible, just as you are, a piece of beautiful nature. Cherish your mind, live fully and openly with all your heart, and let us shine bright like stars through our unrelenting radiating Soul.

There we are, here we go.

No ego, we go.

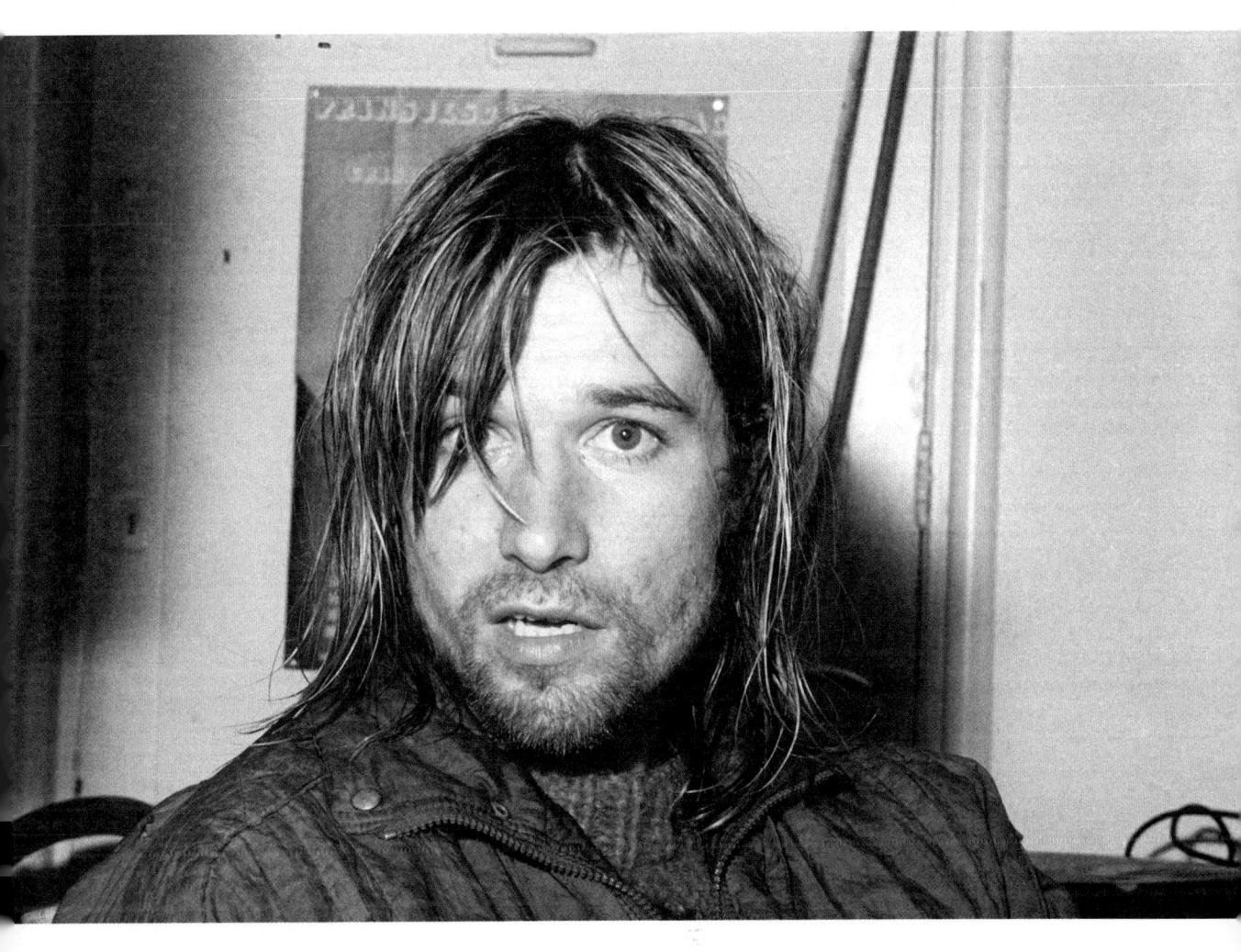

A Note from Henny

I FIRST MET WIM IN a squat in Amsterdam Zuid (south) in the 1980s. We had occupied a former orphanage, and he was already living there when I moved in. You would usually see him sitting in the yard meditating, wearing nothing but a pair of undies, even in the snow. Or nothing at all! He could sit there and stare for hours with his eyes drifting away, softly om-ing. His wife was living in the squat, too. I believe they had had one or two young kids who were born in the squat during that time.

One day, my friend and I decided to have a chat with him. Wim immediately introduced us to some karate exercises and yoga. No one was busy with yoga at the time, so this was all new to us. But Wim was already weaving this into a lifestyle. He was always communicating with everybody, playing the guitar . . . he was just so full of life. Sometimes I'd bump into him

in the park nearby, where he would be meditating or practicing yoga. In the winter, when the pond was frozen, he would make a hole in the ice and then enter the water through it, in nothing but his trunks. At some point, I saw him making two holes with a meter or so in between, and he went from one to the other. Underneath the ice. These were his first steps.

We gradually started doing more things together. We became kind of friends, but more action-minded friends. You wouldn't see us sitting down and having a chat over tea. It seemed something was always happening when we spent time together. That's when I started taking pictures of him. I was a photography student at Rietveld Academie, in Amsterdam, so I was always walking around with a camera. And I sure did find Wim an interesting motif!

I started photographing Wim more frequently in Spain. Wim's wife was Spanish. Many times we'd visit her parents in Pamplona and spend time with some friends of hers living at an abandoned farm in the area, in the middle of nowhere. In yoga terms, Wim decided to make this place his ashram. He started inviting people from the Netherlands, including me. So we drove down to Spain by car, went swimming, climbing, even canyoning. We spent a lot of time there in the mid-1980s. All of the fun and excitement ended when back in Amsterdam our squat was evicted, and we each had to find new homes. Wim and Olaya decided to head to Spain, back to the farmhouse, and I moved south, about ten kilometers away. Although I was sad this part of my life was over, I was so thankful for the connection with Wim in my life then. I wished him well and went on my way.

And then a few years later, Wim appeared on my television screen in some footage broadcast by a local television station. The funny thing was, he was doing exactly the same thing that had caught my attention back in the squat years earlier. It was winter, and he was sitting in a local park in the ice. *So, he's still around*, it struck me. After the eviction, each of us had been going about our own lives and hadn't kept in contact. I was so excited to see him that I found out where he lived, got back in touch, and we continued right where we left off. It was as if no time had passed. We went to Spain, climbed some trees, swam in some lakes, went canyoning. Nothing had changed. I started photographing him again and following him around documenting the many travel outings he'd host for himself and others. We had plans to sell the pictures to papers and magazines, only no one wanted to pay for them.

But it turned out that Willibrord Frequin, a known reporter with one of the bigger local television stations, had seen the very footage I saw and decided they needed to film Wim. So they filmed Wim in the ice, swimming underneath the ice, while I photographed beside them. And that's when things started getting big and the Iceman was born. They started doing challenges with Wim, making him sit in a box full of ice or taking him to Lapland to swim long distances. Wim finally got the audience and attention he deserved. And I was there every step of the way with my camera. I even went with him under the ice in Lapland!

Over the years, I have taken thousands of shots of Wim from all angles and perspectives. We've been to the US, Iceland, Belgium, Germany, Poland, Spain, and France, and probably a few other places. As a photographer, what I find most fascinating about him is that he has this primal element. The way his body is built. Anatomically, everything fits together. He has some kind of a savage aura. But he's also tender, soft, and loving. I've always found the best way to appreciate Wim is in action. That's why many of my photographs catch him in a moment. It's through those actions and moments that you can truly see the power Wim yields, as well as the composure and grace he elicits. I hope these photos stir the same level of inspiration, awe, and possibility in you that I see every time I look at them.

HENNY BOOGERT

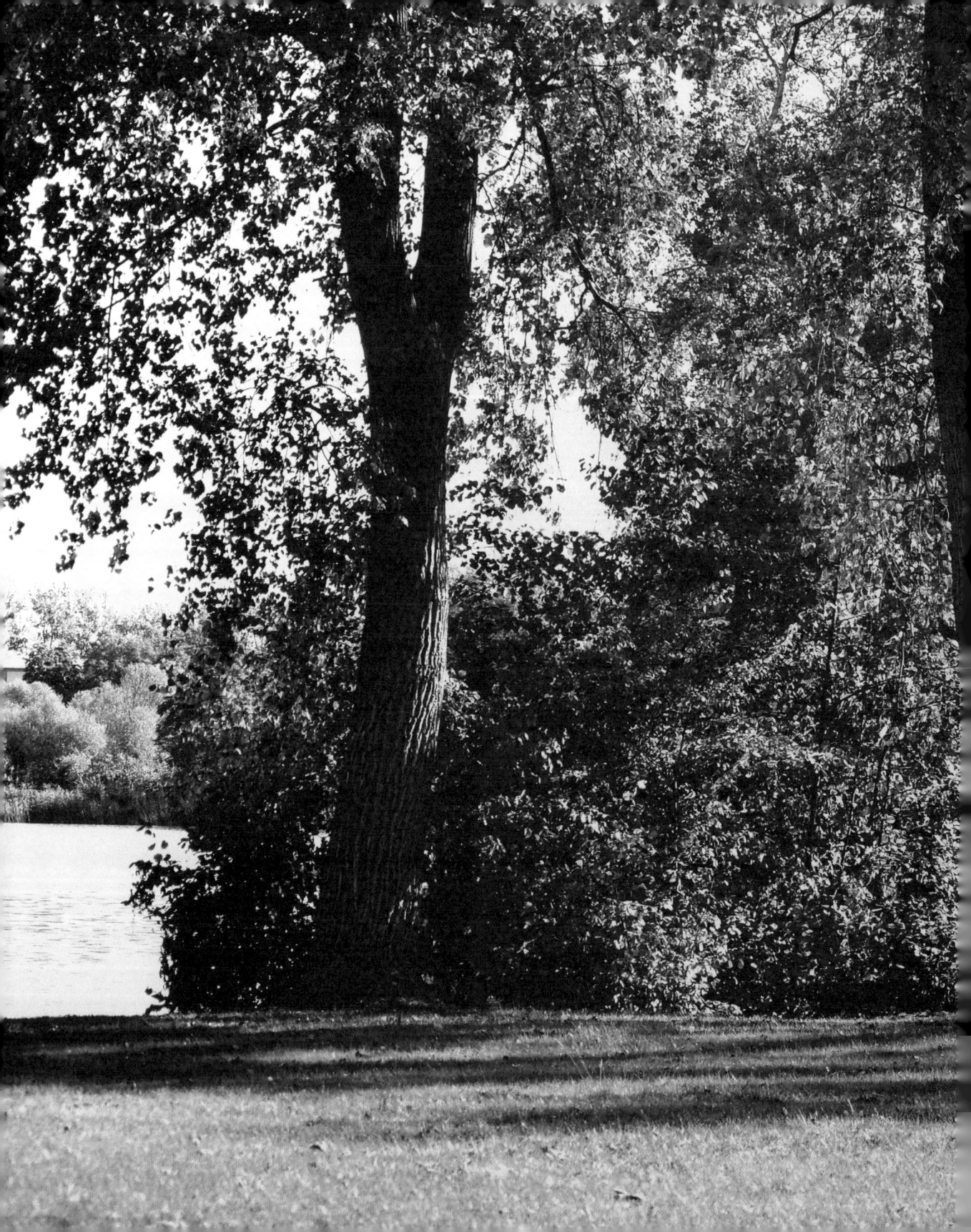

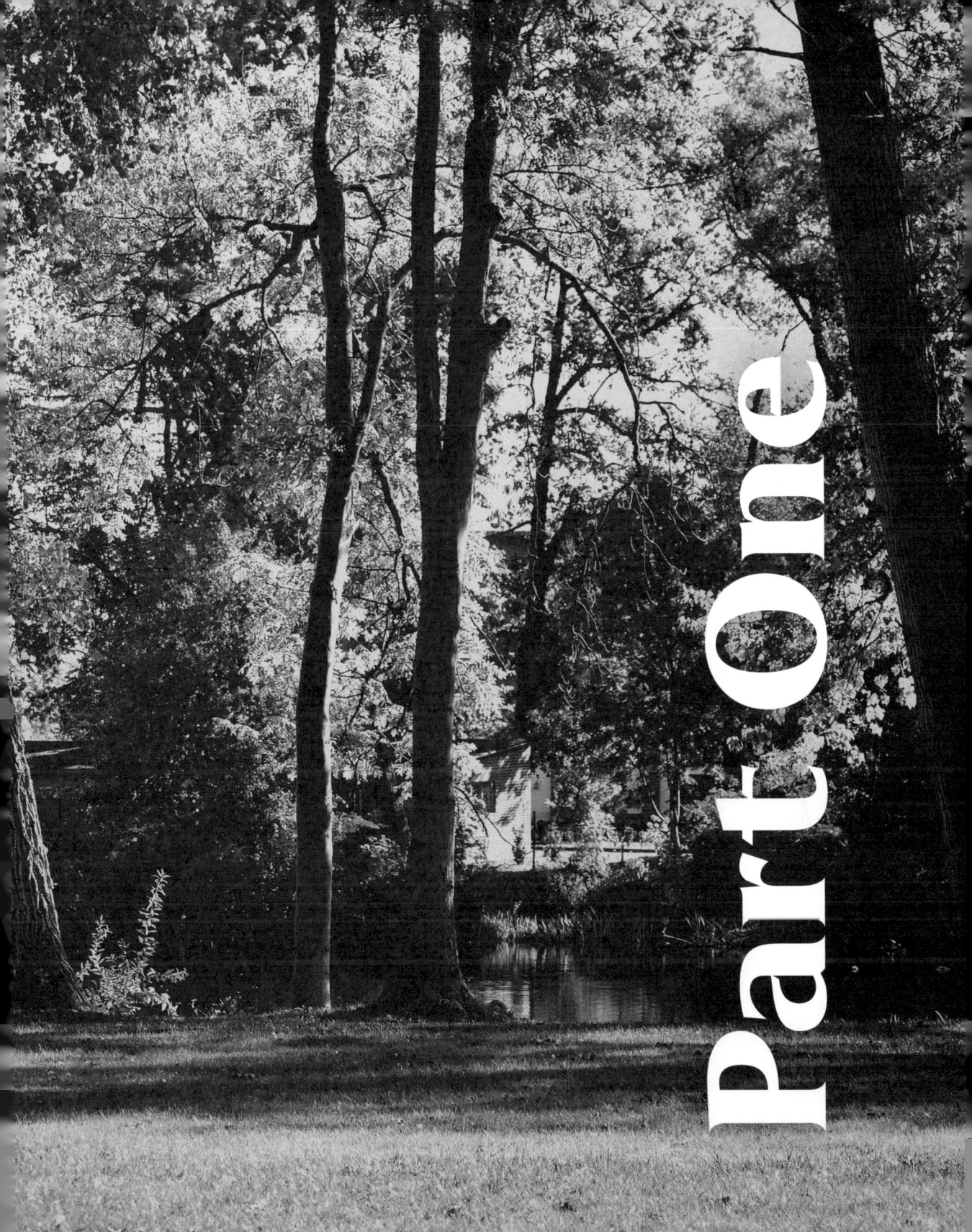

Part One

Revealing Parts

IN 1999, I RECEIVED MY first Guinness World Record in Paris. I sat for thirty minutes, "full body contact in ice," as they called it. This set off a frenzy of appearances around the world, and "the Iceman" was born. I was seen as a daredevil, an anomaly, but these extreme appearances are what led to the scientific discoveries that have since remapped our understanding of the natural capabilities of the human body and mind. Incredible how that all happened! For years I had practiced on my own in the lakes and canals of Amsterdam, a family man trying to make ends meet, and now there is a global movement even outside of the Wim Hof Method.

But I have had my fair share of light and darkness. As you will see in these pages, I have lived many lives. Not being locked into a nine-to-five daily routine, I followed my ideas, the drive to think freely, be free, and realize my dreams. That was always deeply ingrained in my psyche. It has always been a subcurrent and never left.

Looking back, you could say the squat set the course of my life. It was in that neighborhood that I had my first deep conscious encounter with the cold. I met Olaya there in 1980 and had two of our four children there. So much of my thinking was founded within those walls. We lived in freedom. Society was outside those walls. Inside we had space to think freely, without the normal pressures of daily life. That space for thought allowed for natural contemplations. I developed a discipline that was my liberation. The value of that became the foundation of all my philosophical goals. That was where my spiritual destiny sprouted, without me even knowing it. I just went with the flow of it all.

Those times were filled with a lot of idealism and created a founding land to build upon—a kind of heaven in a way. Still, as we were a growing family, when everyone at the squat was evicted, we decided to leave for Spain to build an ashram in the mountains, a place for Souls to meet and live creatively. We had hoped we could do this. But the dream was short-lived. Olaya's condition took a turn for the worse, so we packed up and returned to the Netherlands. That initiated one of the darker periods of my and Olaya's life. A heaven and a hell. From the idealism of the squat and the dream of the ashram to the reality of living in the real world with a small family and a wife who was getting deeper and deeper into the shadows, until she took her life in 1995.

Can you imagine the pain she was in? And I couldn't help her. And now here I was with four children and no idea of what to do. We were helpless. But I just kept going. I had to. It was a very dark period. The through line, the thread that held me together, was one of faith and discipline. Of facing the here and now with heart. The cold and the breathing enabled me to have enough energy to face life as it was, and it made me feel good. I would wake at four every morning to do my breathing. I would practice in the colder months in the lake, doing all my crazy exercises that helped me feel my body and the energy. This let me see through it all to the Soul of the moments right in front of me.

It's easy to succumb to what you think your reality is, to fall into the illusion of it all. The struggle. But I had no space for that. I had to take care of my kids. And I found that my discipline pulled me through.

I took on life! I used anything I could to explore my body and mind. In Amsterdam, I scaled the trees and kayaked in the harbor, climbed rock walls and dipped in icy waters. In the mountains and canyons of the Spanish Pyrenees, the abundance of nature provided me with a testing ground to push past my perceived limits and just bask in the beauty of it all. I'm not encouraging anyone to go to the extremes I did. It's imperative you listen to your body and mind and care for the limits that are right for you. Tuning into your innate energy holds the opportunity to crack you open in all the right ways.

Henny joined me on many of my adventures in Spain and Amsterdam. We lost contact for some years after that, but we picked up where we left off after he saw me on a local Amsterdam TV station doing my training in the cold. From there, he often joined me in the Pyrenees where I took groups to explore with me. We even made it into a couple of outdoor adventure magazines. These early years enabled me to act when opportunity came knocking. I was ready. I had been through it all, and it felt like the energy was ascending.

The Iceman was about to be born.

Getting into Utthita Utthana Padmasana.

Every day I would go to the park and do asanas. Discipline was my liberation. I was a young man but also very curious about everything I could do. I was very focused on that. I trained every day without a pretense of what to do, always following my feeling. It is that simple. I wasn't locked into a certain regime. I just kept at it, no matter what it was. If you keep a discipline, slowly but surely, the reward of that is huge.

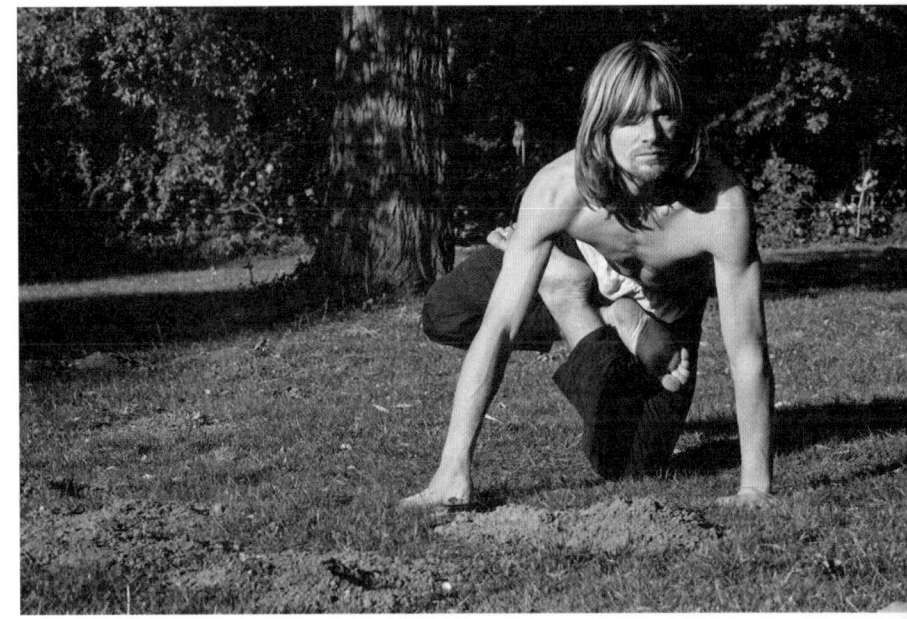

My discipline in the earlier years began with my fascination with Eastern thought. I stumbled across a yoga book in the local library in my hometown and began to make a practice out of the poses. It was about creating flow. Hatha yoga is about decluttering and removing blockages in the physical body. This has an amazing impact on the mind. Perfect!

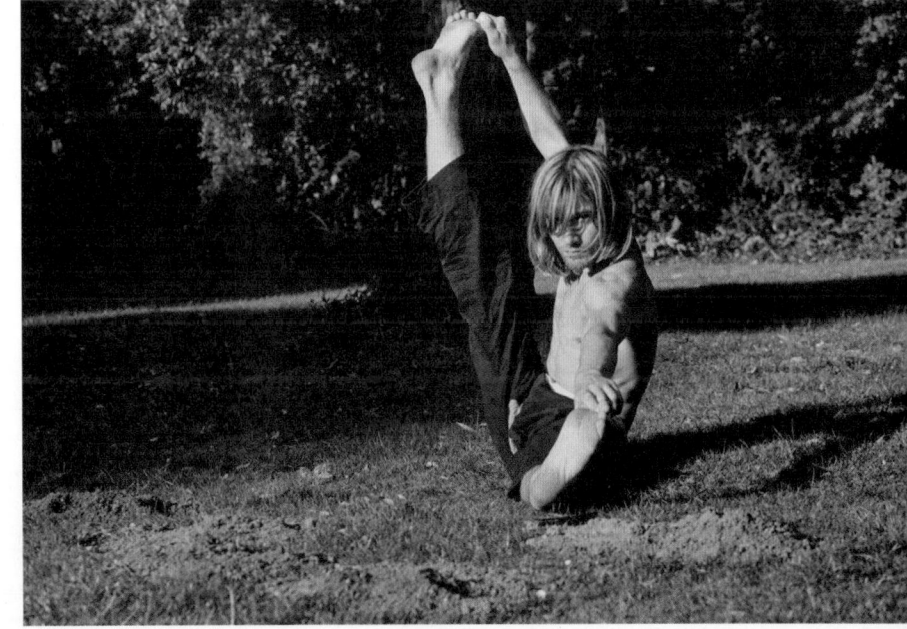

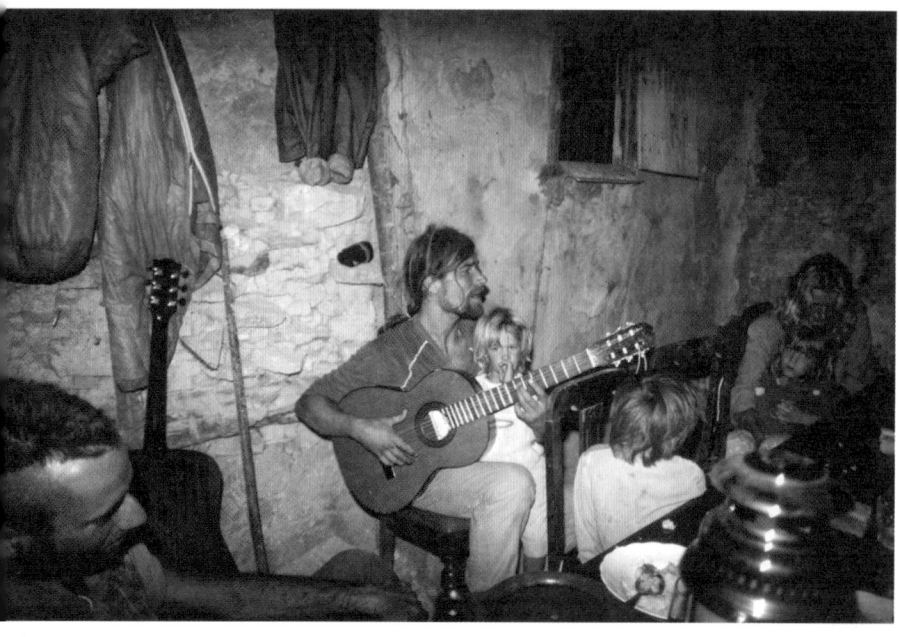

In the kitchen of the old farmhouse we rented, our little ashram. Enahm and Isa by my side.

In 1985, we left the squat in search of a place of our own. We headed for Spain with the dream of creating an ashram in the mountains. Inspired by our freethinking in the squat, we wanted to manifest it for ourselves. We wanted to revive an old farm and make it a community. Just like-minded people, living together, sharing, no individualism.

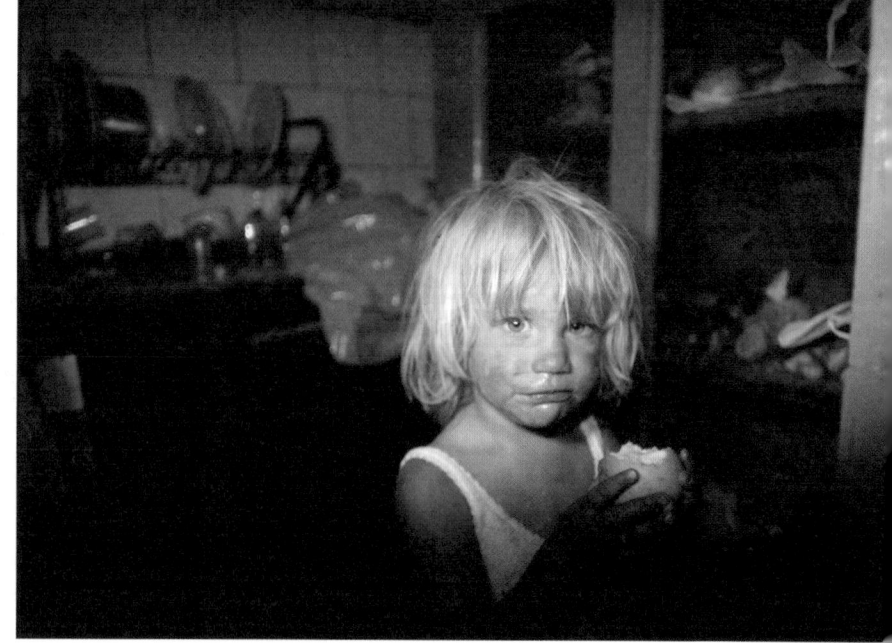

The innocence of children. Isa enjoying an apple in the farmhouse kitchen.

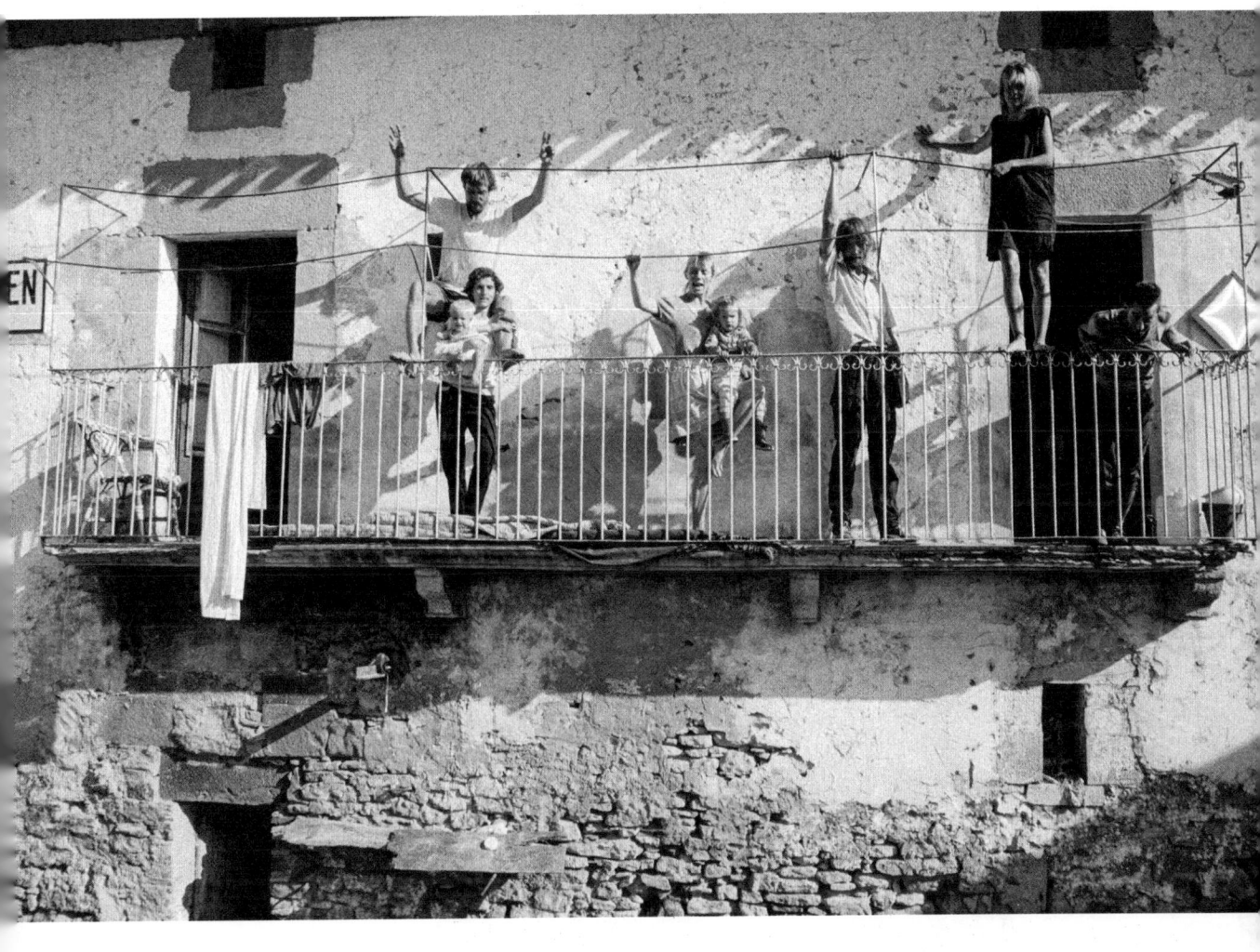

One of the few photos we have of Olaya.
Here holding baby Laura on the balcony.

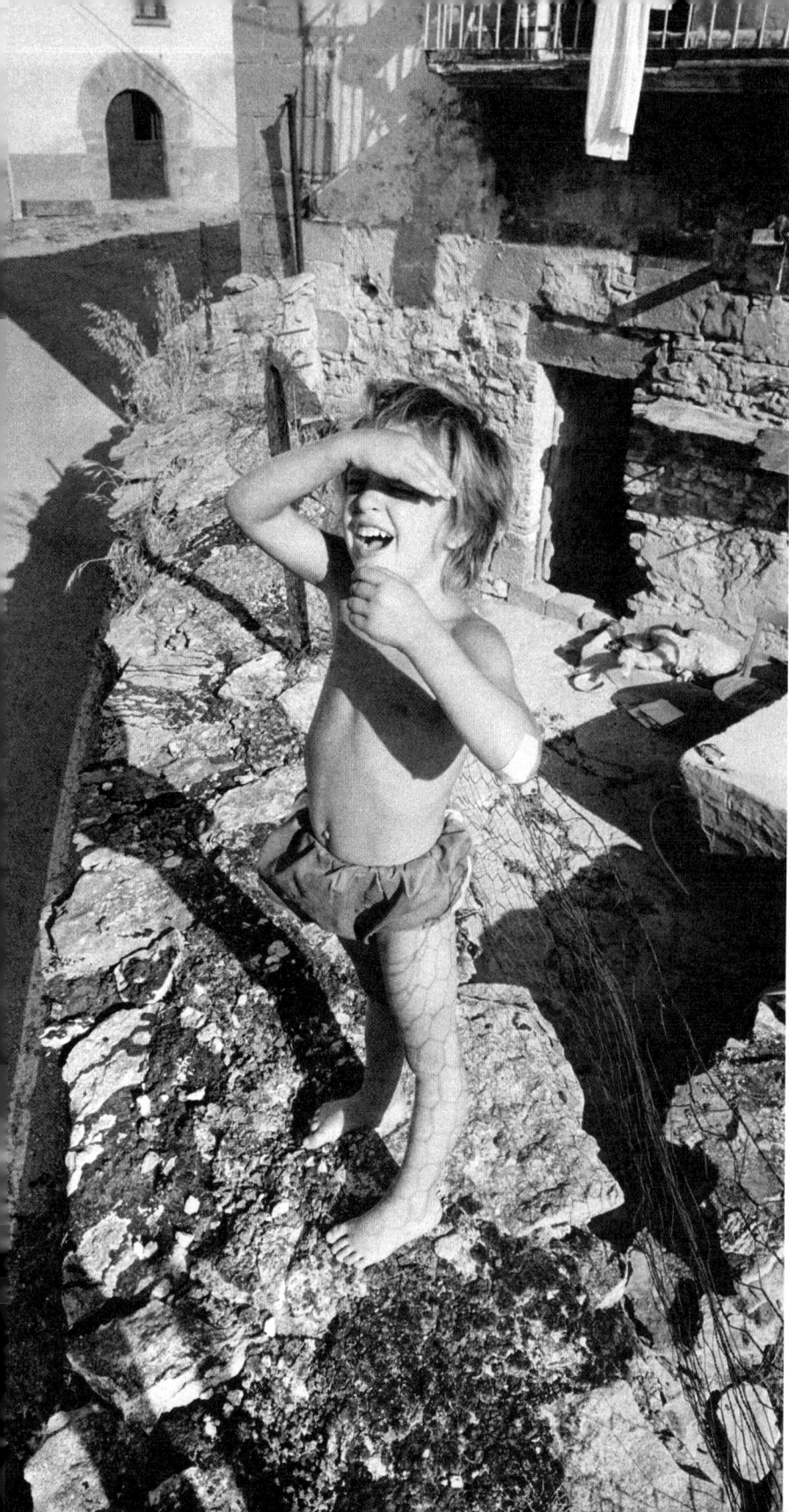

As the firstborn, Enahm had an intimate bond with his mother. Here he is around the age of five or so. An energetic kid, he was always pushing past himself. He developed his distinct identity very early on.

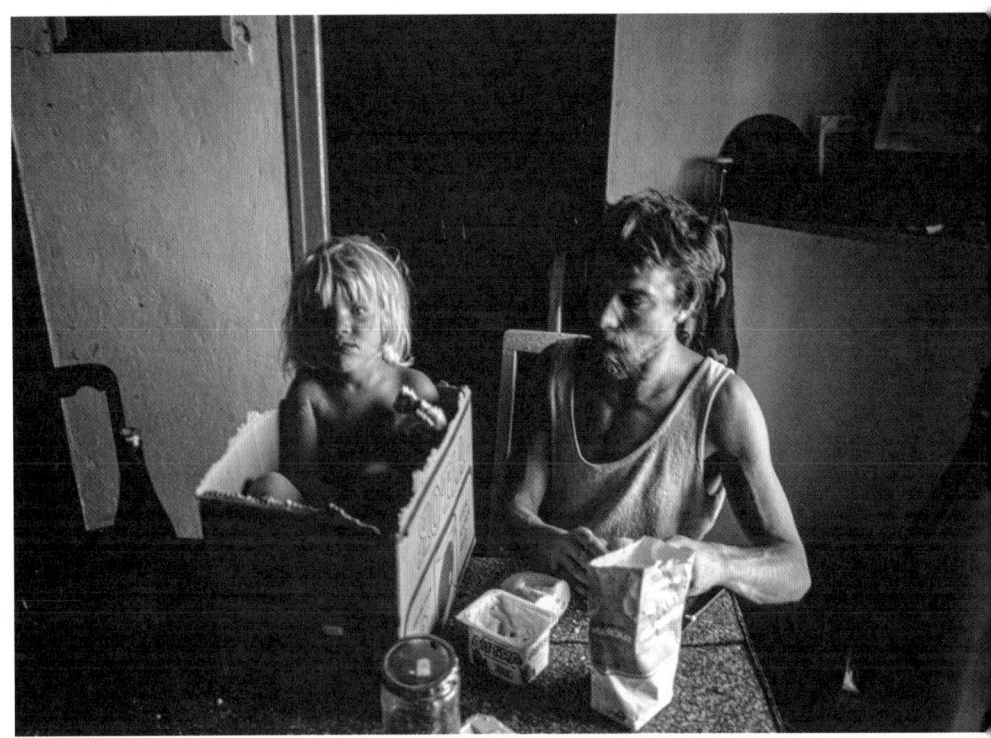

Daily life. Little kids and boxes. Classic. The simple pleasures. Love binds it all.

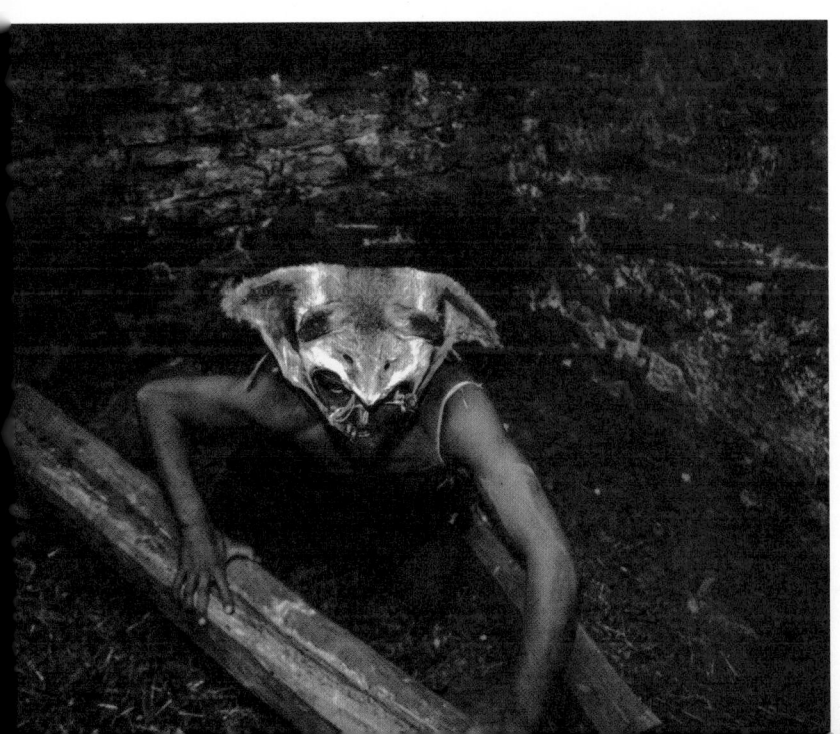

We found this fox skin when we were building the ashram. Just playing the part.

TURTLE

As fast as a slow turtle

Signs

Science

Patients patience

Where stress becomes second

Time has gone

Until its done

Results in publishing

Patience exercised

Patients helped

Bless the stress

That made this possible

As fast as a slow turtle another hurdle

A leap of consciousness

Factual awareness

Where stress is channeled

Into oceans of understanding

That I know nothing

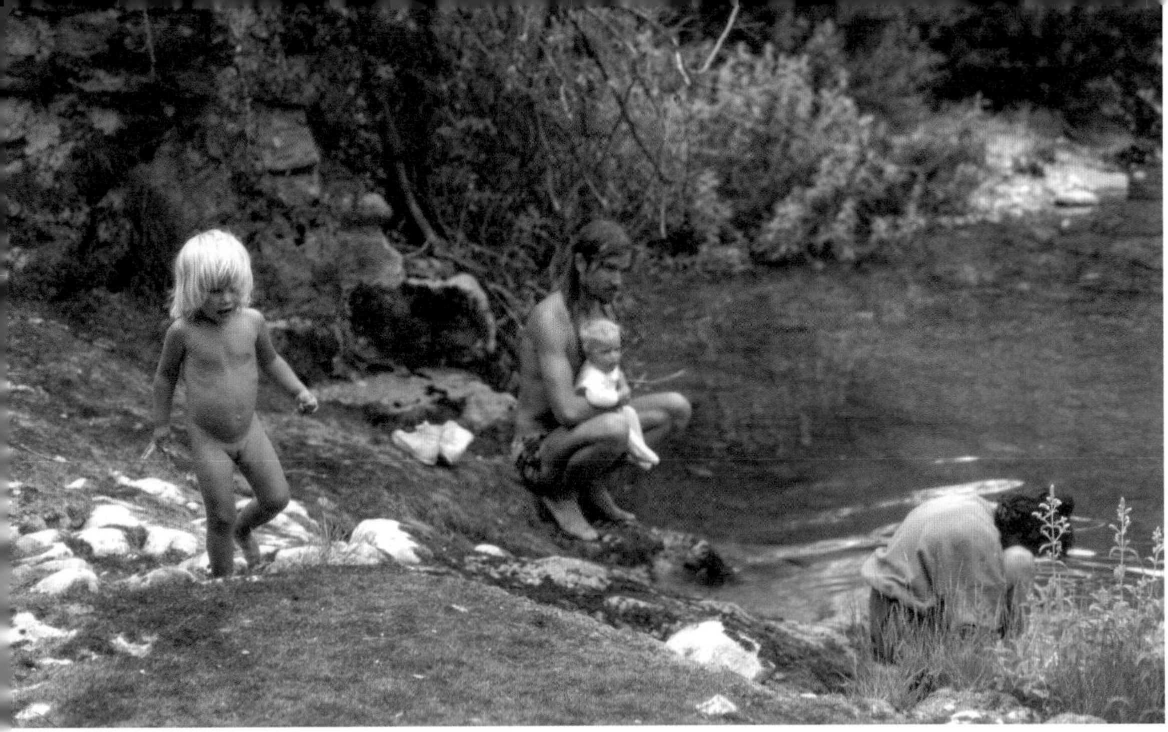

Here we are in Burlada, Spain.

I have Laura on my lap, and Isa is there also. Olaya by the waterside. By that point, we had tried everything and anything to help Olaya get out of the shadows. Nothing worked, and it became difficult to uphold my own emotional and mental state with the children. It wasn't long before we decided to go back to the Netherlands, and I set off on quite a downward spiral trying to find more safety and stability for the children. I lost contact with Henny. But I always continued to keep my discipline, exercising, and I had my idealistic, utopian ideas somehow frozen.

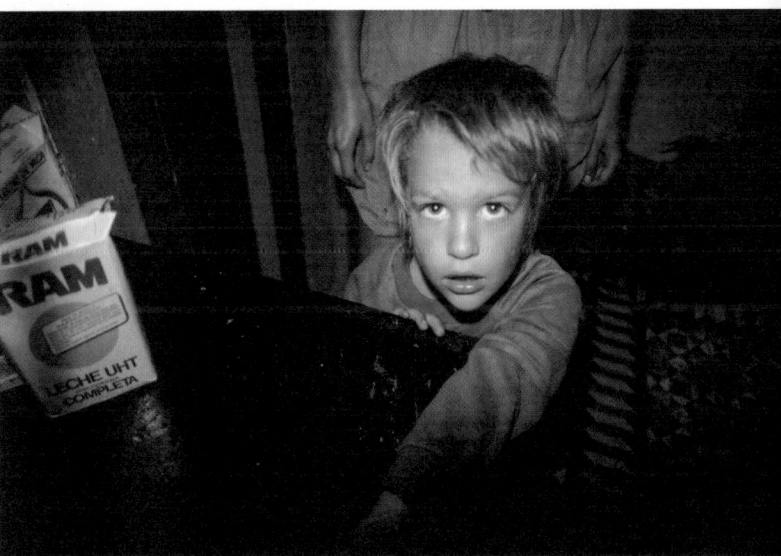

Enahm at five.

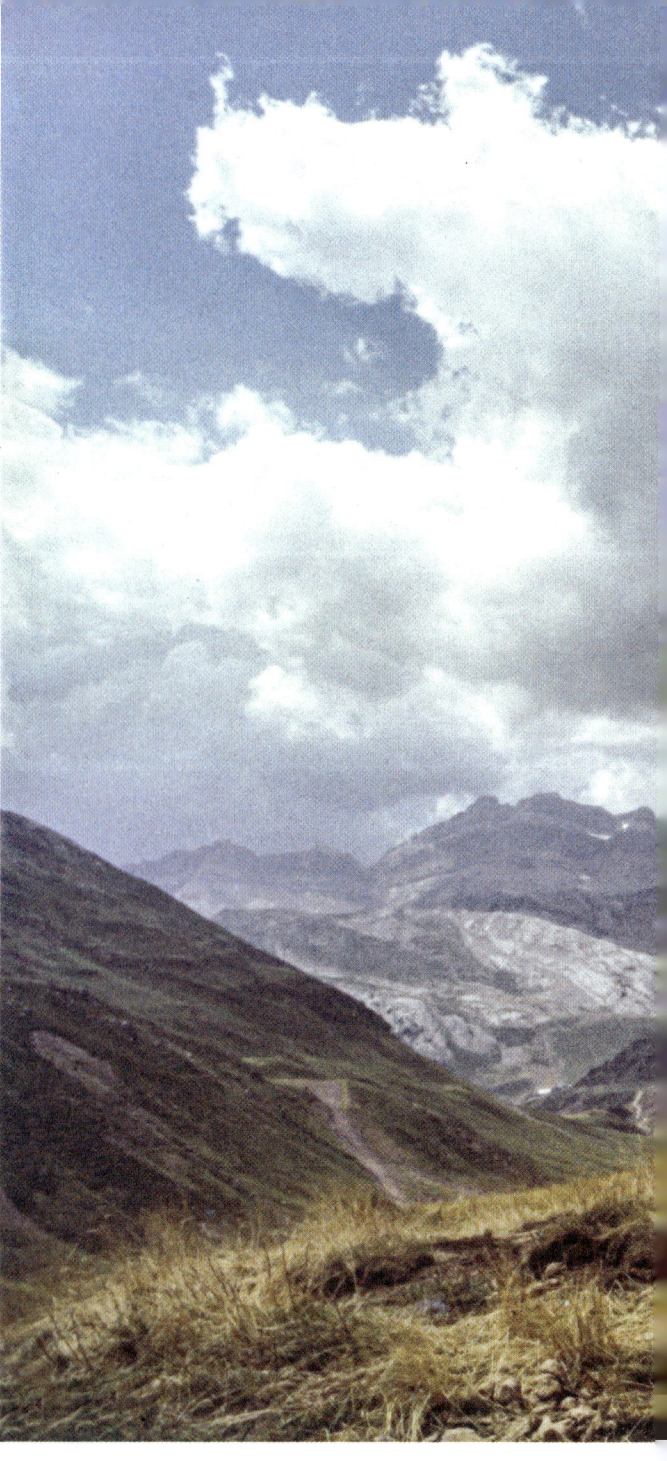

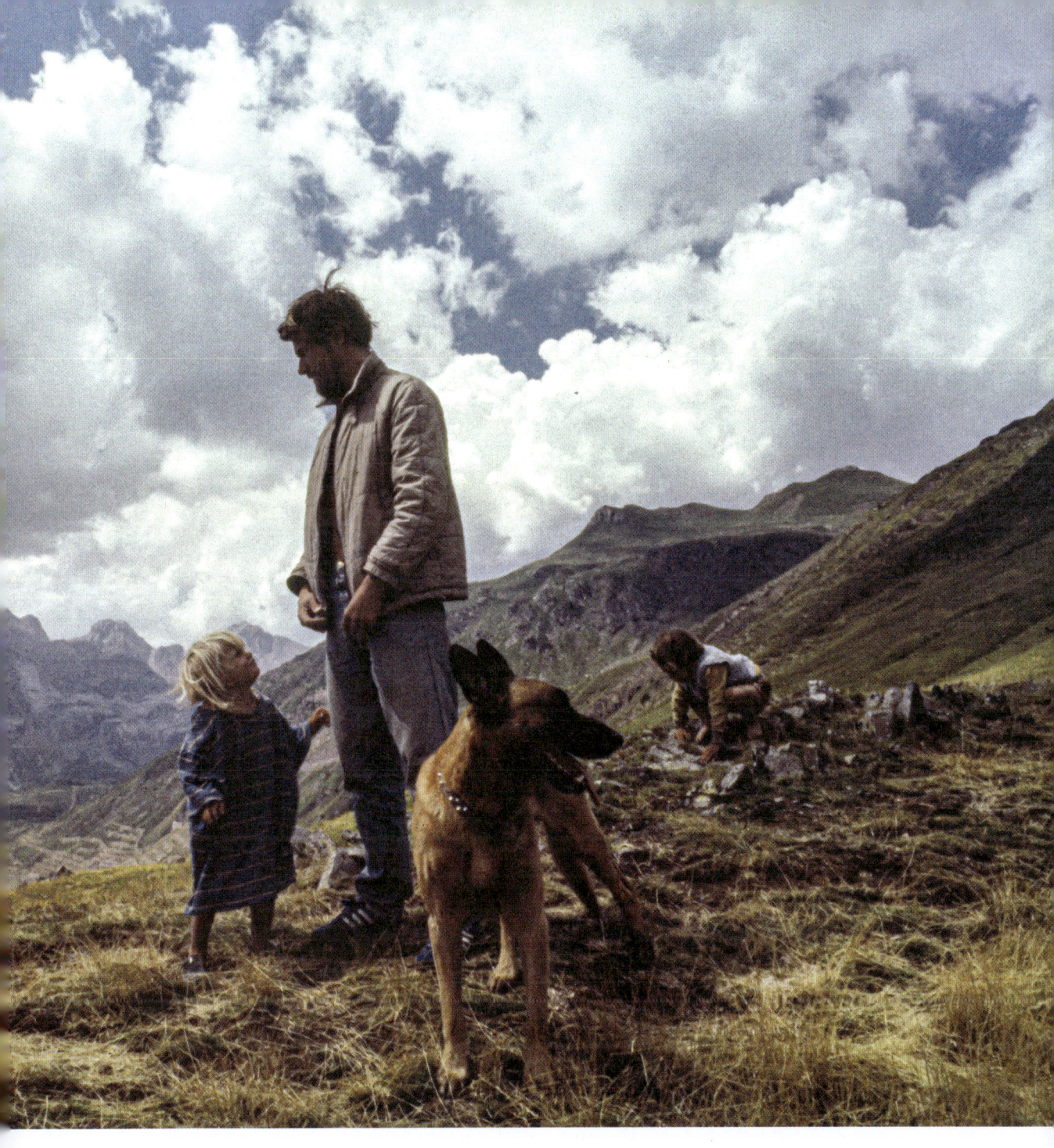

I remember this moment very well. I was troubled, worried. Enahm was there exploring, and small Isabelle was asking for attention. I felt the weight of it all. Small children and a mother who was fading away into despair.

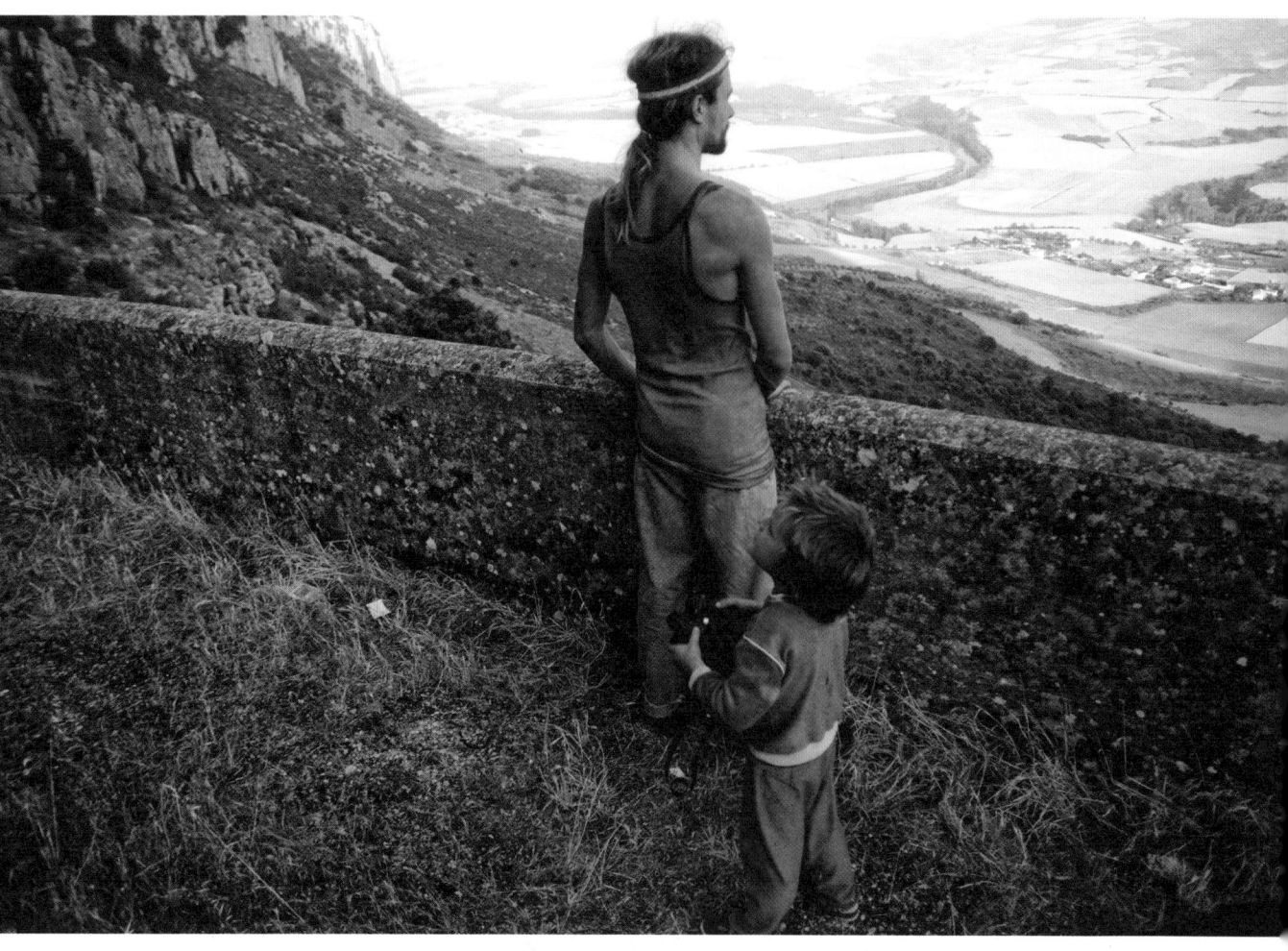

Puerto de Echauri. Spanish Pyrenees.

A place of rocks, heights, and nature.
My refuge to think. Contemplate. Stare.

TRAUMA

A HIDDEN DRAMA

BEYOND WHAT WORDS CAN TELL

EDITING US FROM INSIDE

TO BE FREED FROM THE OTHER SIDE

DEATH, TRAUMA, WE DON'T KNOW

WHAT IF WE FOUND A KEY TO THAT CALL

OUR SPIRIT CAPABLE TO GO PAST OBSTACLES FROM HELL

ACCOMPANIED WITH THE BREATH, REOPENING THE

WELL

CALLED SOUL UNIQUE FOR ANYONE

DIFFERENT AND THE SAME, LIKE DAUGHTERS AND SONS

UNFORGIVEN GREAT POWERS COMING FROM OUR CARE

AND LOVE

SO LET'S CLARIFY ONCE AND FOR ALL WHAT COMES FROM

ABOVE

CONNECTION THAT NATURALLY TAKES SHAPE

WHEN RELEASING FEAR OF DEATH, THROUGH THE

BREATH, AND TRAUMA OUR DRAMA

IS WHEN WE LET GO AND THE SOUL TAKES CLEAR

SHAPE

UNFORGIVINGLY THERE

THE BEAUTY OF LIFE TO ADHERE

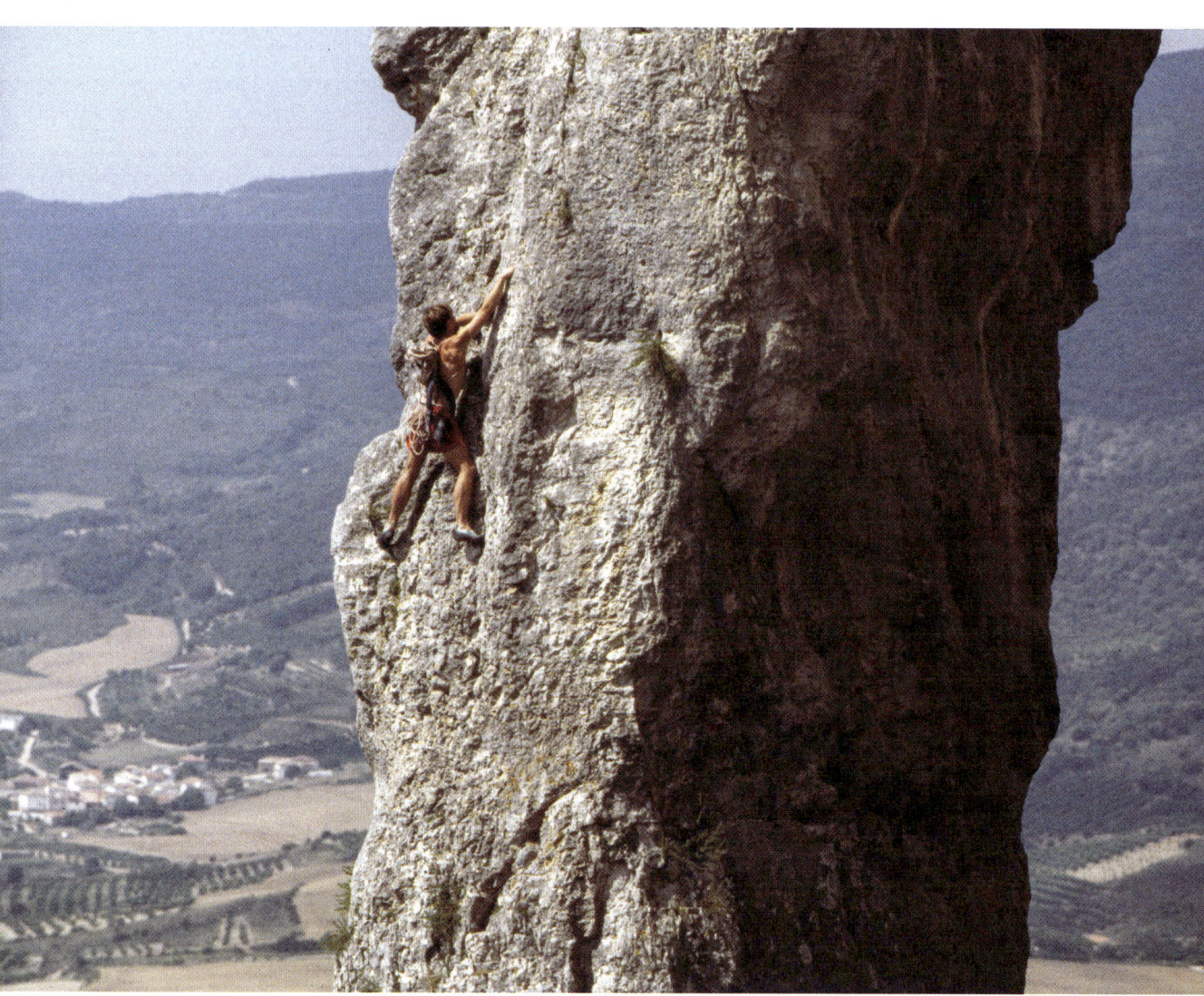

Climbing without gear became an obsession for me. As an asana
practitioner, I was flexible and knew my body's capabilities well.
Climbing is about control, down to the millimeter. Everything is on the
line. And that is a feeling, not a thought. You recognize it in your gut. As
long as that feeling doesn't leave you insecure, you just go with the flow.

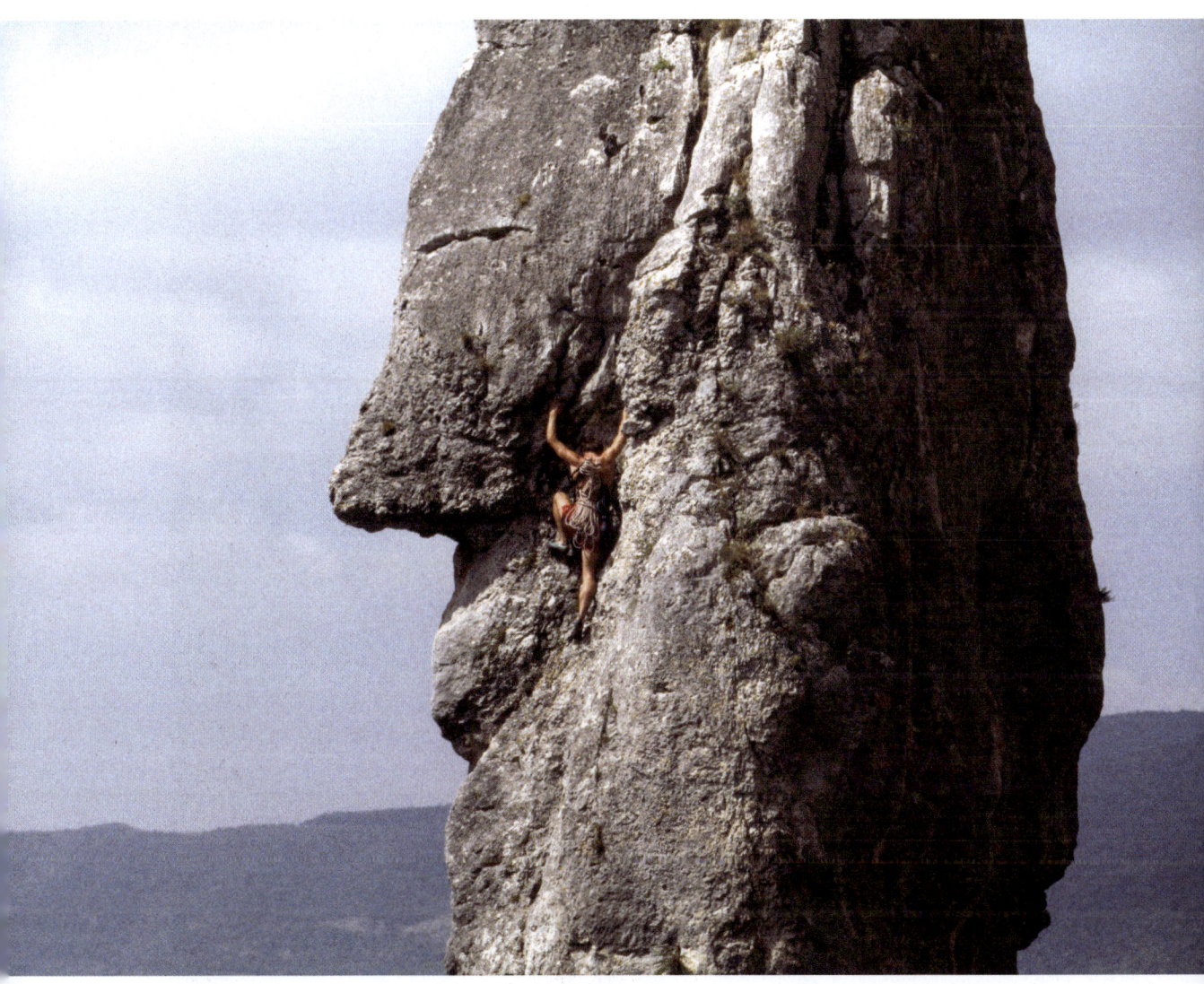

It's almost inconceivable that I laid my life on the line every time
I climbed free solo, but it gave me such relief from the ongoing struggles
of our home life. Climbing was a refuge. This was how I gained control of
myself again. I got energy from this. I could not help Olaya. Through
nature I was guided back. It held my hand and guided me through.

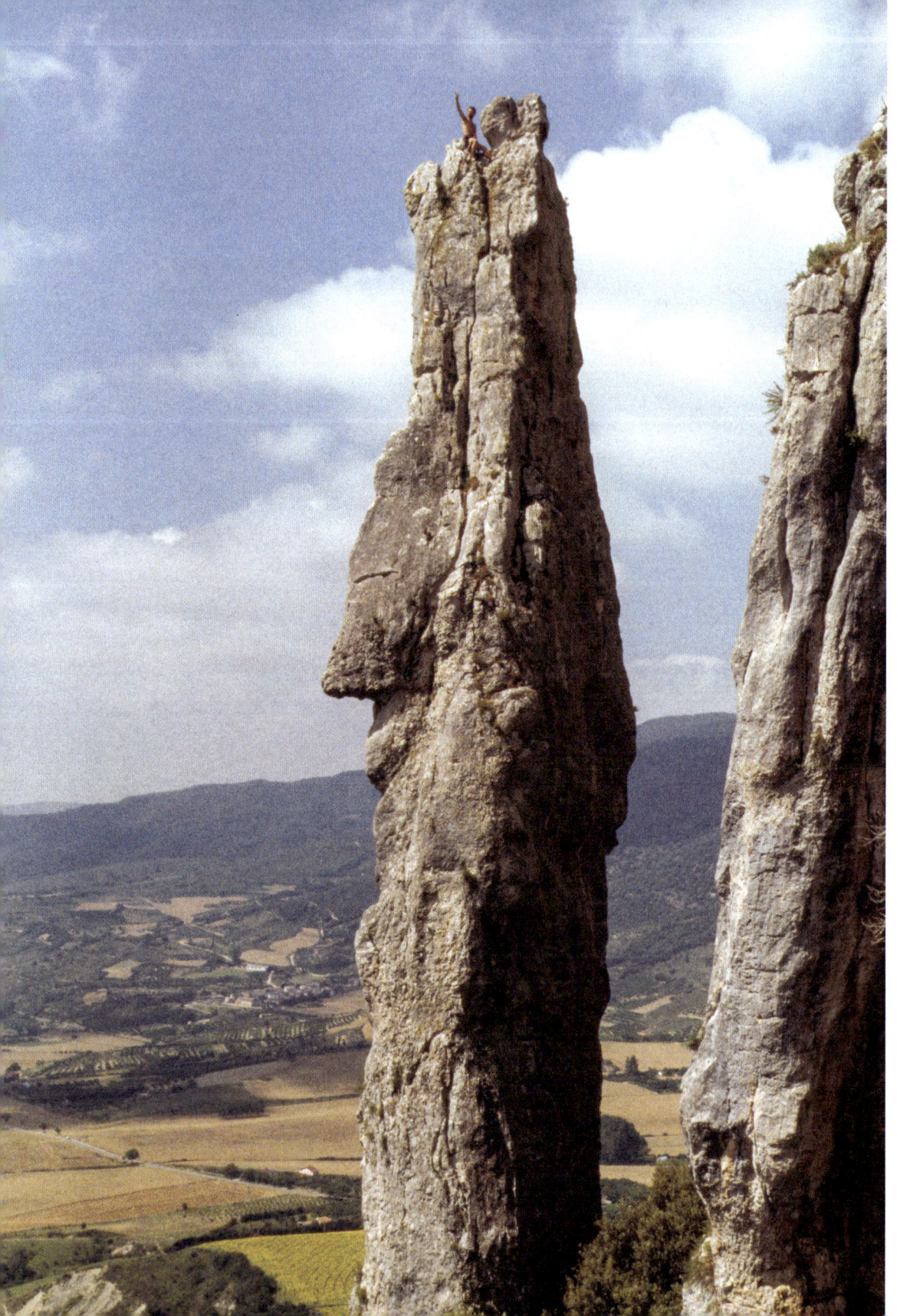

Challenges in nature were shown to me by intrigue. I was attracted, magnetized to it. My body was trained. Flexible. That preluded the climbing. When your body is highly trained, it's as if it seeks a mirror. Something to reflect back the obstacle. It wants to overcome something. There was an urge to climb, a magnetism to mirror my psyche through my body. This is not about competition but expression itself. The body wants to express, wants to move with the mind as one. It gave me peace. It colored my life. And only you as a person are able to see that, to feel that. It is a deeply personal and intimate moment with your Soul. The sanctity of that intimacy is what I sought out. I found it within nature, within nature as a mirror. I could go deeper and deeper, and it was never done. It just kept on giving.

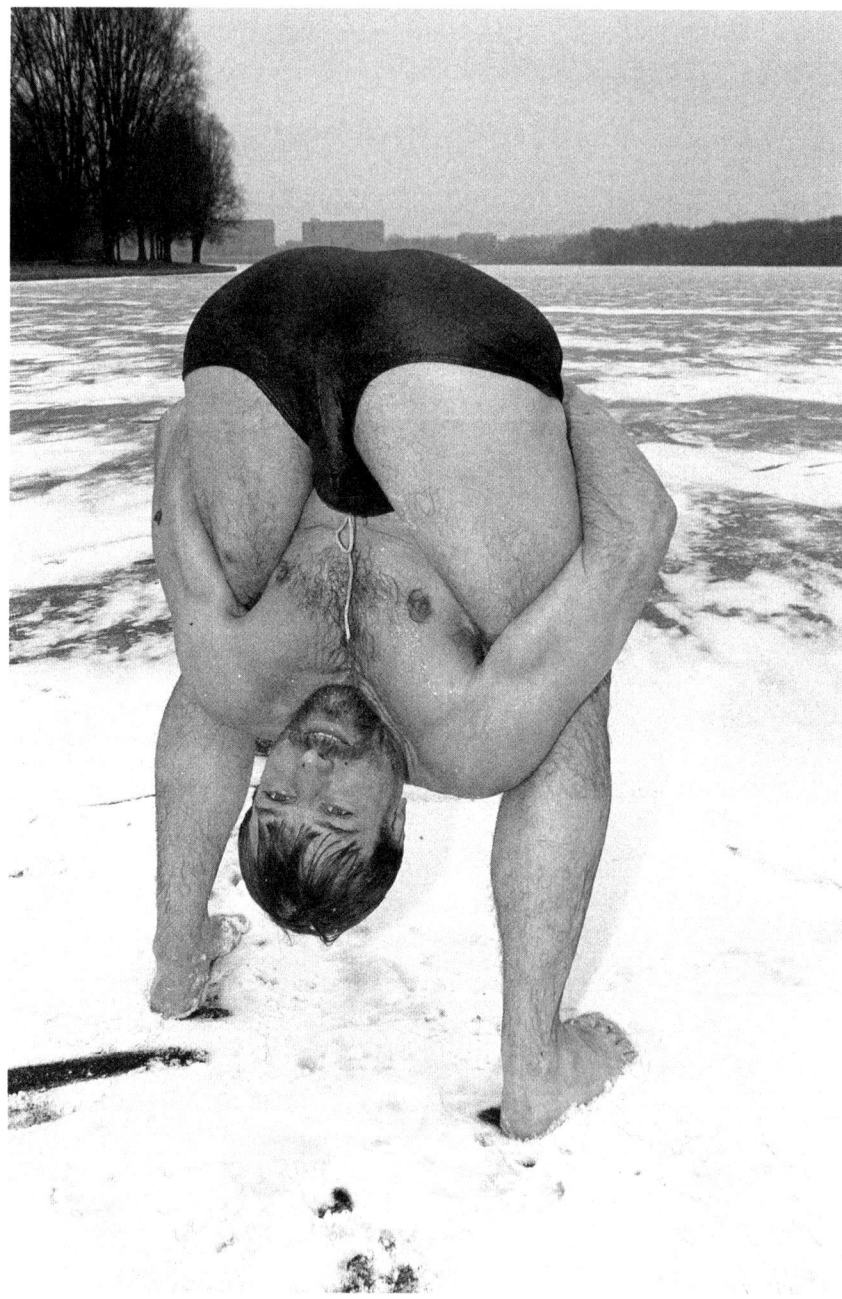

Winter training. Sloterplas, Amsterdam.

I was always out there doing crazy stuff. The common understanding of
the cold's effect on human flexibility is that it stiffens our bodies. This is me
after ice bathing on a frozen lake where I lived nearby with my four kids.

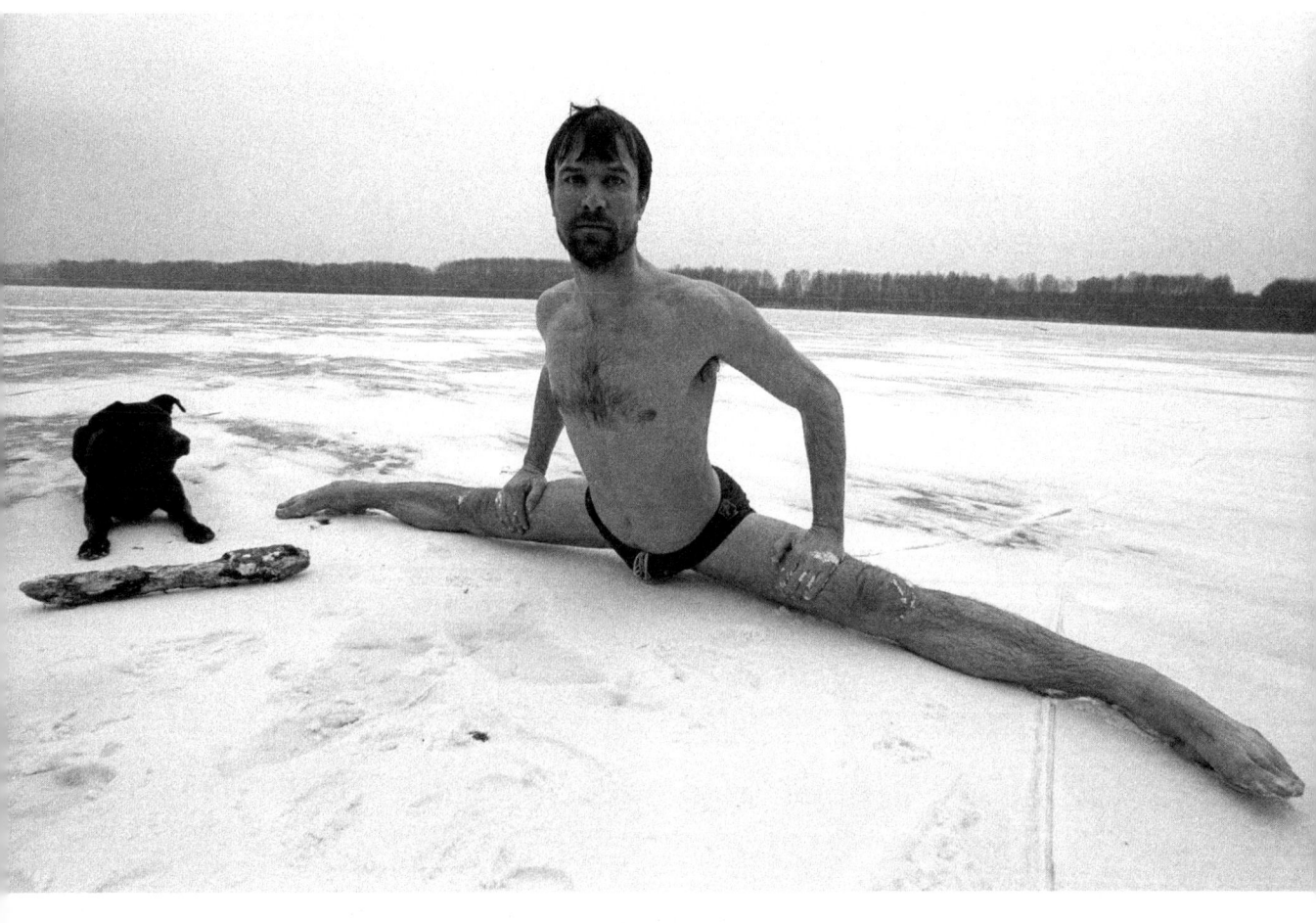

The body and its level of conditioning is really serving a greater good. Expression. It's all an expression. Throughout my life I didn't feel I could fully express who I was. That pushed me to the limits of my capabilities physically and mentally. And it still does. Only now, I can contemplate it better.

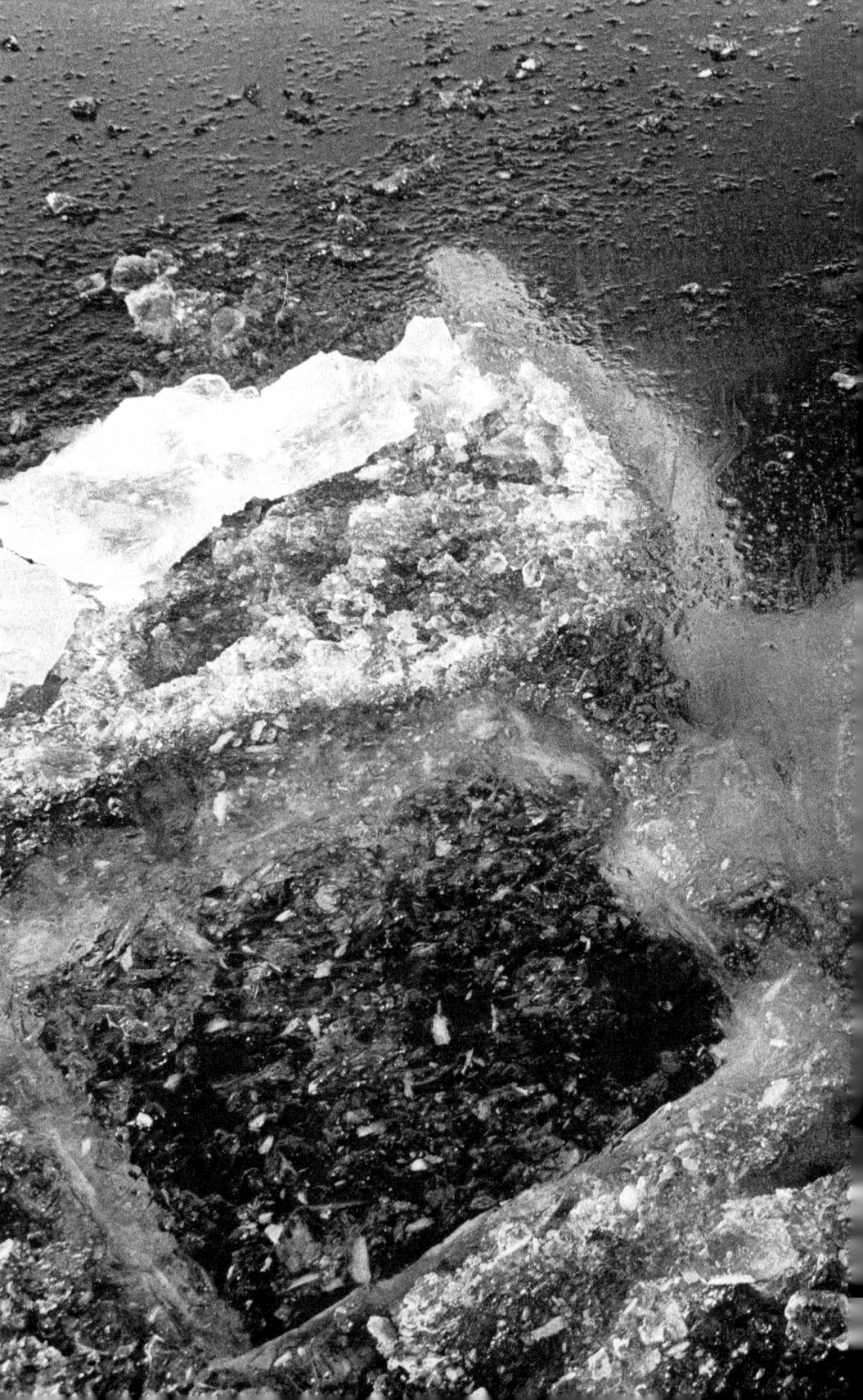

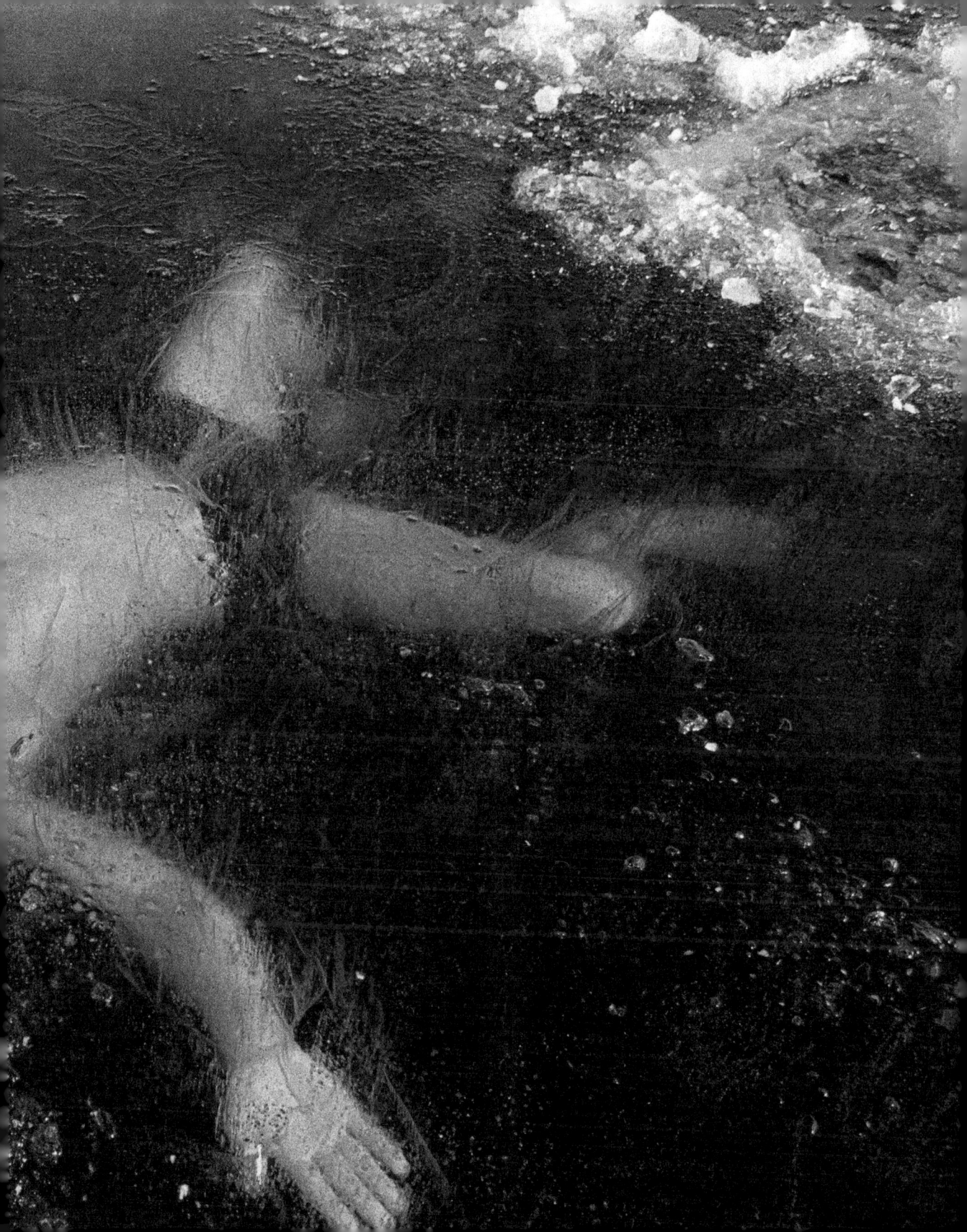

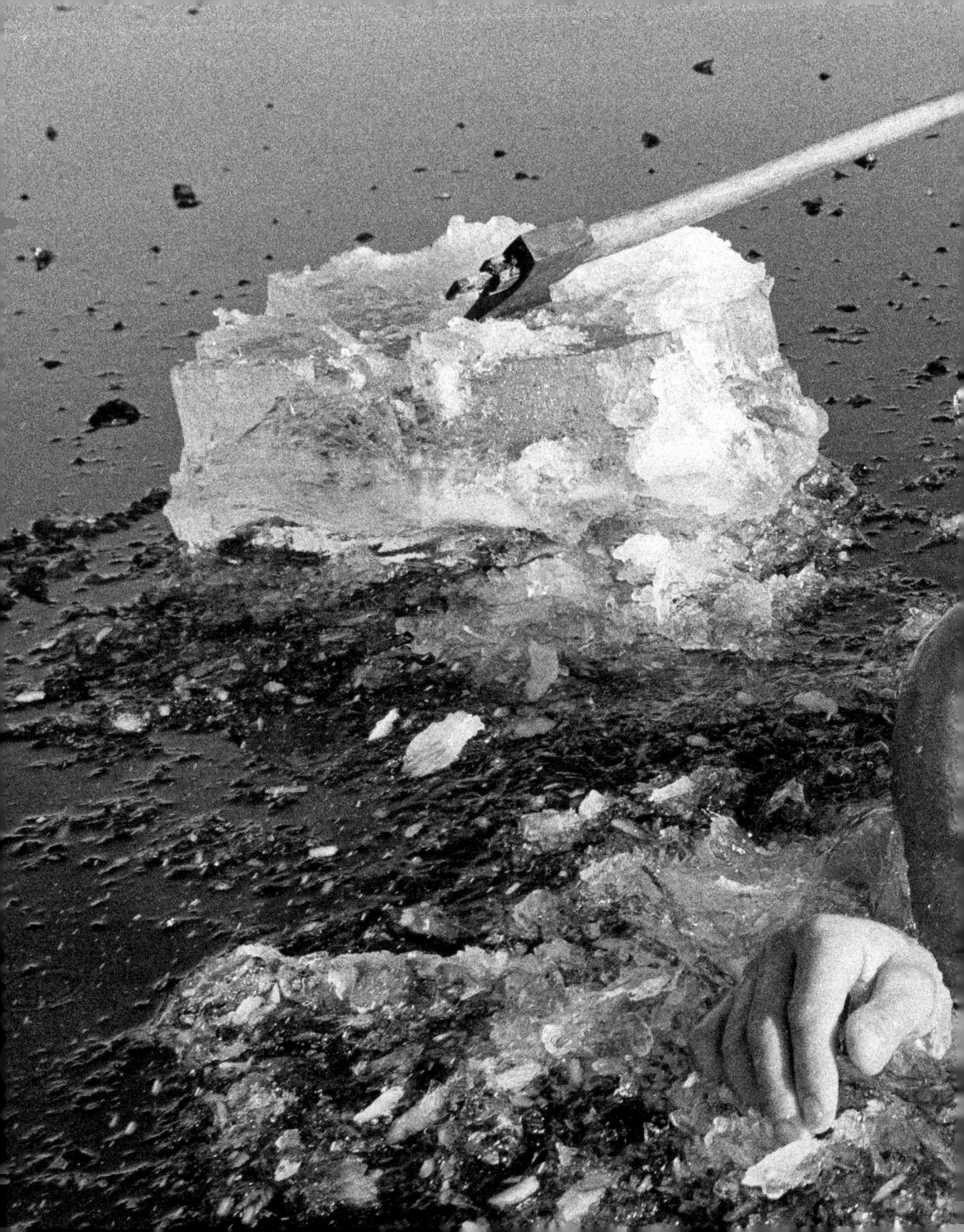

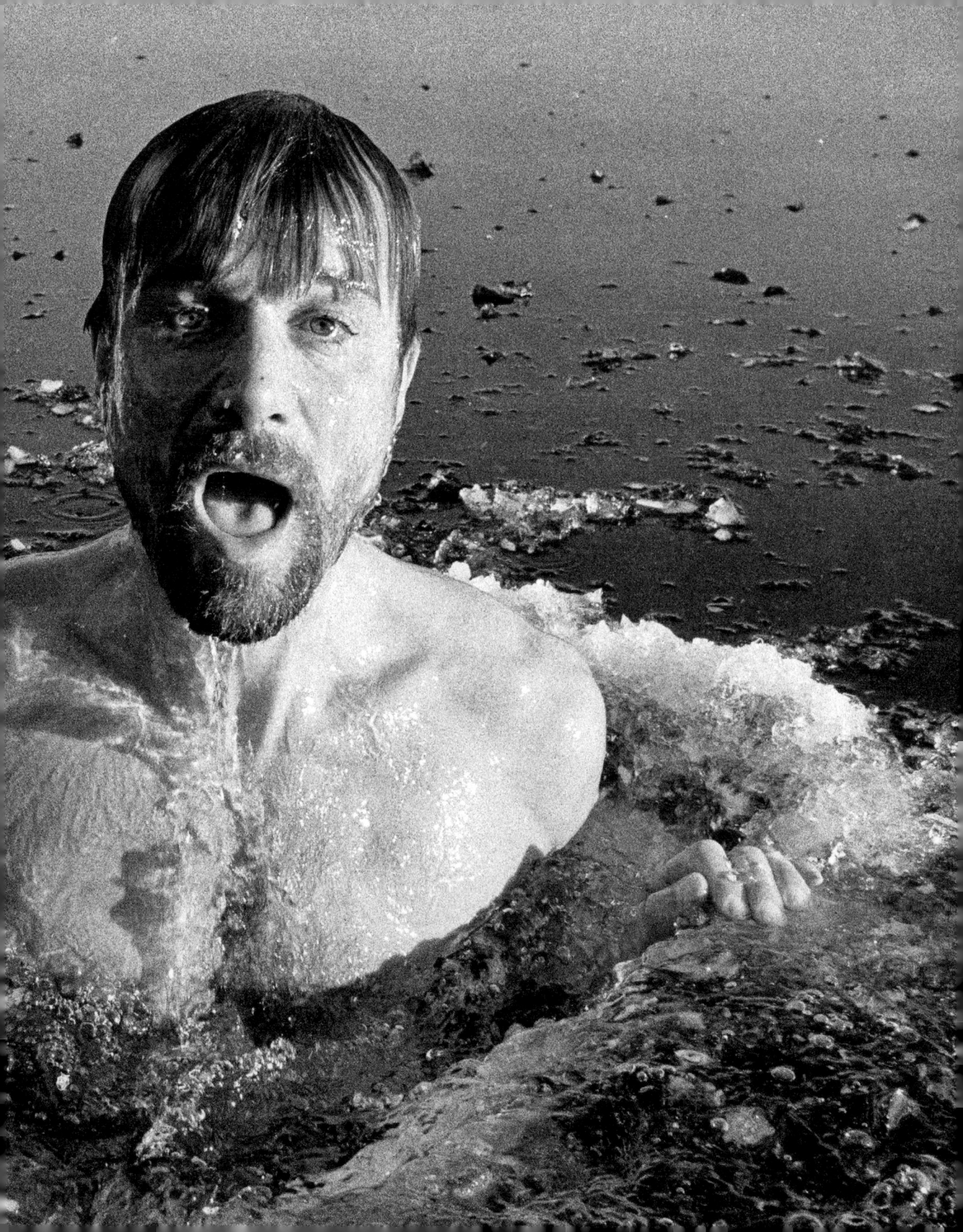

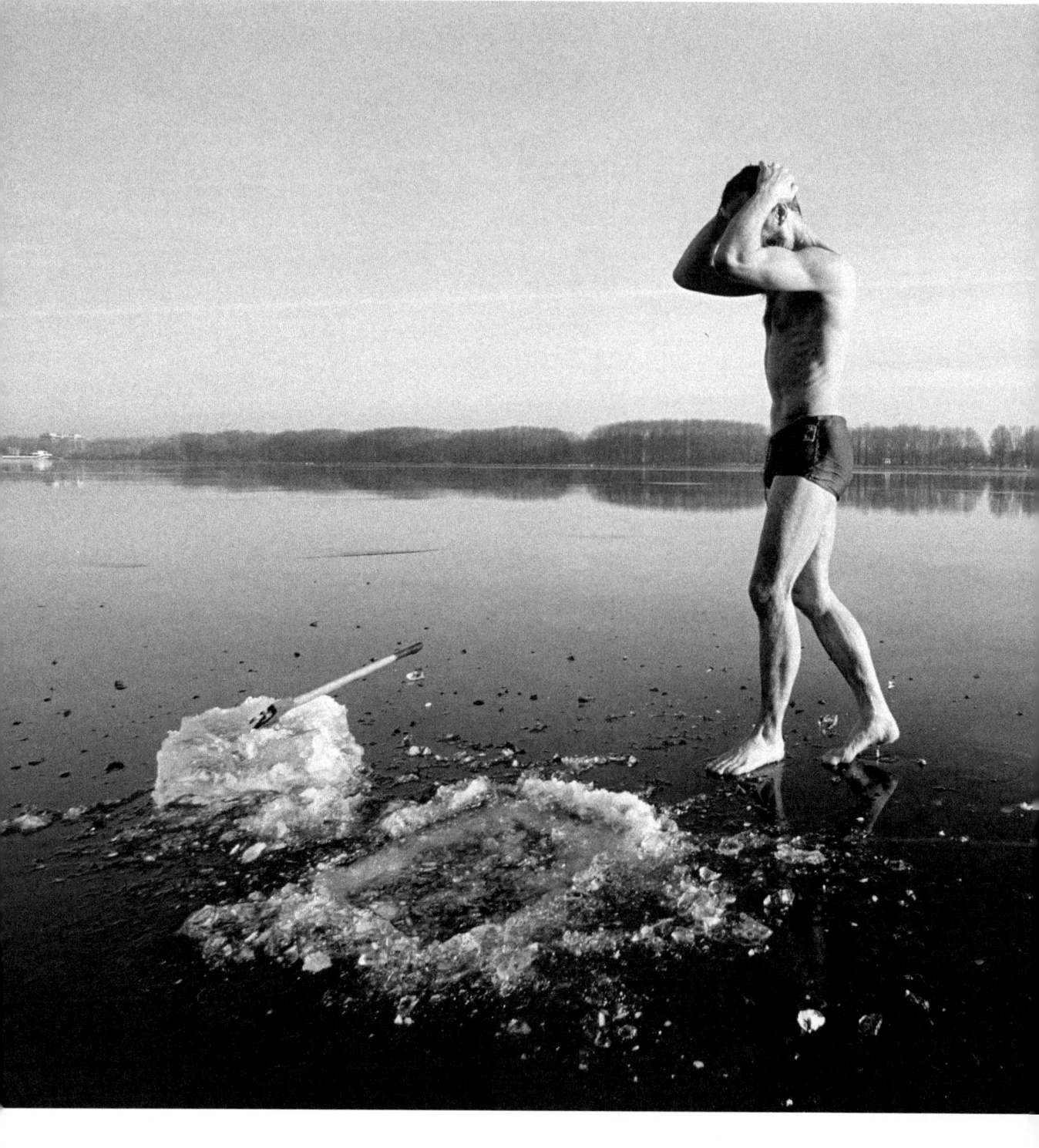

The cold helped me overcome my emotional loss. It was the only way to stop the thought loops I experienced. Why did she do it? Why am I all alone? Why me? Doing these things became my lifeline. I had to see how far I could go, and something to strive for was exciting. When we experience grief, anxiety, or depression, it's so important to find something to hold on to. Nature was the principle for getting out of my maddening loops. I challenge you to use nature to break your own loops and patterns of thinking. You don't have to be extreme. I had to seek in the dark; you can seek in the light. Take the shortcut. Just going for a walk outside in the fresh air can improve your perspective.

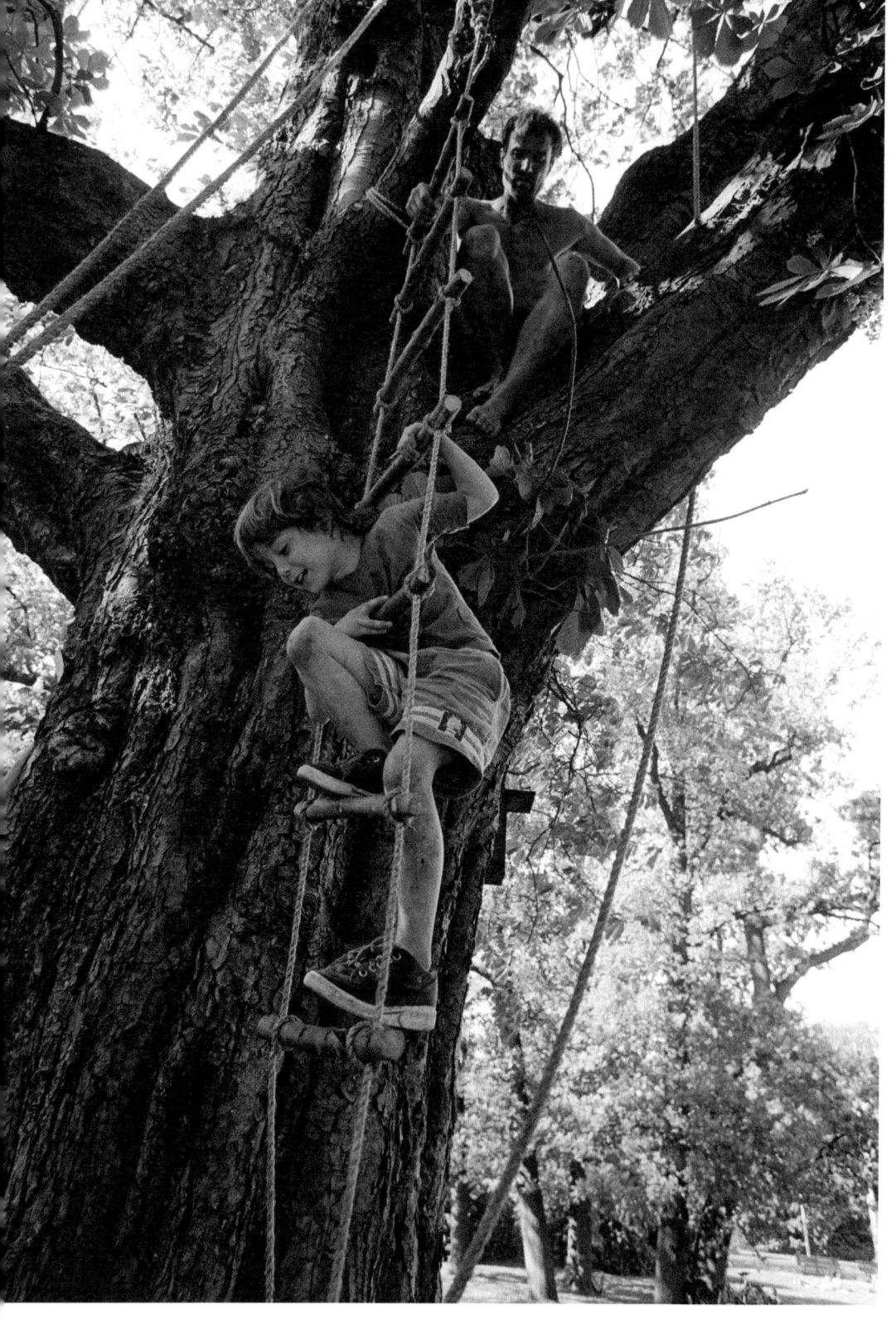

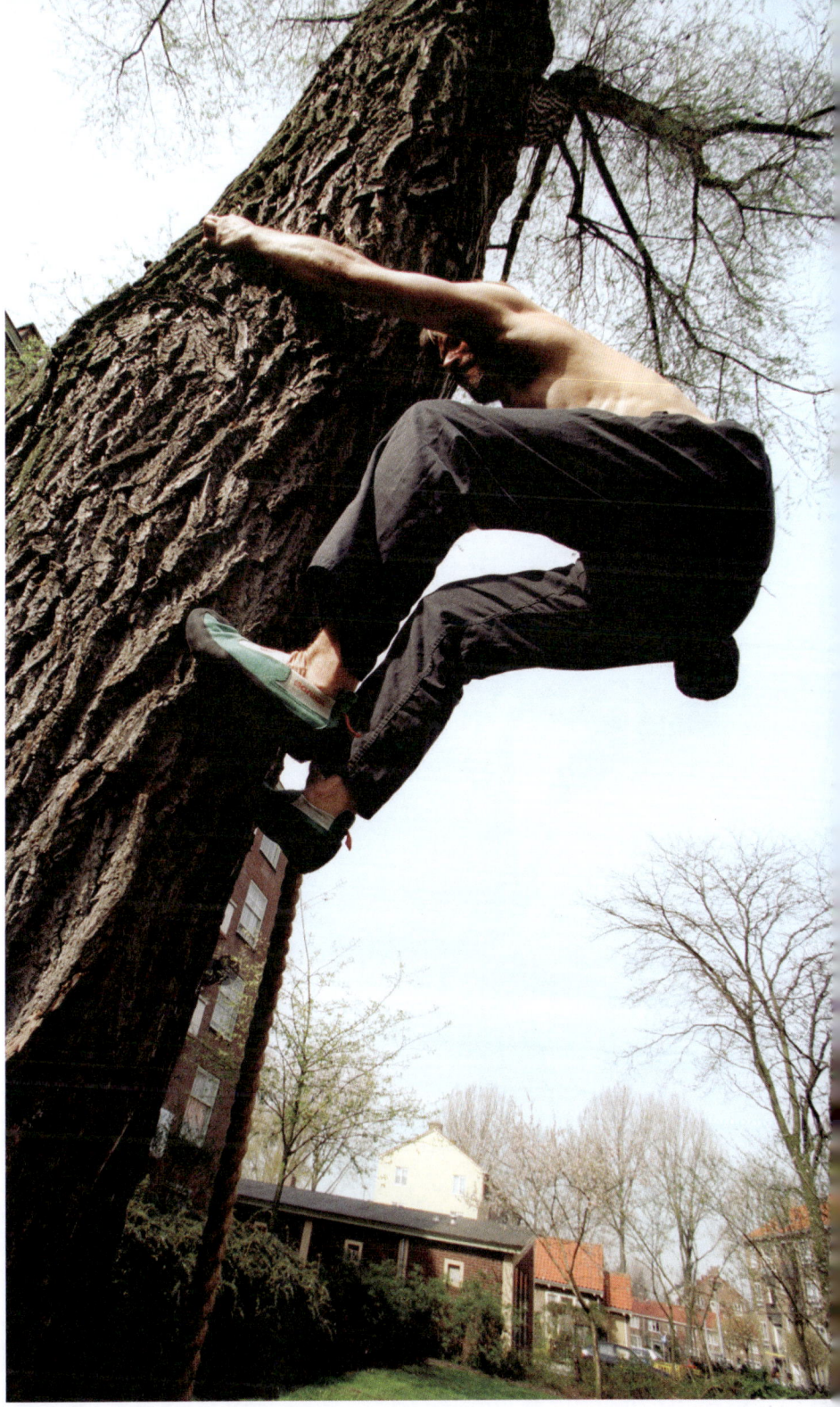

The Netherlands is flat as a coin, but I could experience the same feeling I had in the mountains by scaling trees.

We were living in social housing in Geuzenveld, Amsterdam. There was a space in front with a tall schietwilg tree. I just started climbing it. I took on anything in front of me as a challenge. Playing in nature gives me energy. I had no money, but wow! did I have some energy.

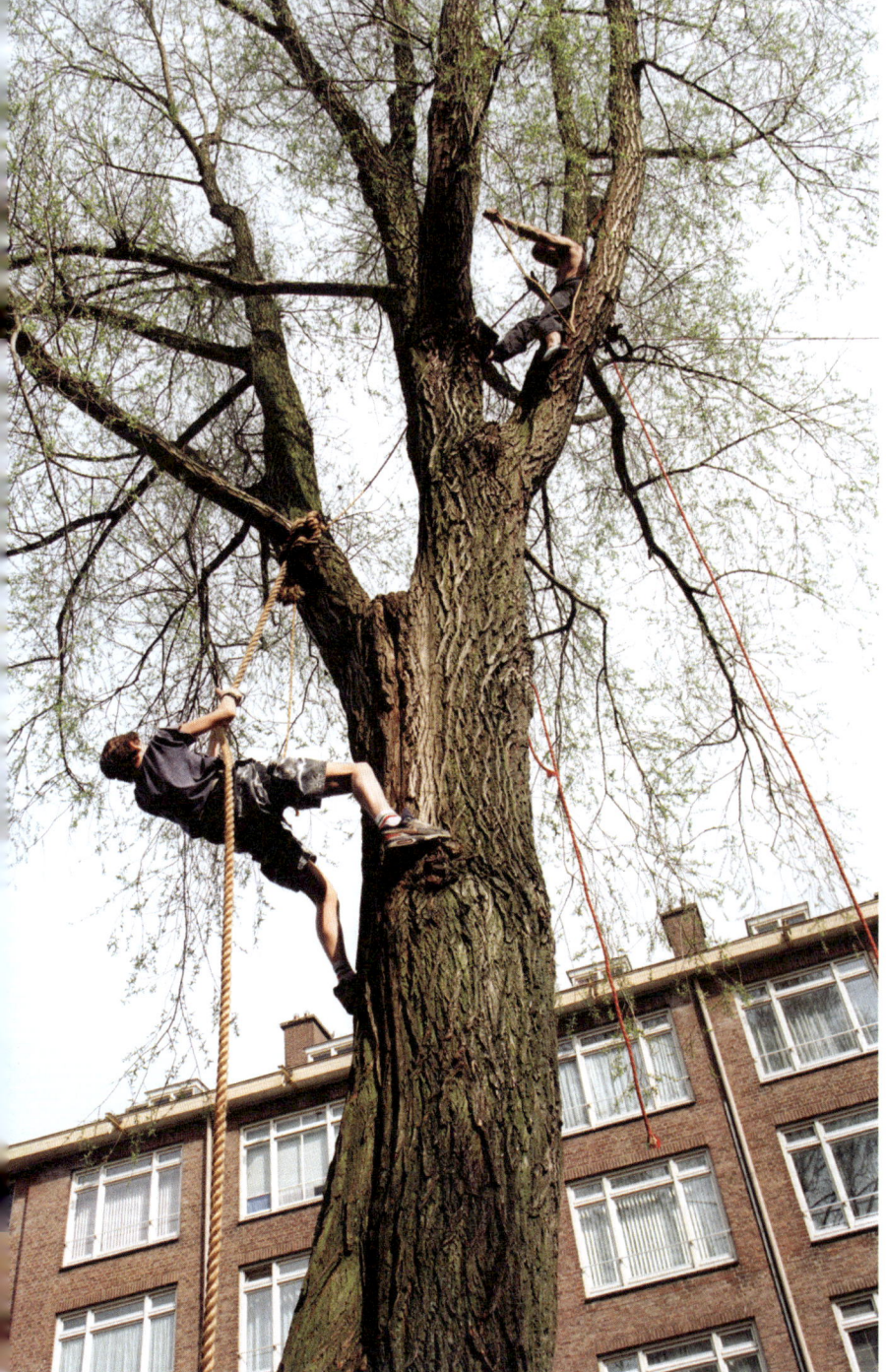

Enahm and me. As a father, I was very unorthodox. I think sometimes my children wanted me to be much more like anyone else. I was abnormal to others, but I think nature does that to you. You don't mind what others think. You just go. I was in my flow, an open, happy guy in the neighborhood. I played more outside than most of the children there!

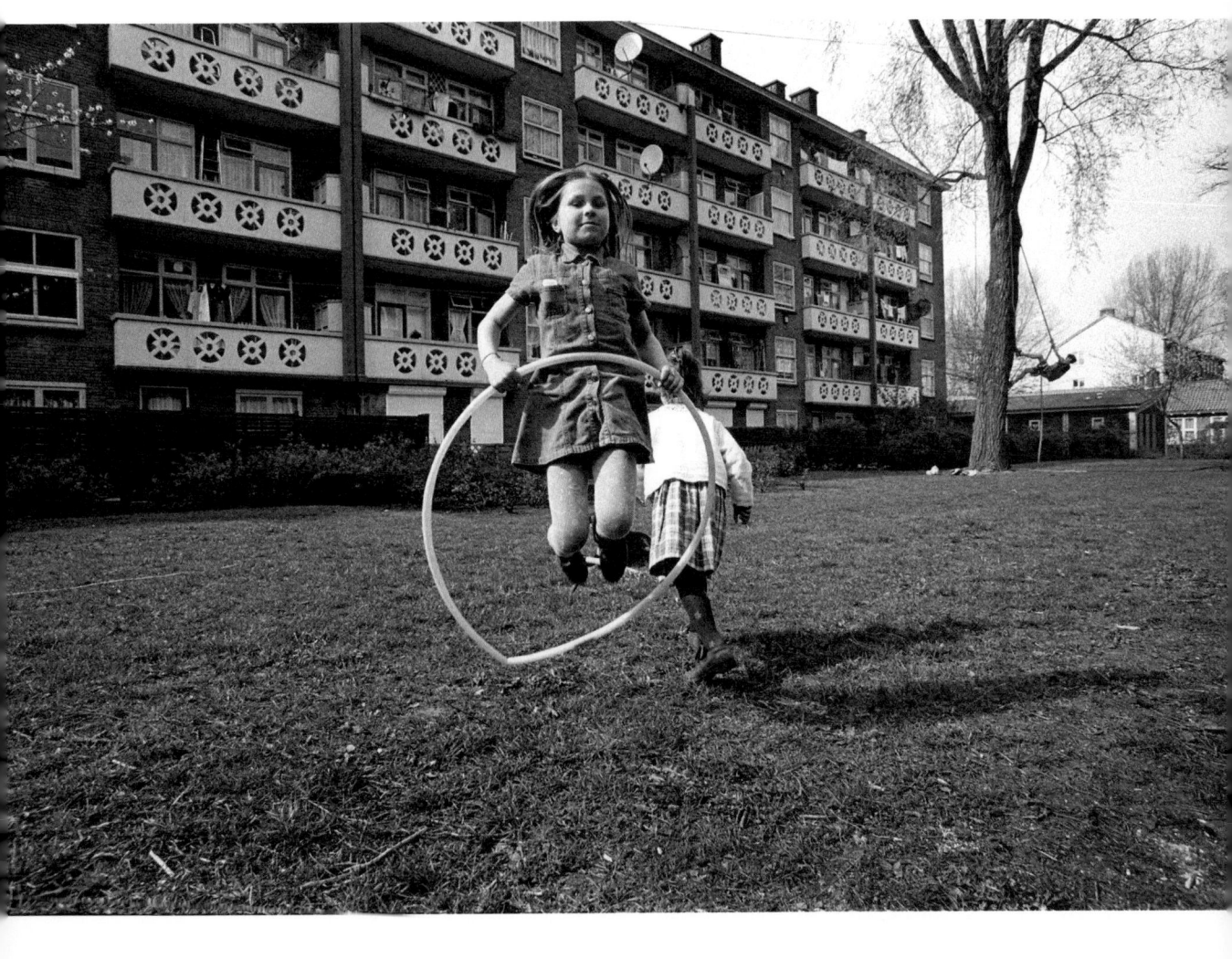

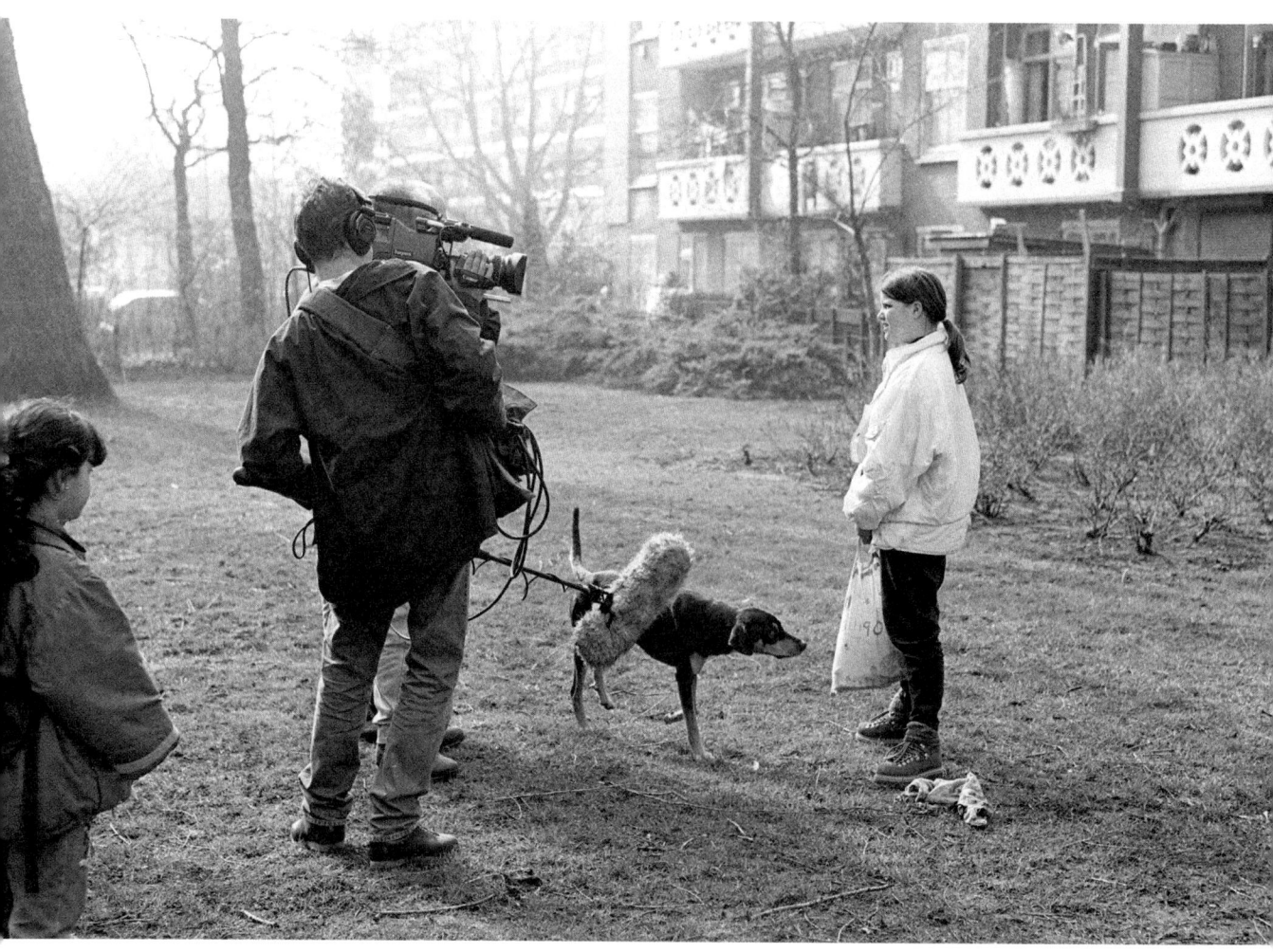

Laura at nine years old, outside the apartment block, being interviewed for a Dutch TV program. I was starting to gain some attention for my strange behavior, from tree climbing to ice swimming, and the local TV and newspapers were taking interest.

GARDEN OF EDEN

The Garden of Eden
Eruruata, eruruata
Step by step, we set foot in Paradise
Where the fear subsides into another presence
Because divine Mother Nature
Is there
Becoming aware,
I dare
That I am one in Mother Nature's care
Doubt is weakness, taken out
The lions piercing eyes, a deep roar
A shout
I am here, humbled to the core
There is no time, waste is gone
Walk in the garden,
Eden has come
Where King Lion
Is da right on
According to the Bob Marley
Authority in the field
It is the love that makes us one
Until then the lions rage on
To show us the Garden of Eden
Should be our daily song.

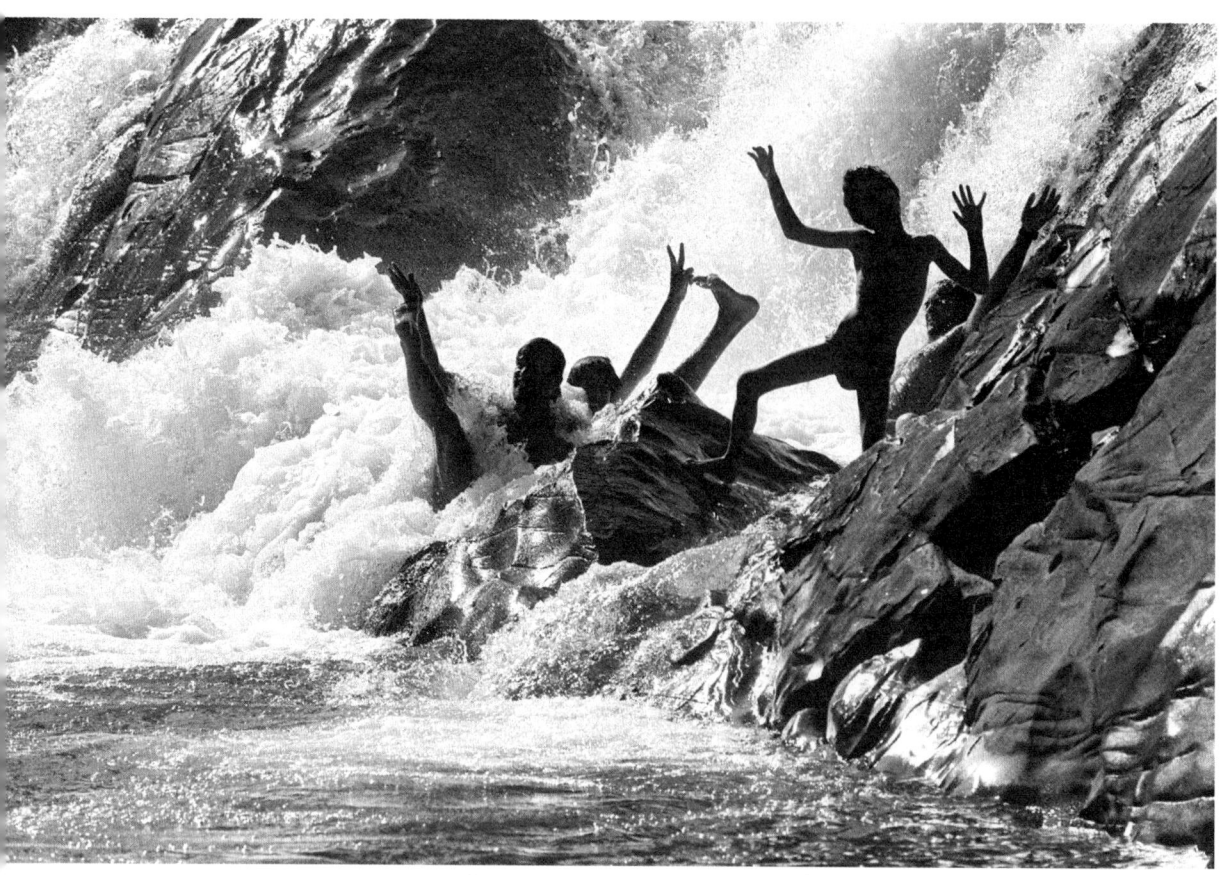

In Spain with the children. Always in nature, in the rivers, trees,
mountains. Olaya was from this region. It's a mesmerizing place.

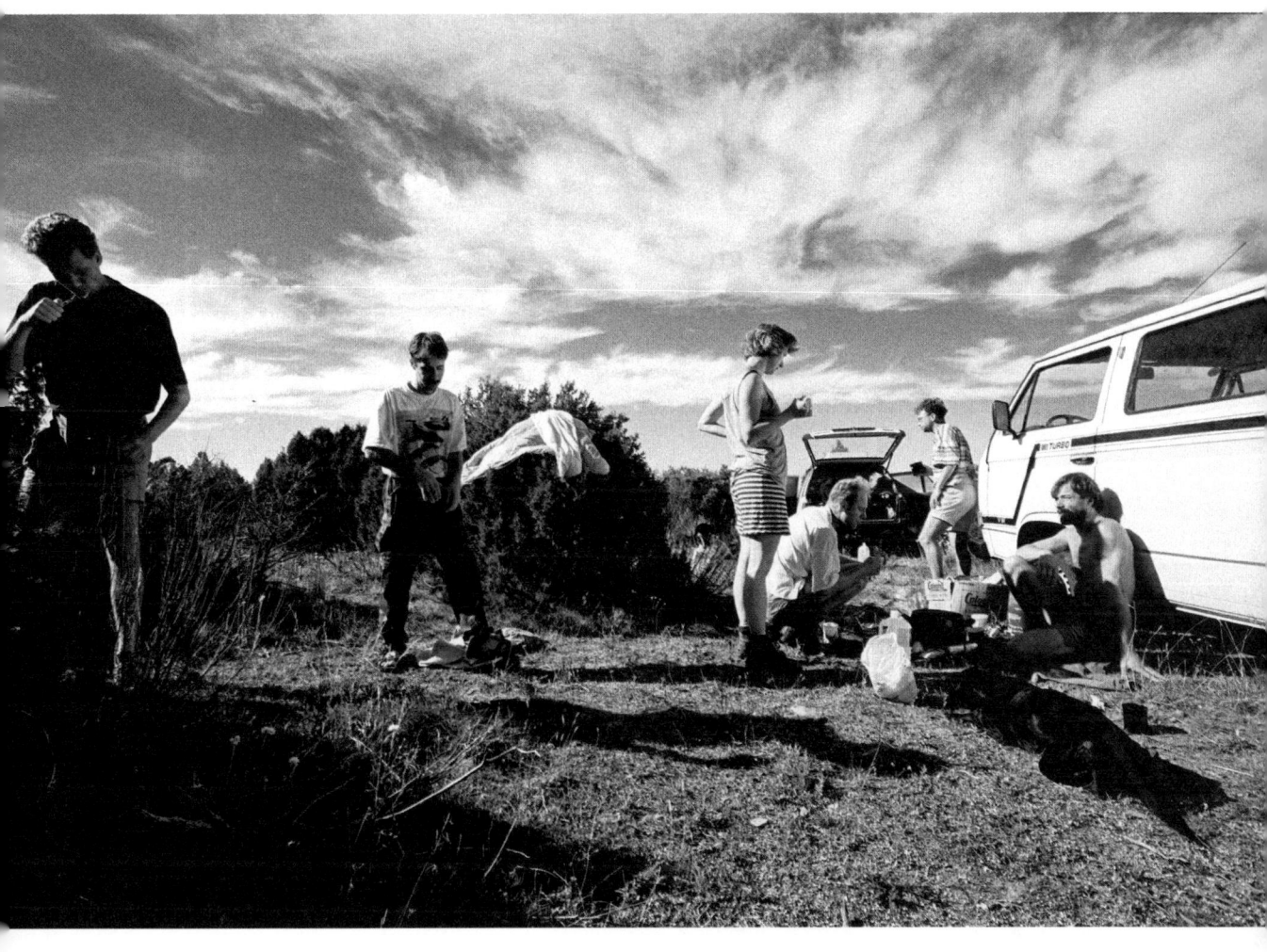

First I went with my friend Javier into the mountains. I met him through Olaya. He was a lovely guy. We did canyoning when it was much less known. It was one of the most impressive, detangling experiences I had while I was with Olaya. I felt life again, the wonder of life again. I began to do it more and more, and soon we began to organize travels to the Pyrenees.

We tried to get things up and going but found little traction at first. We found a Belgium travel company that had a vacancy for a guide, so we came in and first had a small group. We arranged the food, travel, and guiding. You have to persist. If you don't go on, it falls apart. It took me about three years to get this going with very small groups, and then Javier parted because we could not make a livelihood out of it. But I continued with another friend of mine, Rob.

Barranco (canyon) del Furco.

I trained a lot in cold water by not wearing a wetsuit while guiding people through the canyons. There are hundreds of canyons in the Pyrenees, all kinds of shapes and sizes. It was beautiful nature, to become one with her amazing forces every time. You can see the rock plates are layers being tectonically pushed from the bottom of the sea to the surface. I was mesmerized by this.

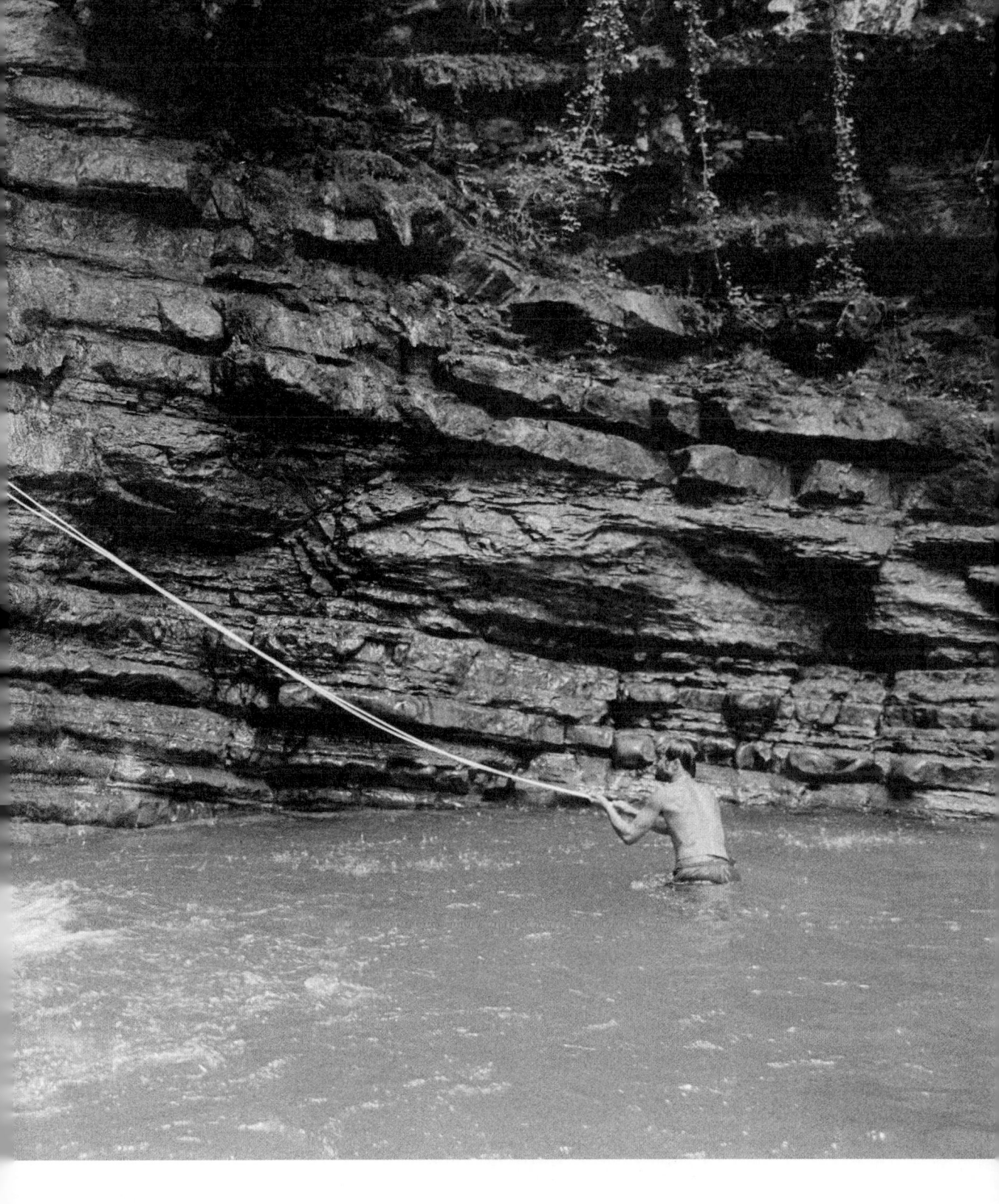

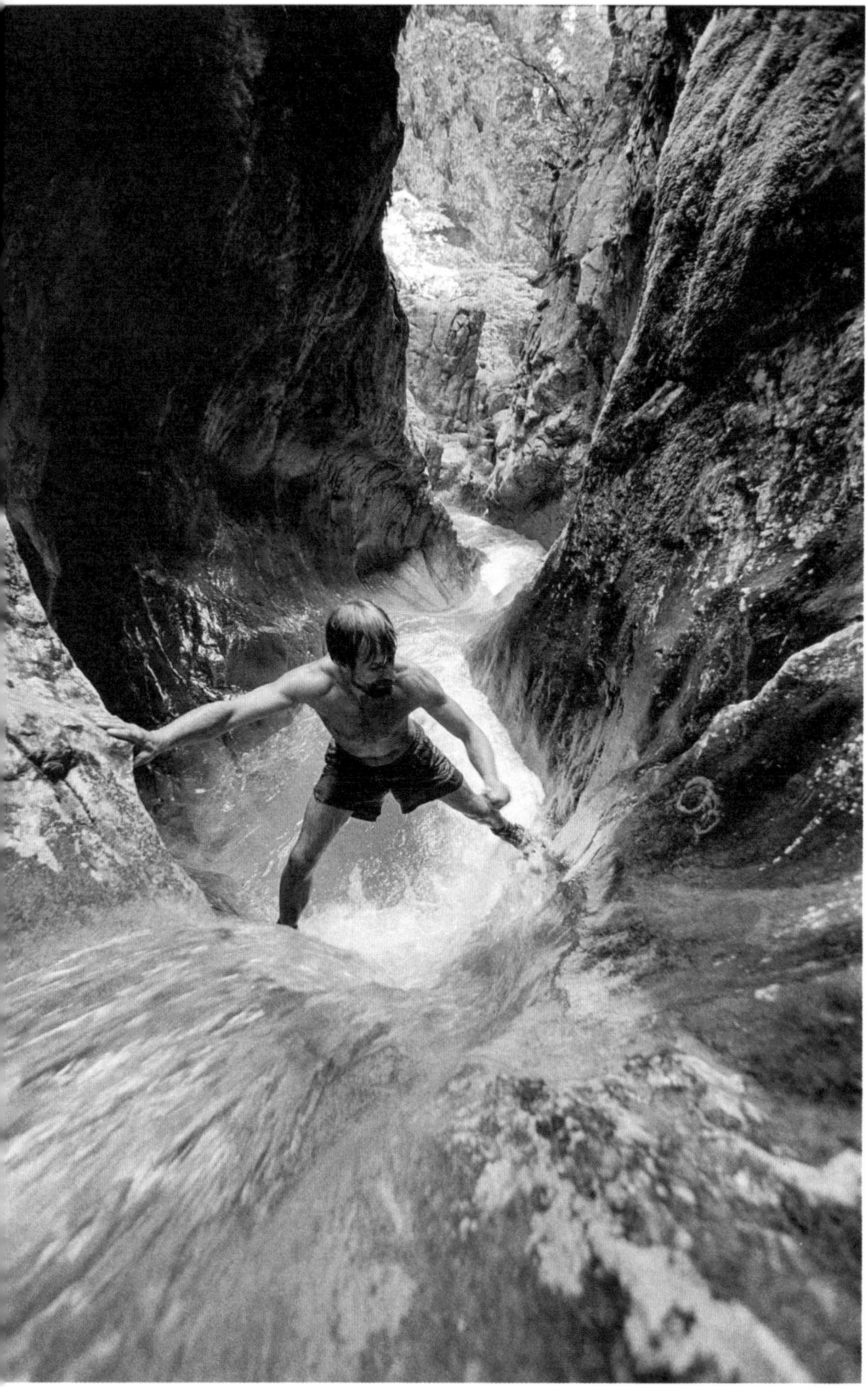

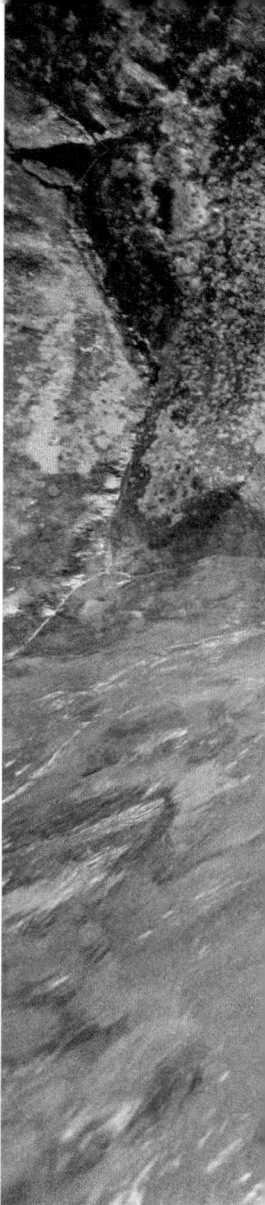

Once you get out of the
water where the canyon
becomes broader, it is
a primordial pleasure
to be heated under
the rays of the sun.
Really, it is only when
we go to the extremes
that we appreciate
being alive. So good!

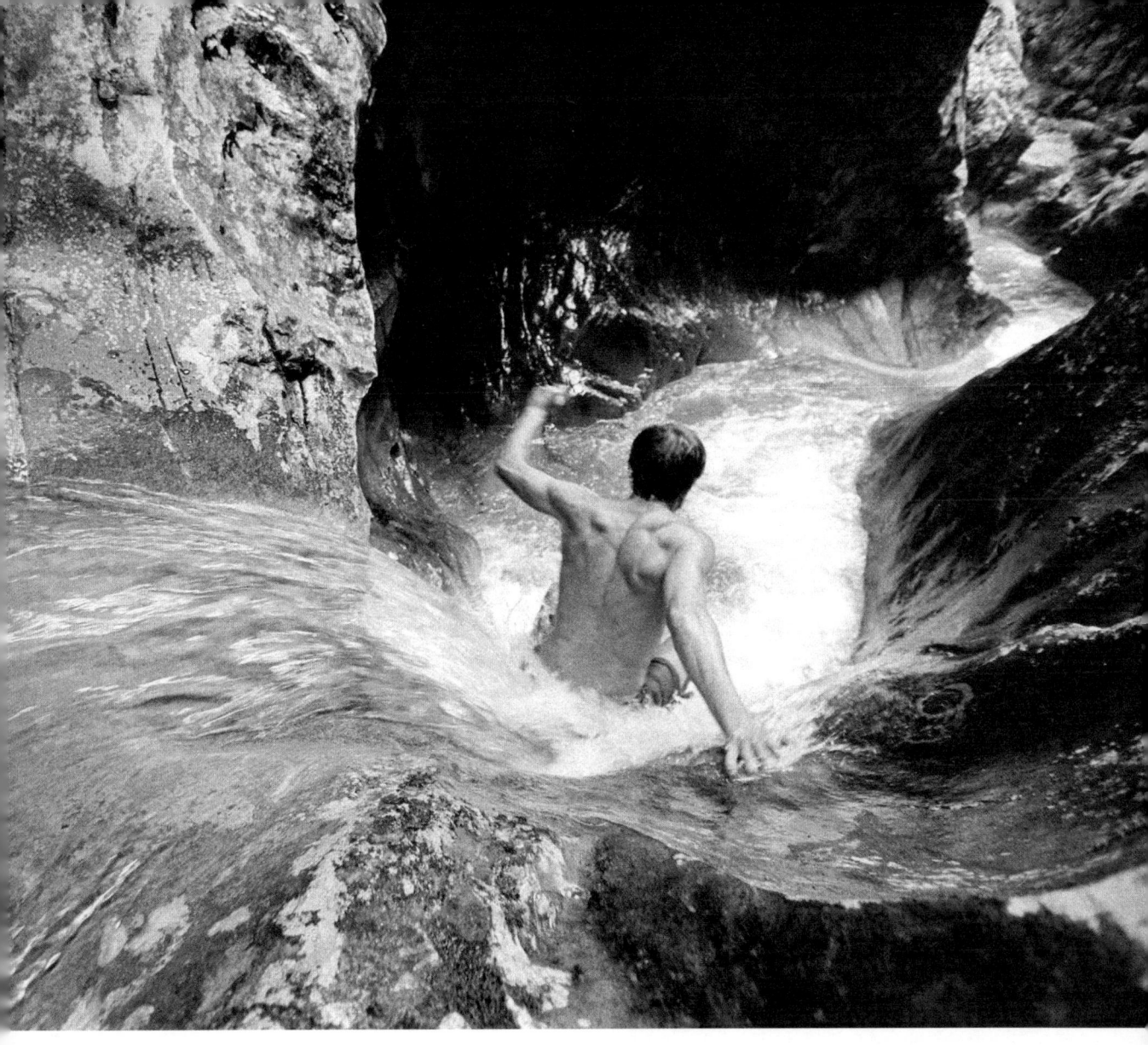

Nature's playground.

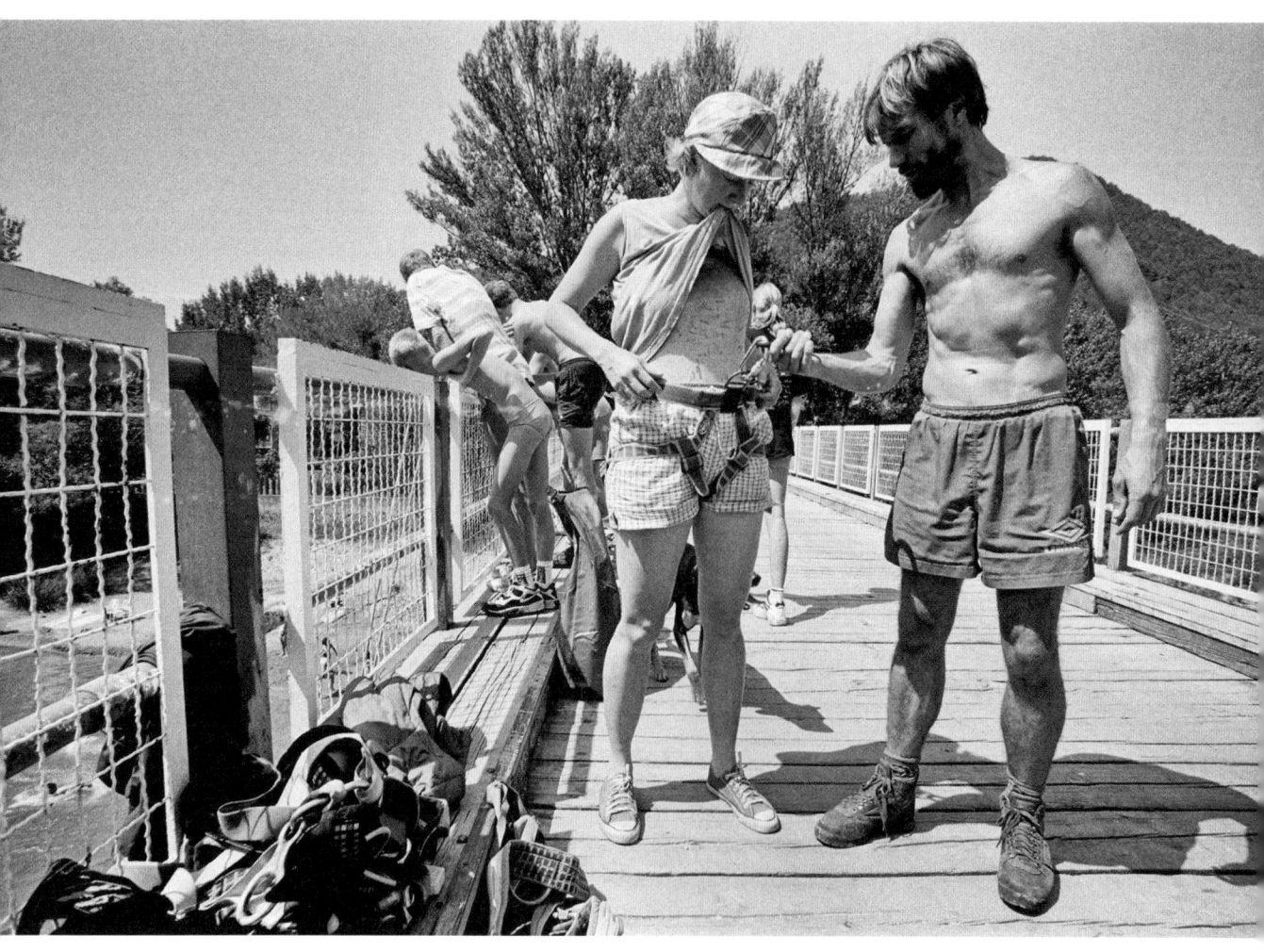

Instruction in abseiling/rappelling before going into the wild. In the canyons you need to be prepared and know the tools of the trade.

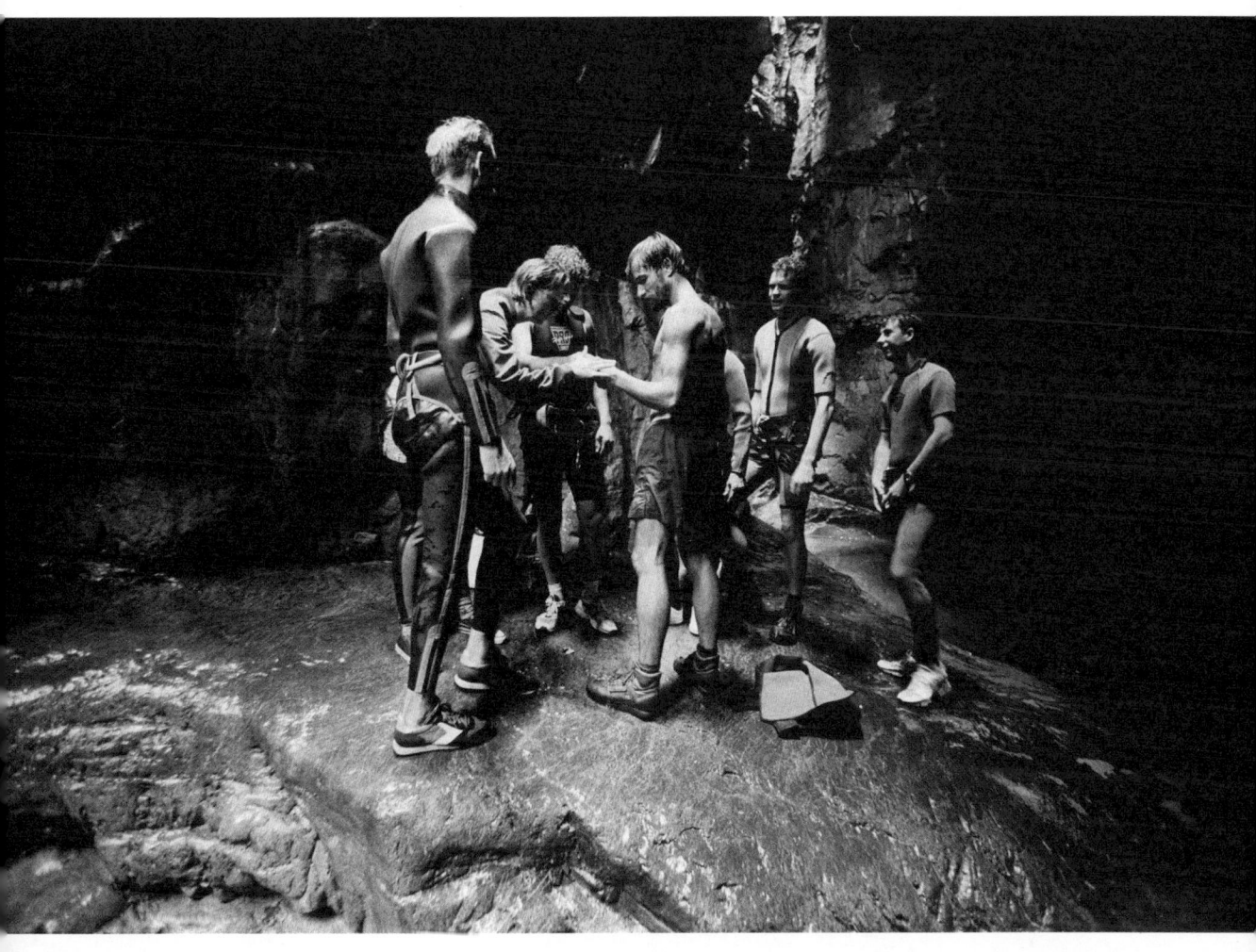

Checking on a safe spot before entering the
narrow dark passages. Excitement.

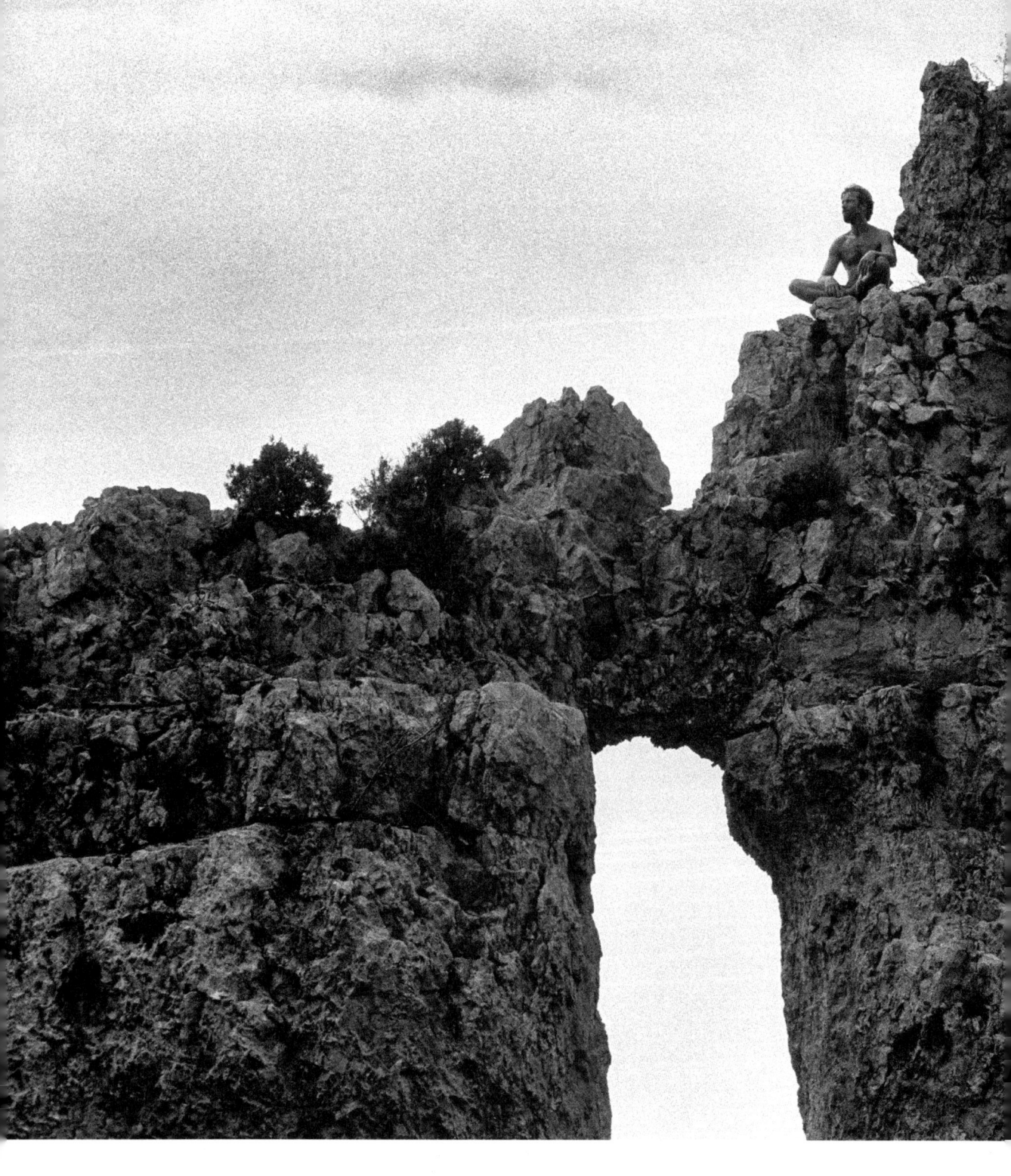

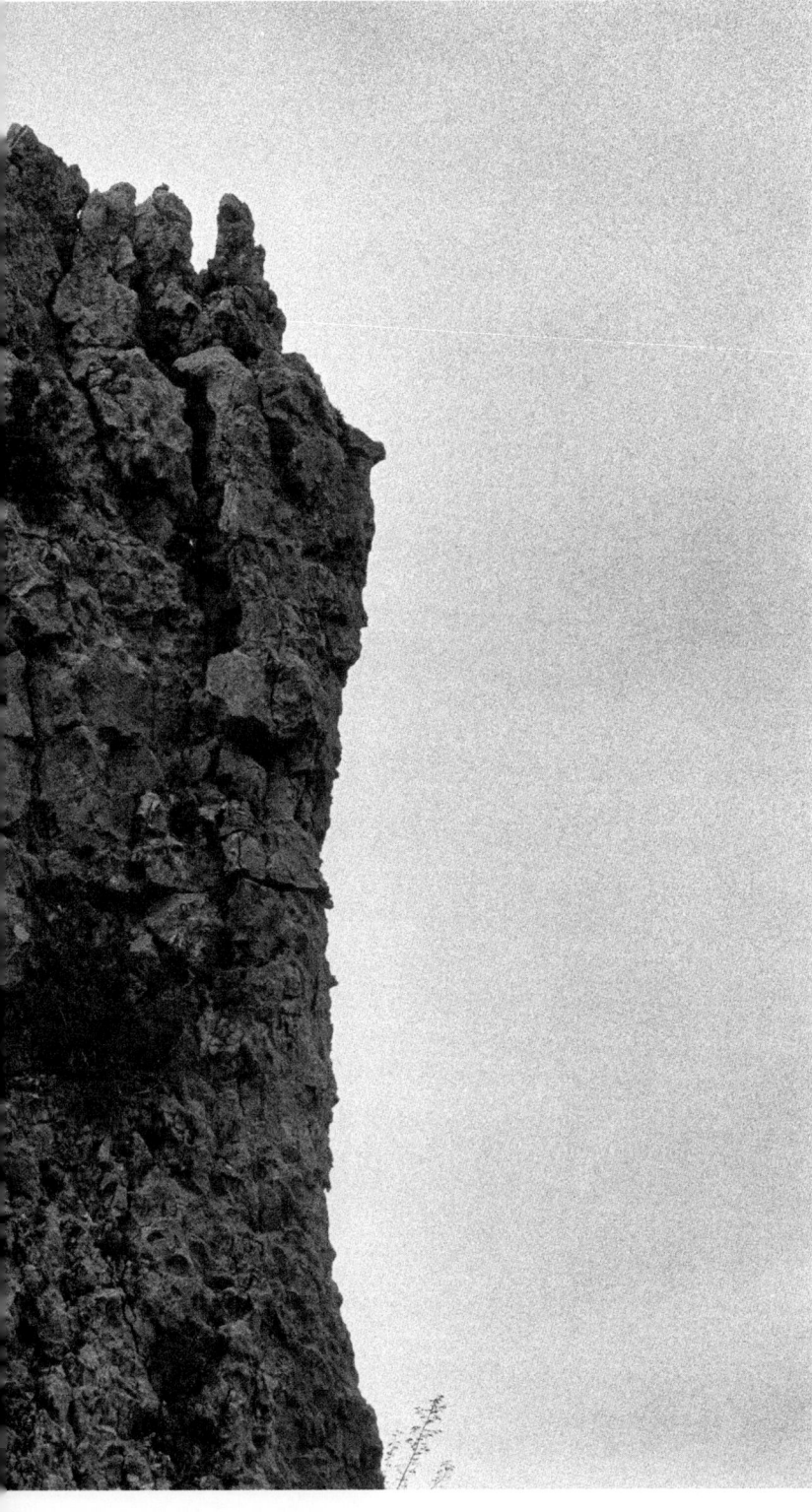

Nature invites us to sit down
and contemplate how little we
actually are. Feeling great.

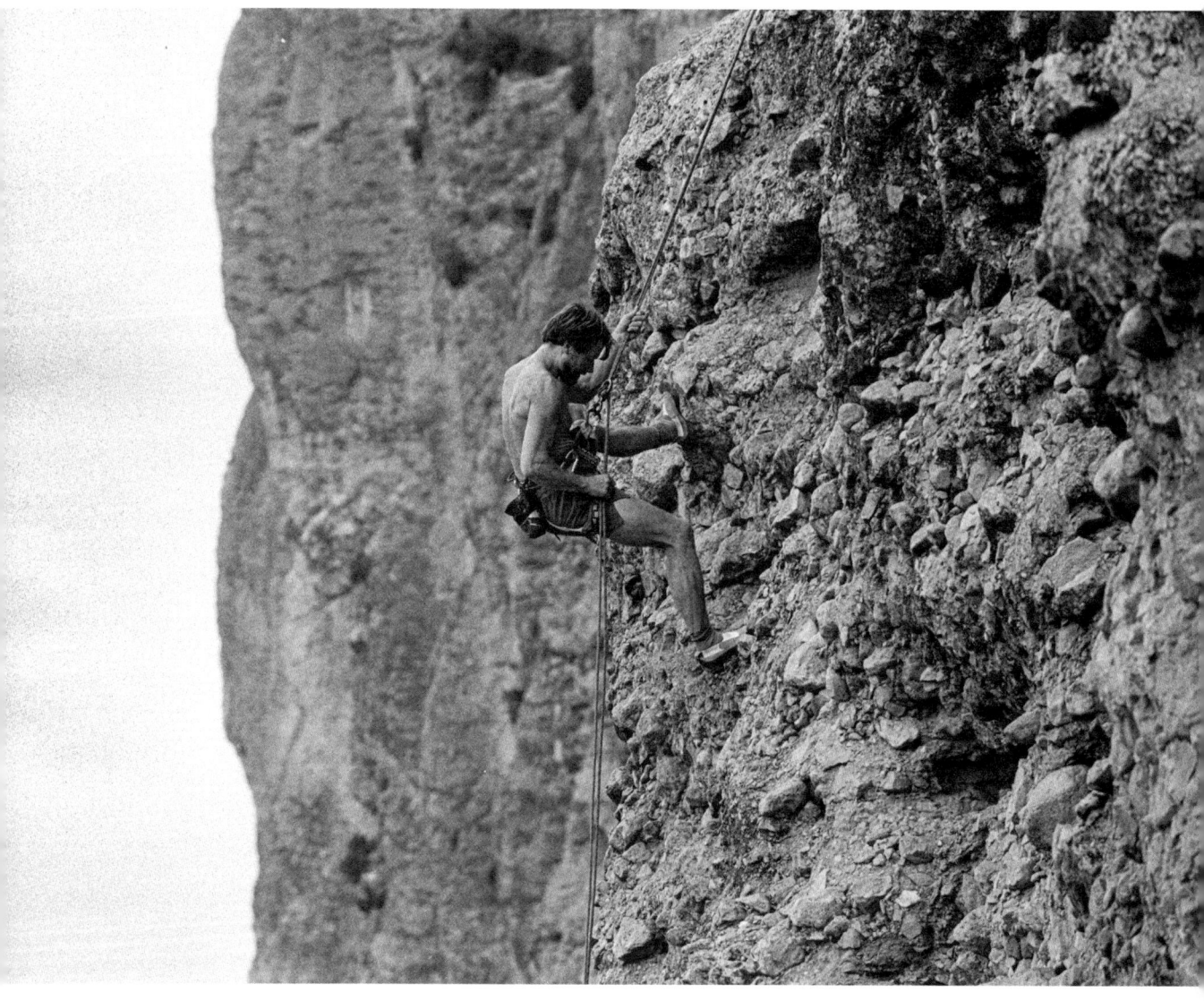

Rocks are beautiful, full of energy. I always found myself feeling
the best of myself in the mountains. Out there. Just being.

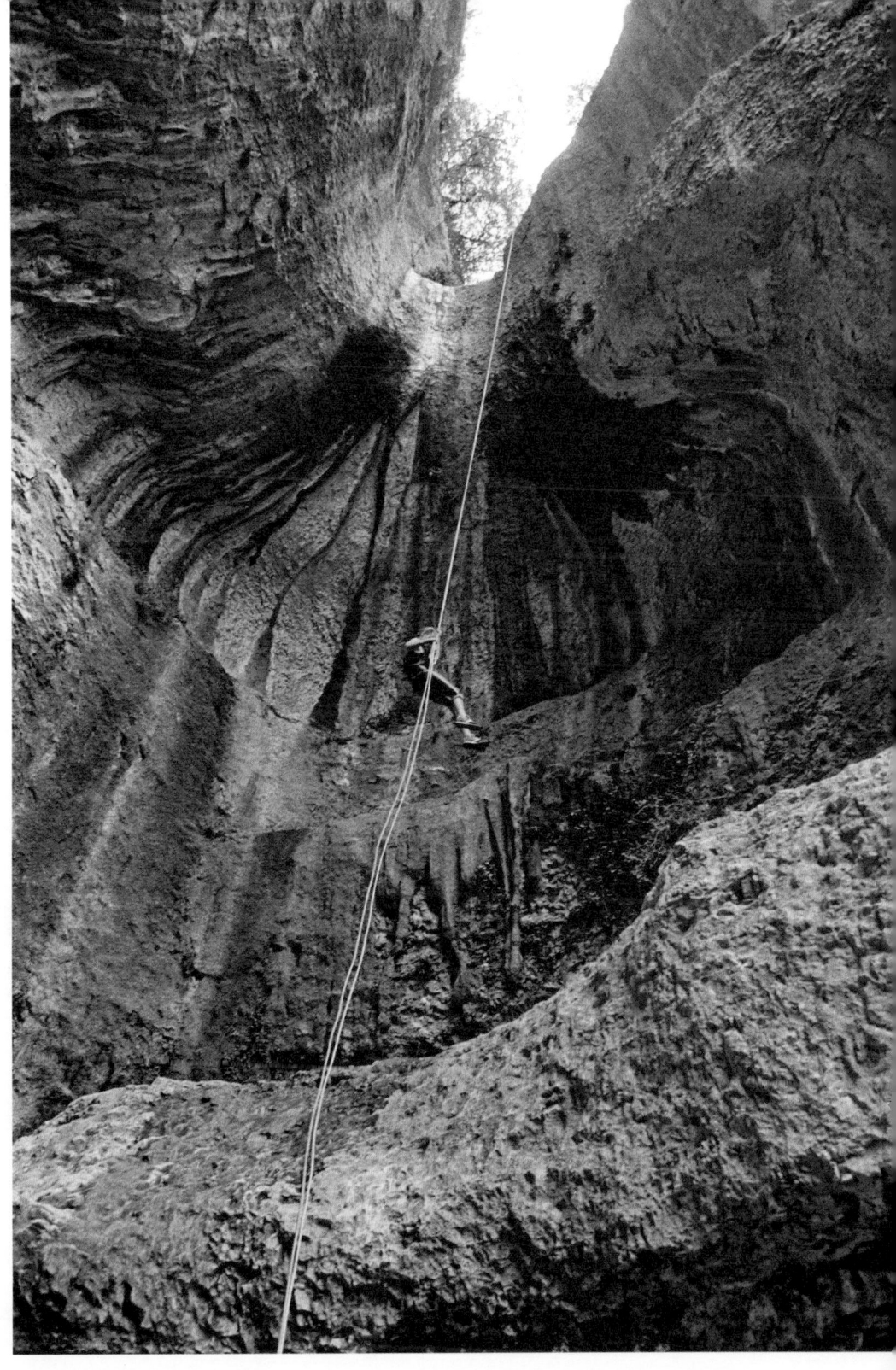

Nature is a
sculptor.

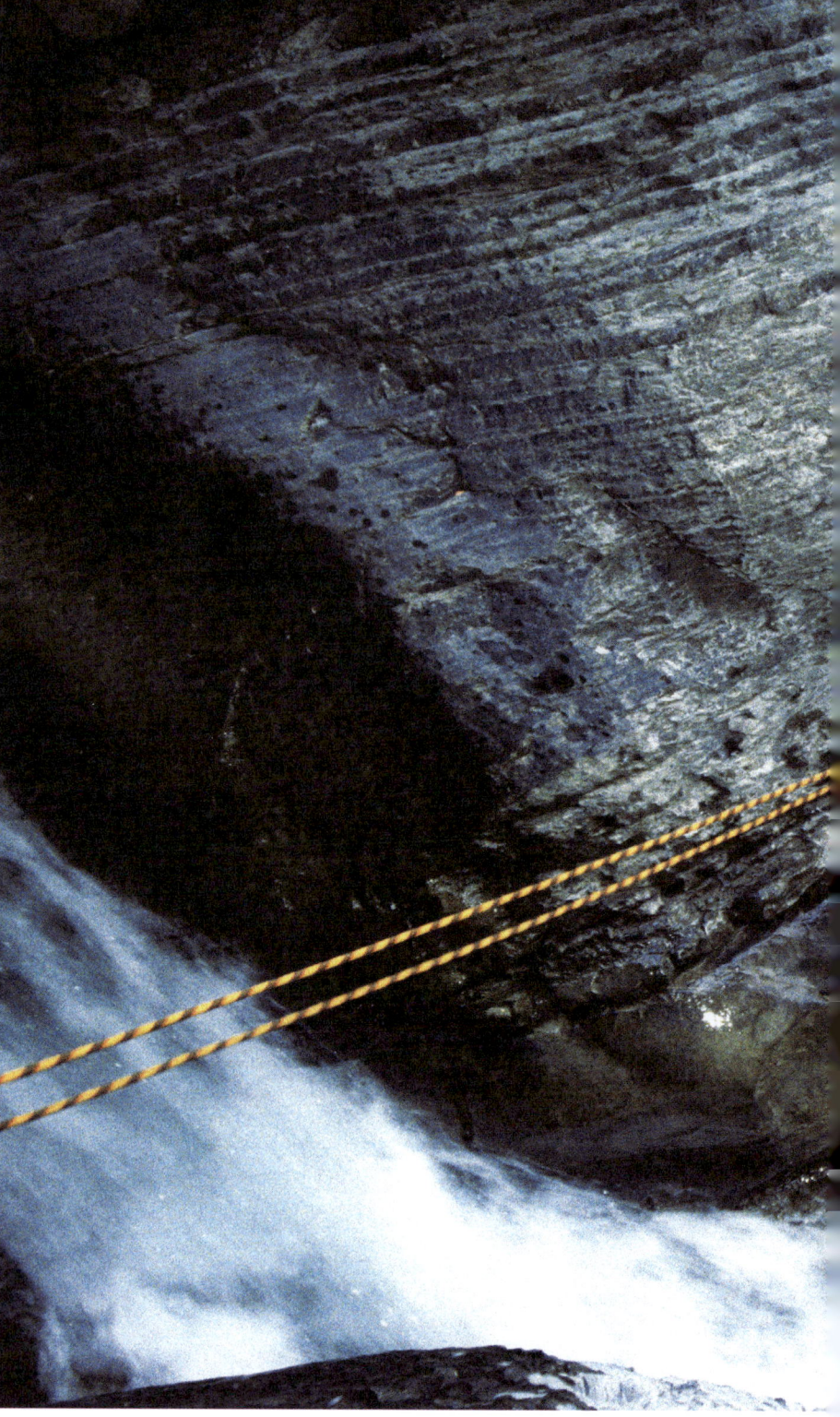

To take groups into the wilderness you have to be alert at almost every step. Danger is always lurking. Nature has a different order from a city.

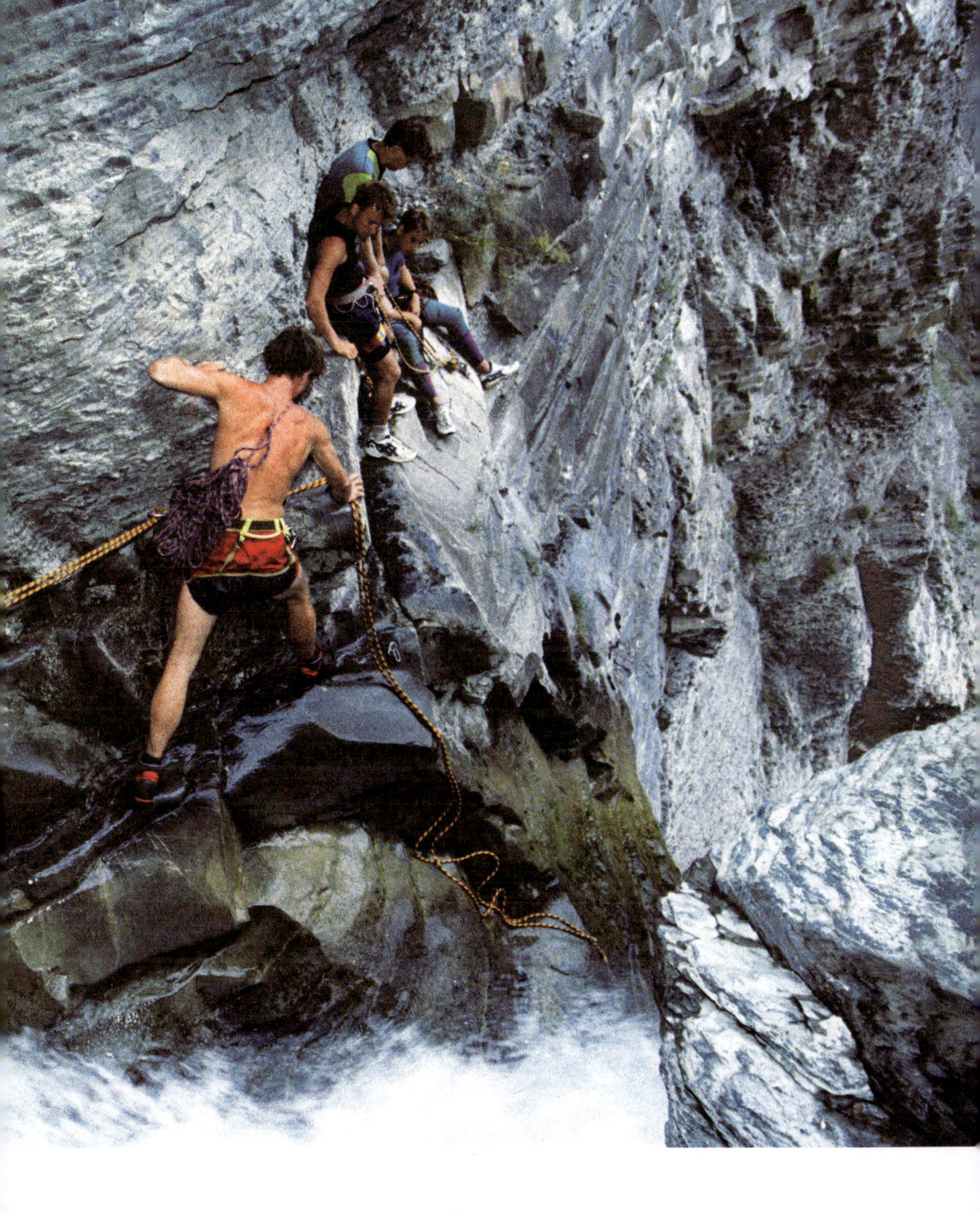

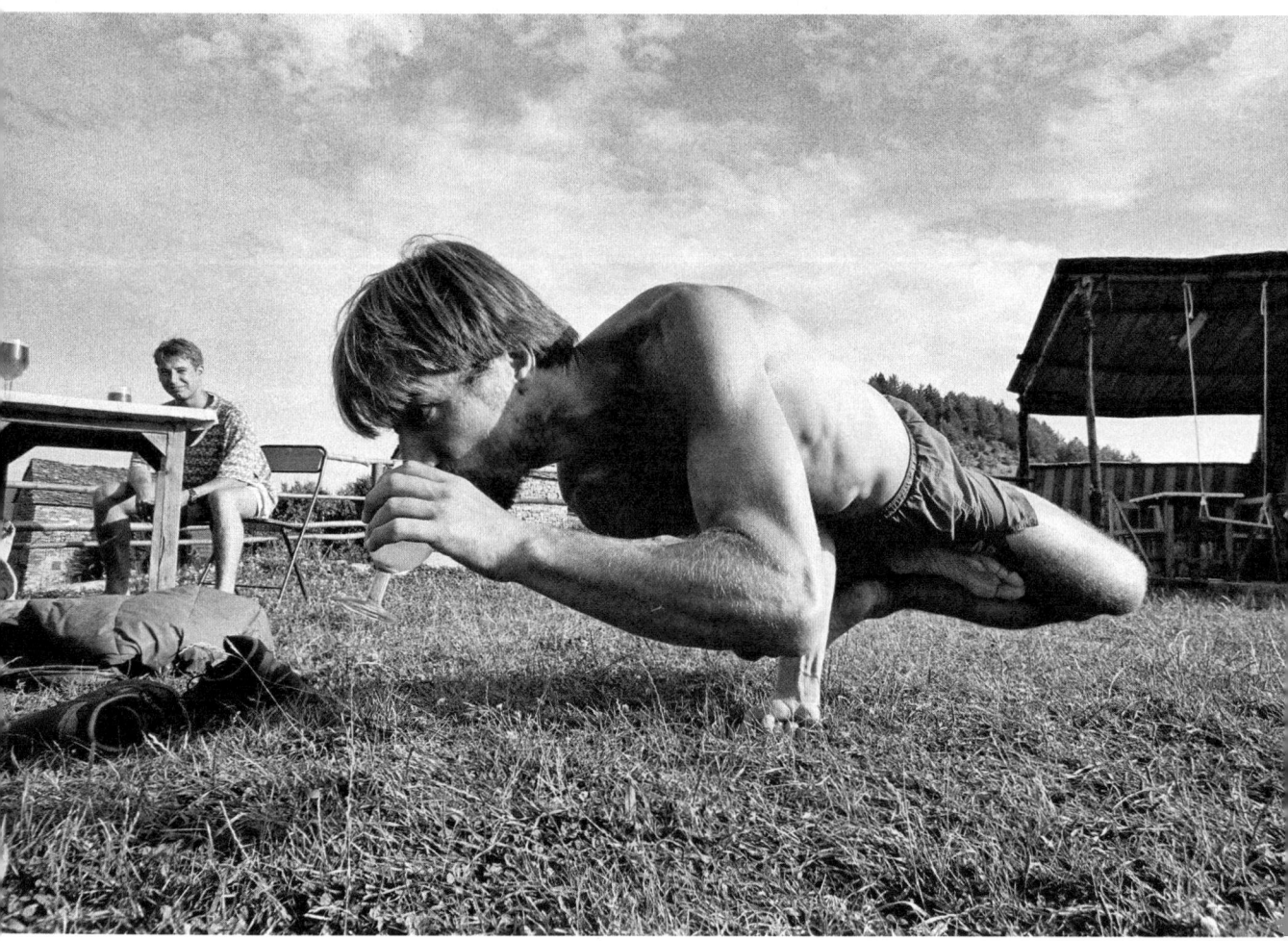

East and West meet in strange ways sometimes. Here I am doing one
of my daily postures, Eka Hasta Lolasana, or One-Limbed Crab Posture,
while sipping on a drink somebody offered me. Having fun after a
trip well done. Sometimes it also serves to be funny with it all.

DELIVERANCE

When the anchor is gone
Life keeps drifting as in a
Song, going along
My kids, innocent
And demanding
Even though troubled
My mind, finding
Purpose in being
present, for them, for me
A new reality you see
They are my eyes of the
Soul, does not make it
Easier at all
Yet unconditional following to serve
You will get what you
Deserve
Exactly tailormade, irrational
Perfectly fit for your fate
Not too early not too late
Right in the moment
An open gate
Eternity is never gone
Do not worry, it will
All be done
Be the love, be the
Gate
Your beloveds become
One with your fate
The mother knows, nothing
Is lost
Be here at all cost
Because when it all comes together
You'll be in heaven, no less, forever
Take it easy, full force

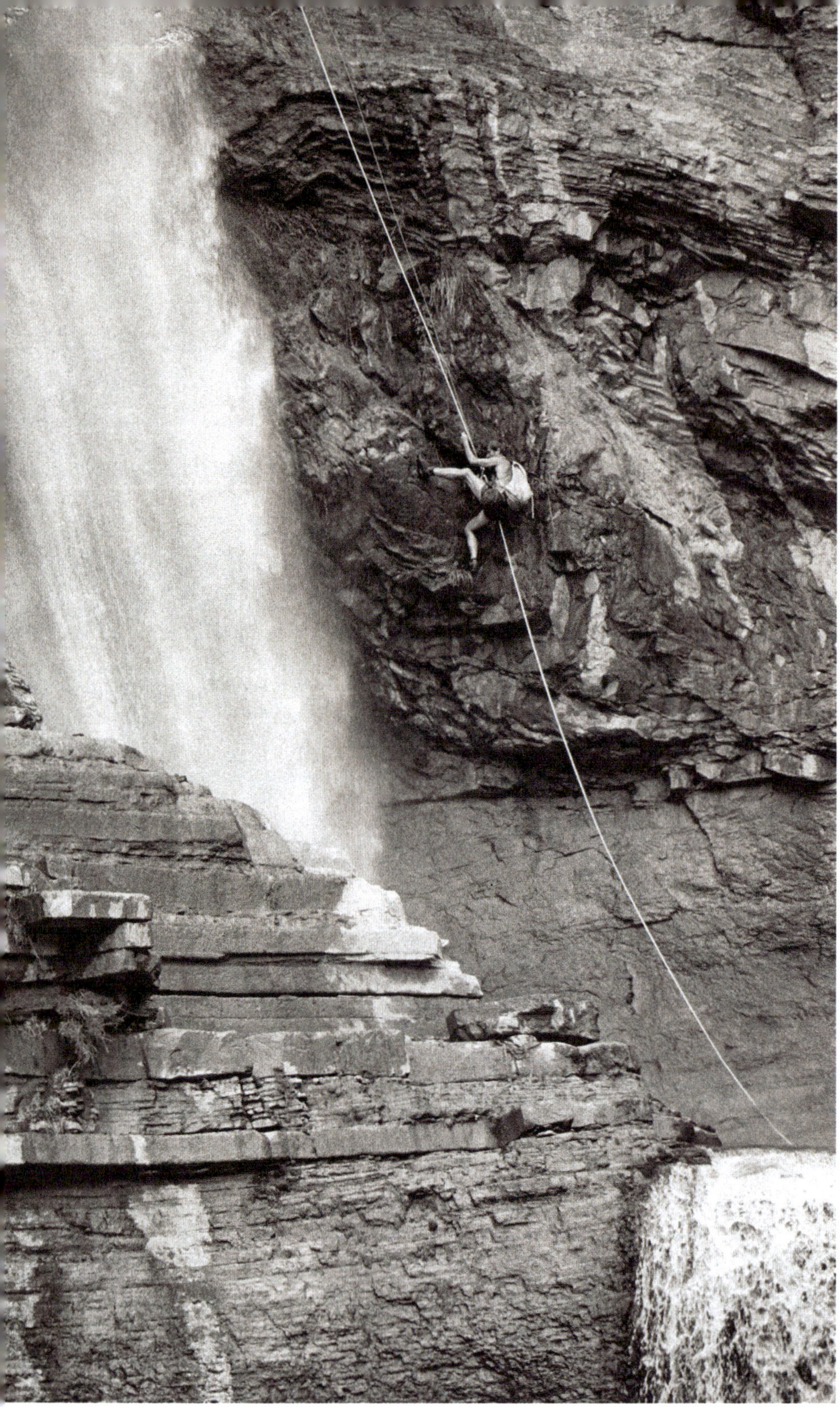

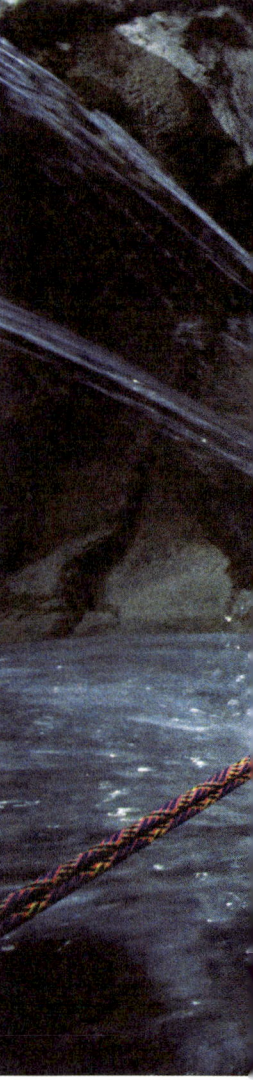

Calculate well because you are part of the calculation. My body was trained in nature, so much so that my instincts and intuition were something I greatly relied upon, especially in the mountains.

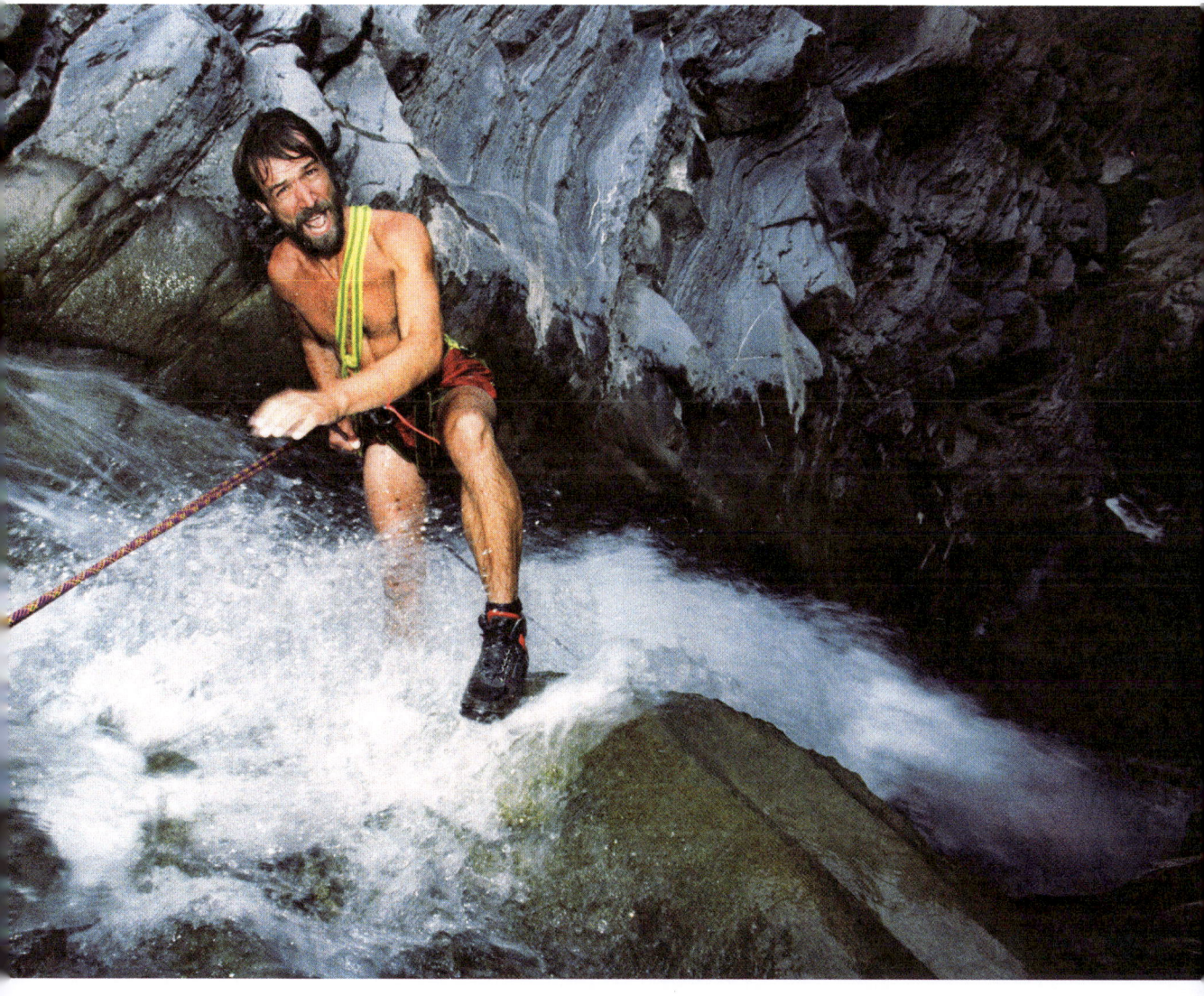

Henny joined me on many of my trips to Spain. We regained contact after Olaya died when he spotted me on Dutch television. We picked up right where we left off. We even made it into a couple of adventure magazines with pictures like this.

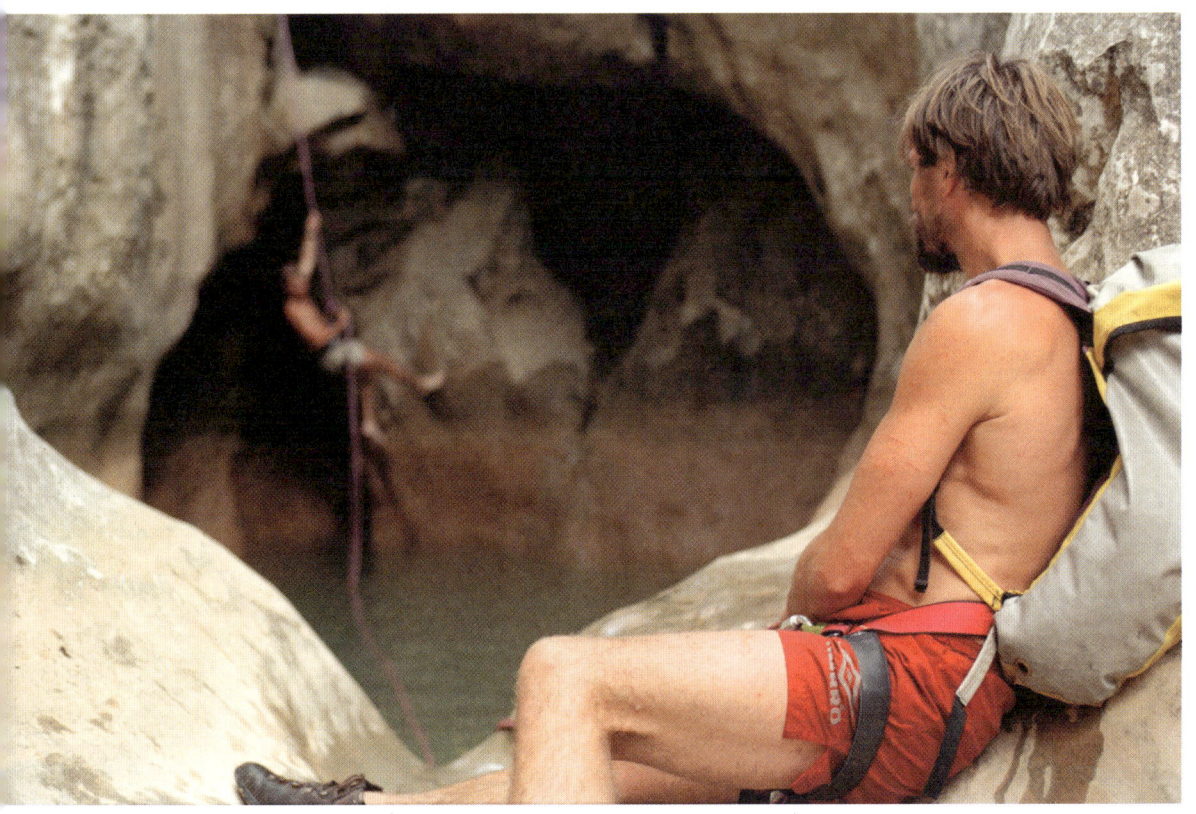

Watching in the labyrinth, the Oscuros, part of the
great Mascun (Arab for "place of spirits") Canyon.

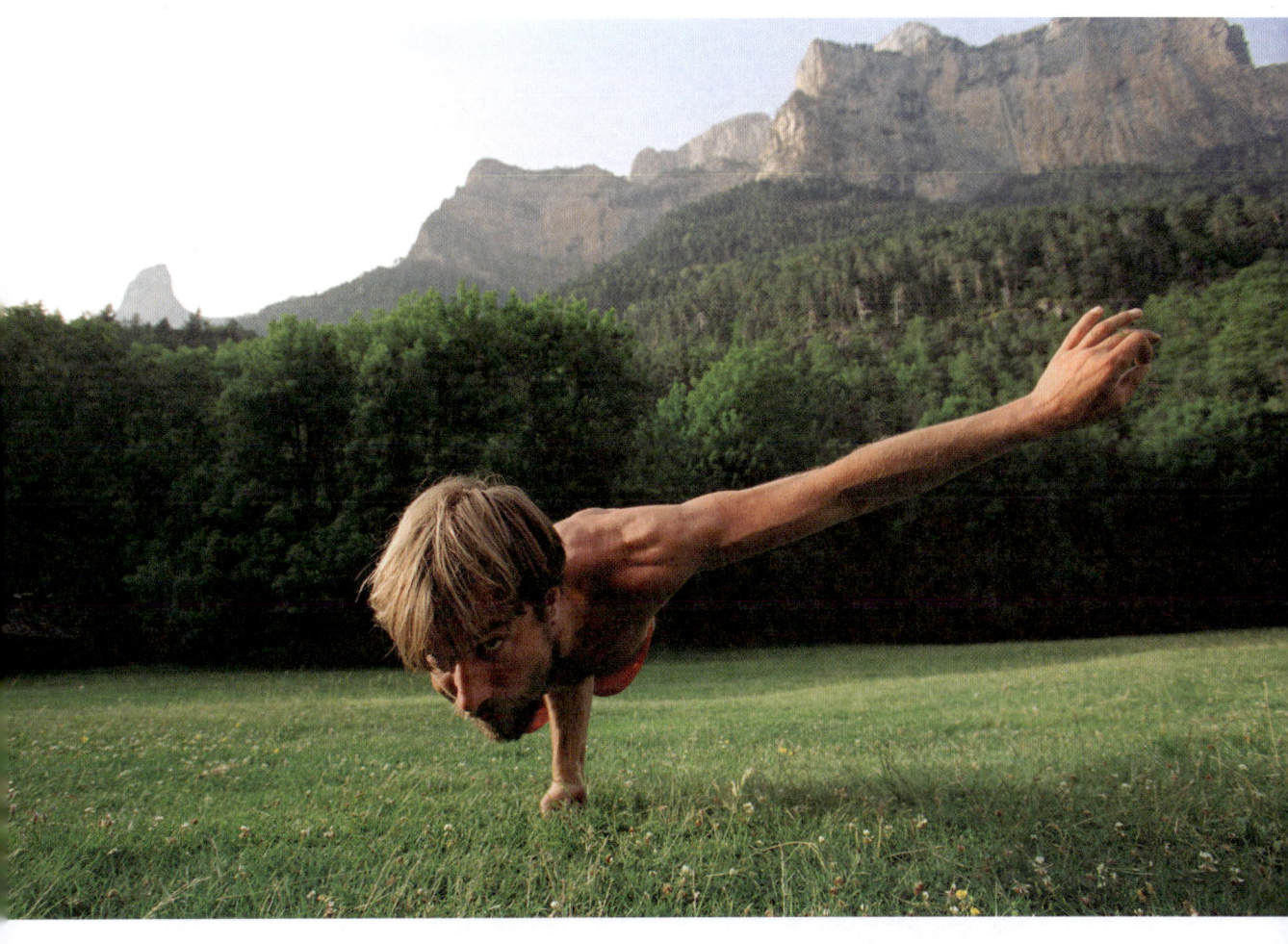

Behind the great walls of the Bujaruelo, part of
the Ordesa Valley in Huesca, Aragon.

This is one of my exercises. I know Sanskrit from learning the sutras of
Patanjali and all the postures, so I just came up with a name for what
I'm doing here: Eka Hasta Sarira Uttanasana, or the One-Armed Bandit
Posture. Yoga as a principle is nondogmatic and not rigid. New things can
be added. It is good to learn principles but even better to have your own.

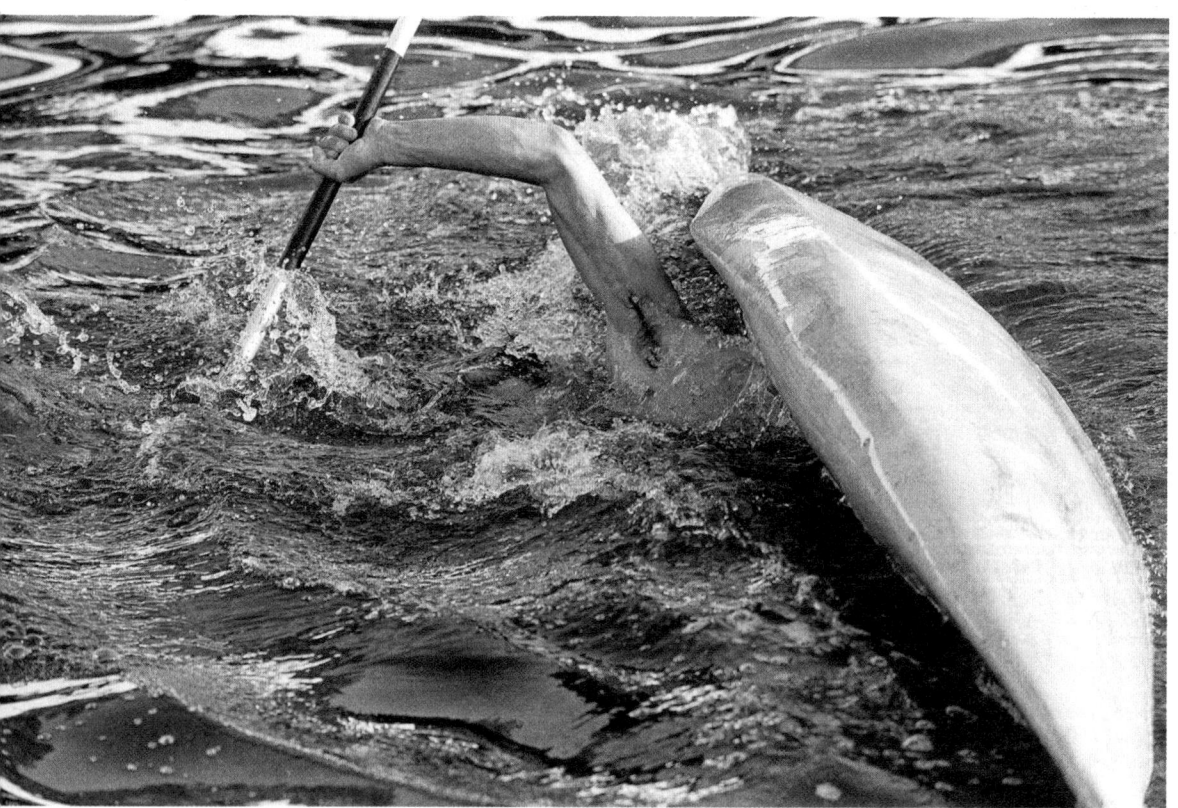

A full circle. The Eskimo roll. Back in Amsterdam.

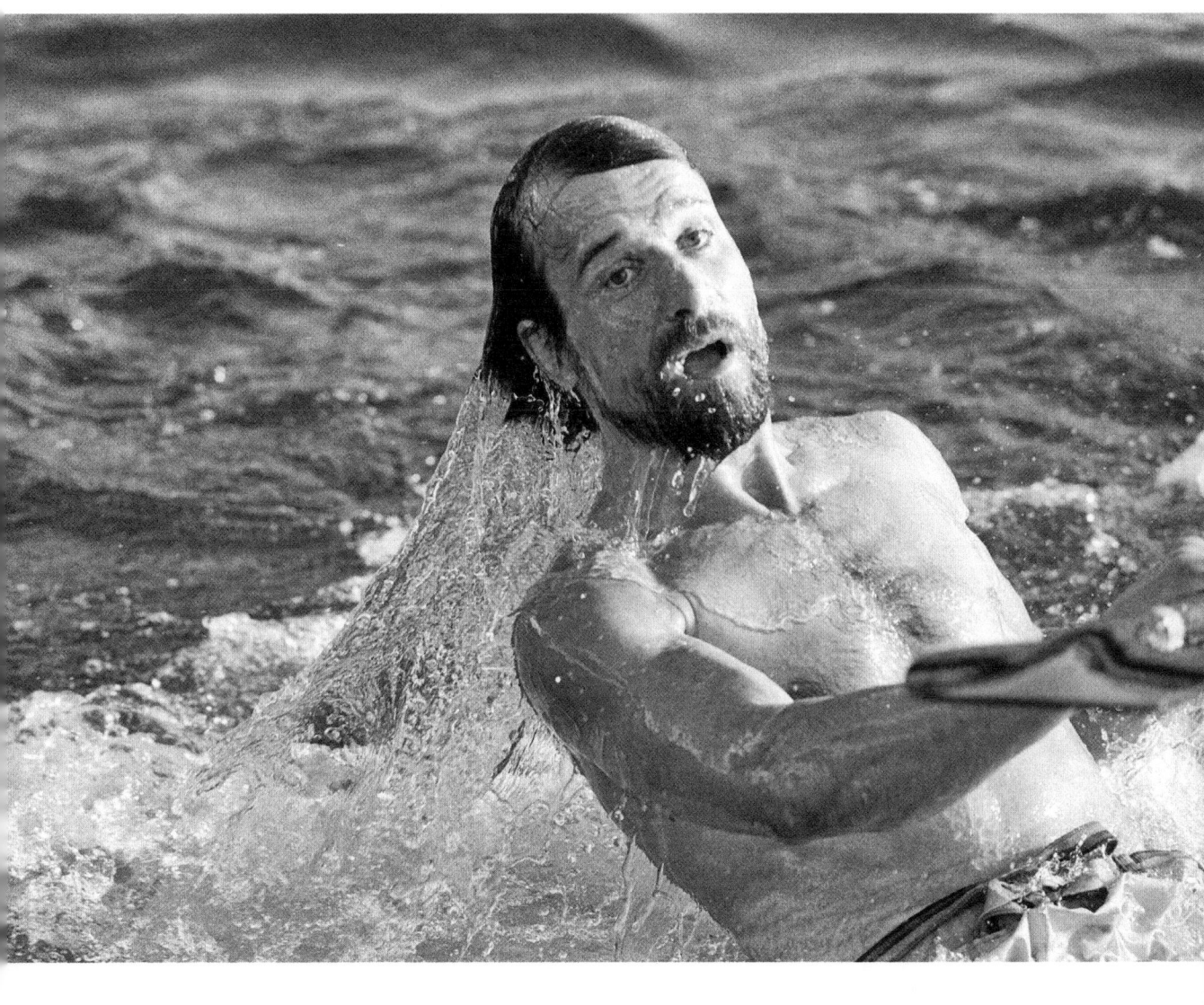

RIVER

The perfect swimmer rests on the tide of the water

Peace in his mind, no clutter

As his mood flows past the turbulence of time

Having cleansed and care for his inner shrine

He brought what was really mine

Golden

Brilliant

Modest, just fine

More than okay, because of an unconditional state

Of being, seeing

It all

Without claiming anything, but equanimity

Of the Soul

Friendly and observing life

While the universe manifest its strive

To bring and see

That there is plenty for all to be

Golden

Brilliant

modest, just fine

Where the river flows

Divine.

To me, the mountains in the Netherlands are its trees and bridges, and its stony shore walls are boulders. While I was kayaking in the waters of Amsterdam, I wanted to challenge my body and mind, so I used Amsterdam as my fitness room. I would take on anything, the bridges, the waters, the trees. I saw opportunities to train and exercise anywhere in the city. Mostly, I did things on my own. I knew what people were thinking: What a crazy guy. What an idiot. Hey, that's dangerous. Hey, you can't do that. I didn't mind seeming like an outcast. It didn't stop me from doing things my way. It is amazing how differently you can look at a city. Consciousness is everything. It is pure alchemy.

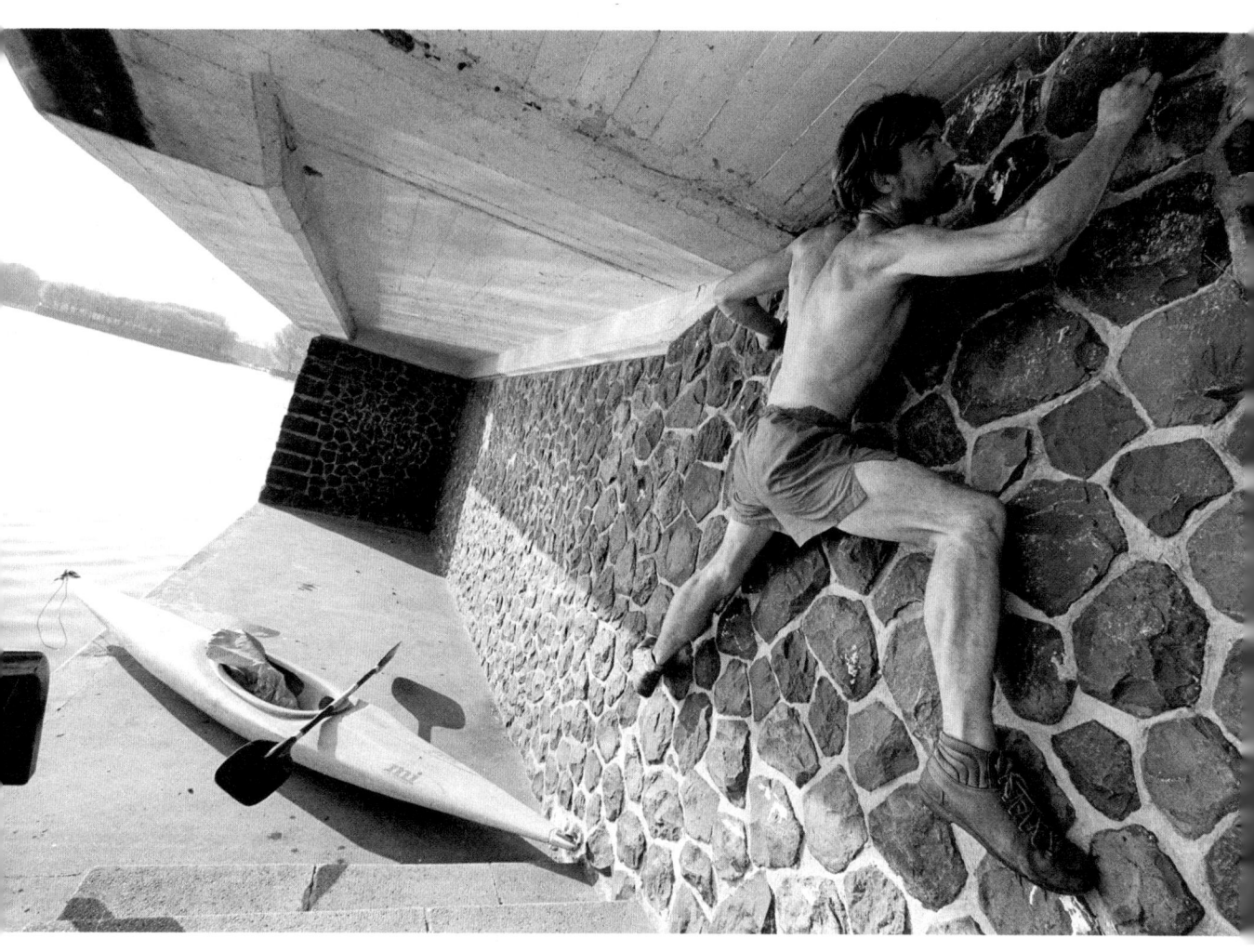

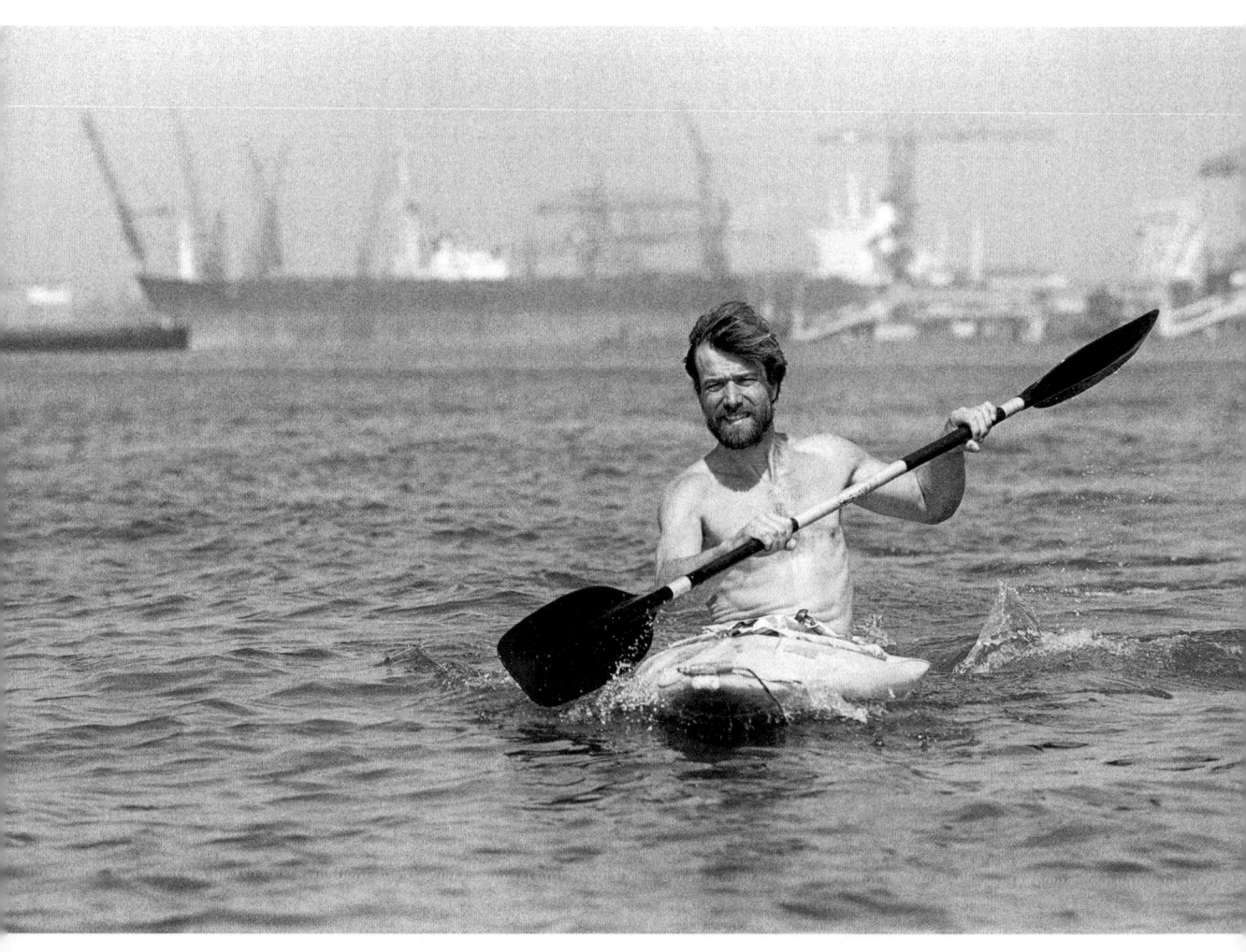

Dutch harbors, big ships, little canoes, great experience.

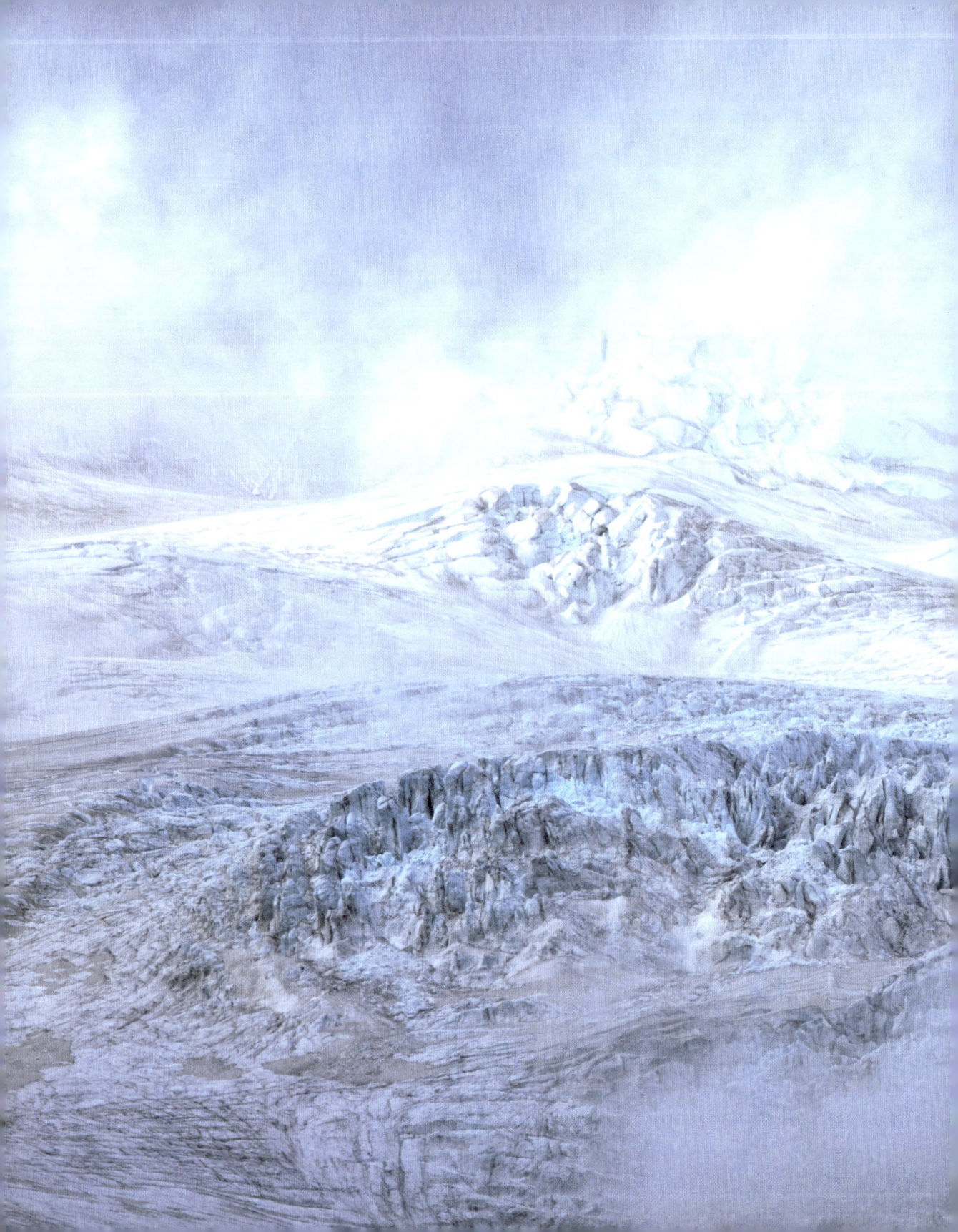

Part Two

Fully Exposed

THERE IS OFTEN A TIME in life when you don't see anything growing from your efforts, yet something is growing. In the bewilderment of emotions, you can become lost, your energy drained, and it can appear as if nothing is happening. No movement. No growth. But growth is happening. You have to trust in that. Life put me in certain conditions, and I had no choice but to act, even when I felt I was failing. But without my knowing, those earlier years made way for this particular future. You get what you serve, not what you deserve. Life throws lessons at you, and you have to face it as it comes. An identity greater than I ever thought possible emerged out of all those crazy and often sad times. You see what I mean? I embraced it all. All of the challenges I took on were part of my learning to finally arrive at a discipline

that supports my life, and now many others. I kept my discipline, and everything I experienced became the fuel for that much more.

All the world records and TV appearances came as a whirlwind of energy, pulling me out of my daily life. I found it exciting. To challenge my body, to come out from the shadows. It was all ascending energy. And I was ready for it. After over a decade of just surviving, there was suddenly a spark, and I went for it. I pushed the limits more and more. But pushing the limits isn't without certain unforeseen dangers. I've lost my way under the ice, been caught in a whiteout on Mount Everest, and endured cramping while climbing without gear. I went to the extreme, but it doesn't mean you have to.

But what I learned from these challenges is that we are capable of doing more than we think. That could be climbing a mountain you never thought possible or embarking on a creative endeavor that is slumbering inside of you. We don't give ourselves enough credit. It was through all of these challenges and challenging myself that I found the different dimensions of what we as humans have deprived ourselves of through modern-day life.

The importance of that far outreached any physical challenge. If I had not been so inviting to the harsh lens of scientific scrutiny, I would have remained just a spectacle, a circus artist, someone to watch from afar. Now, all over the world, people are getting out there and experiencing the power themselves. My mission is to show we have far more power to control our lives, through science and sense.

I challenged the accepted physiological understanding. Shifting the paradigm became my goal. I will always go back to that nature, the core of our strength and our true vulnerability. That is the heart of it all. It brings the unexpected to your awareness, which normally stays deeply hidden. It gave me an unearthly, deep confidence in my ability to cope with exposing myself in merciless nature.

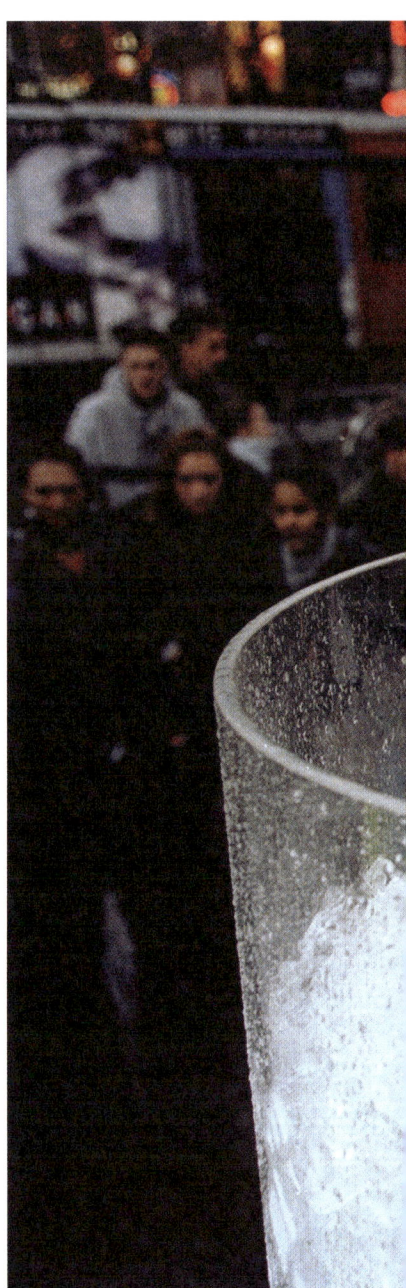

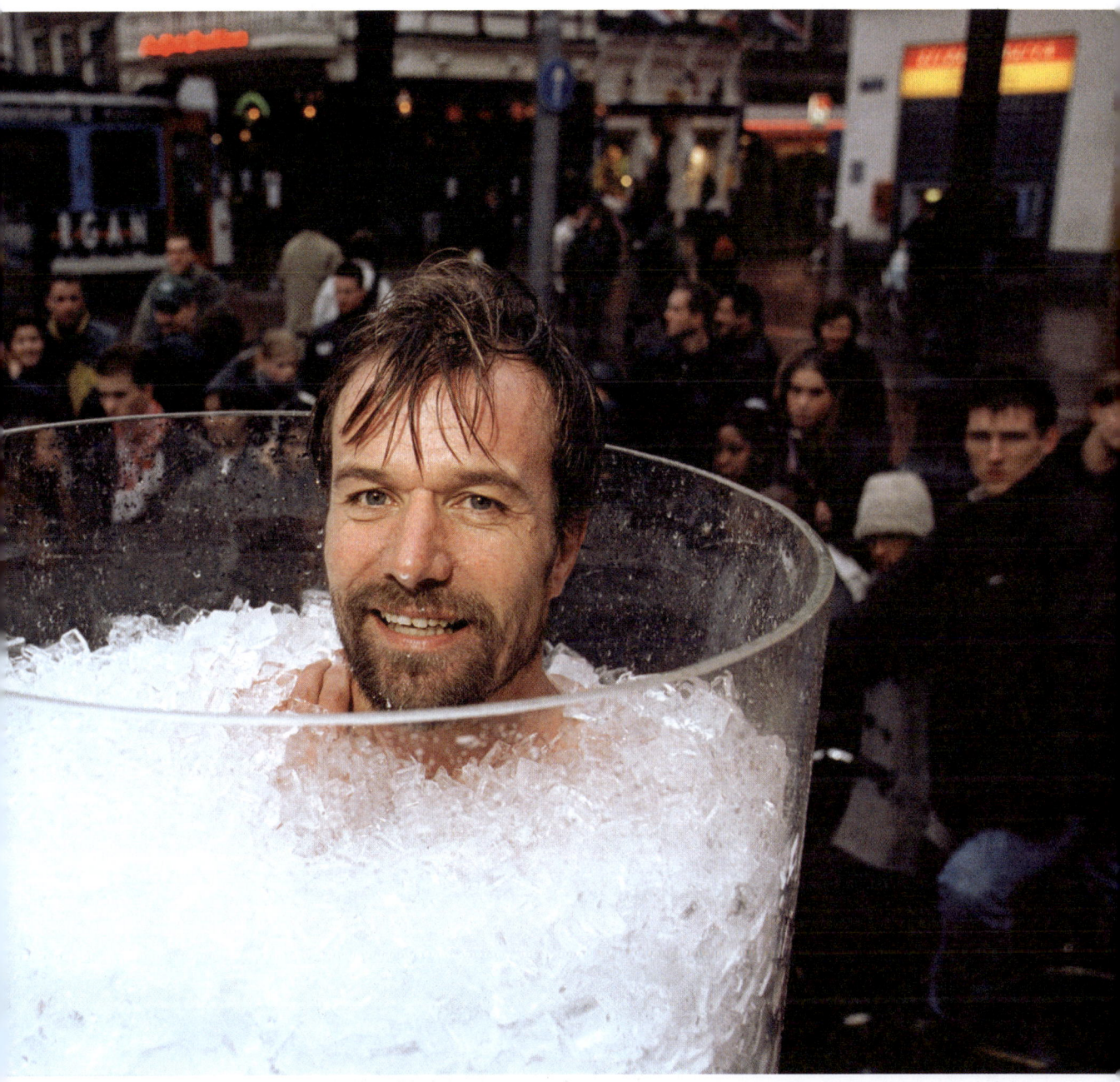

One of my first appearances in public for American television. I was building a
name for myself. I was just enthusiastically going with it all. So, every time I did
these things, it took me out of my daily routine. I was excited to do all that. Imagine
yourself in an icebox in a main square of a city somewhere—I loved it!

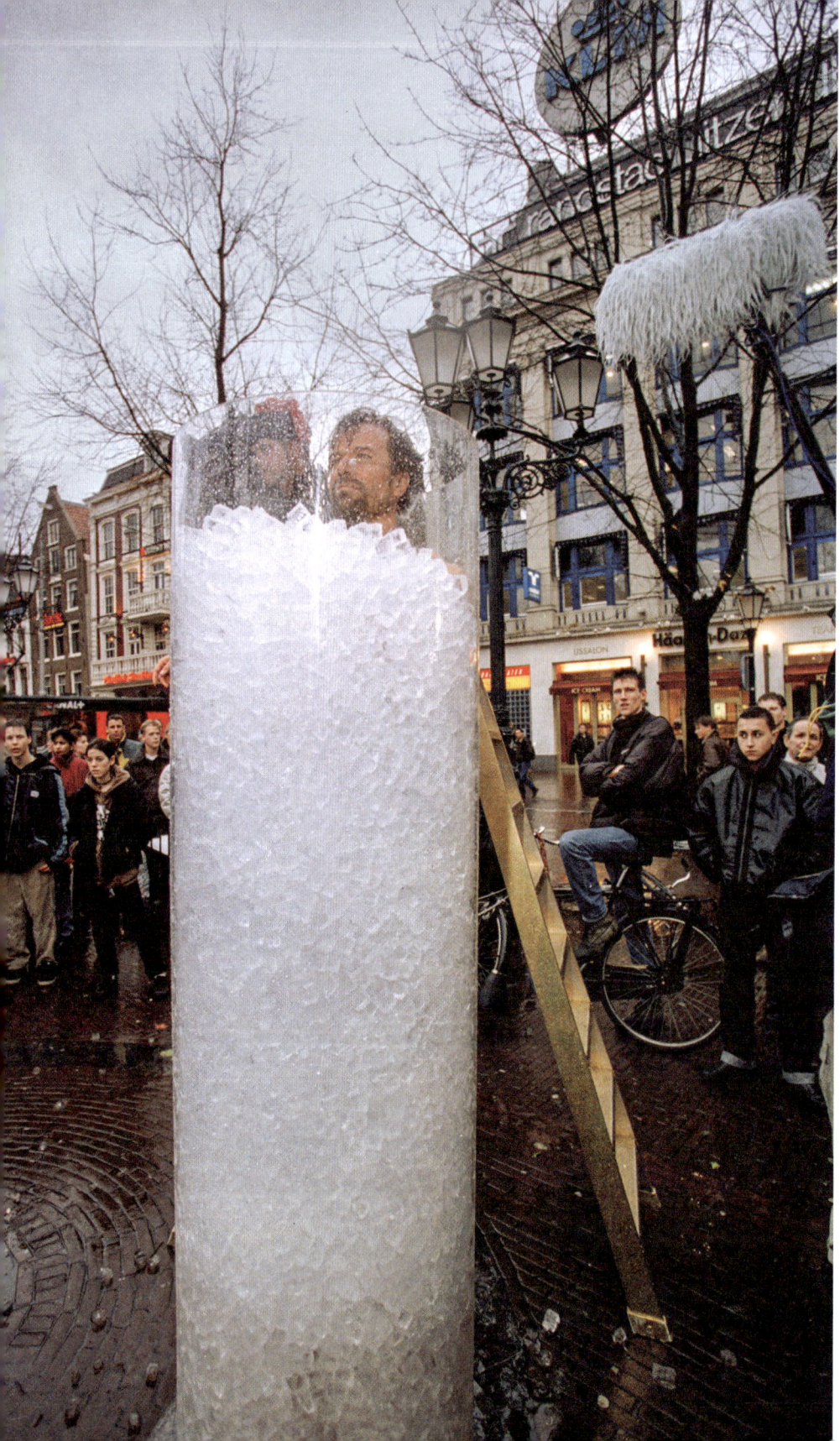

I felt the attention of the public, the audience of spectators, but when you are in the cold, you go to the core and stay there! This is where one learns for oneself to focus on the body and going inward. In neuroscience this is called "interoceptive focus," the eighth sense.

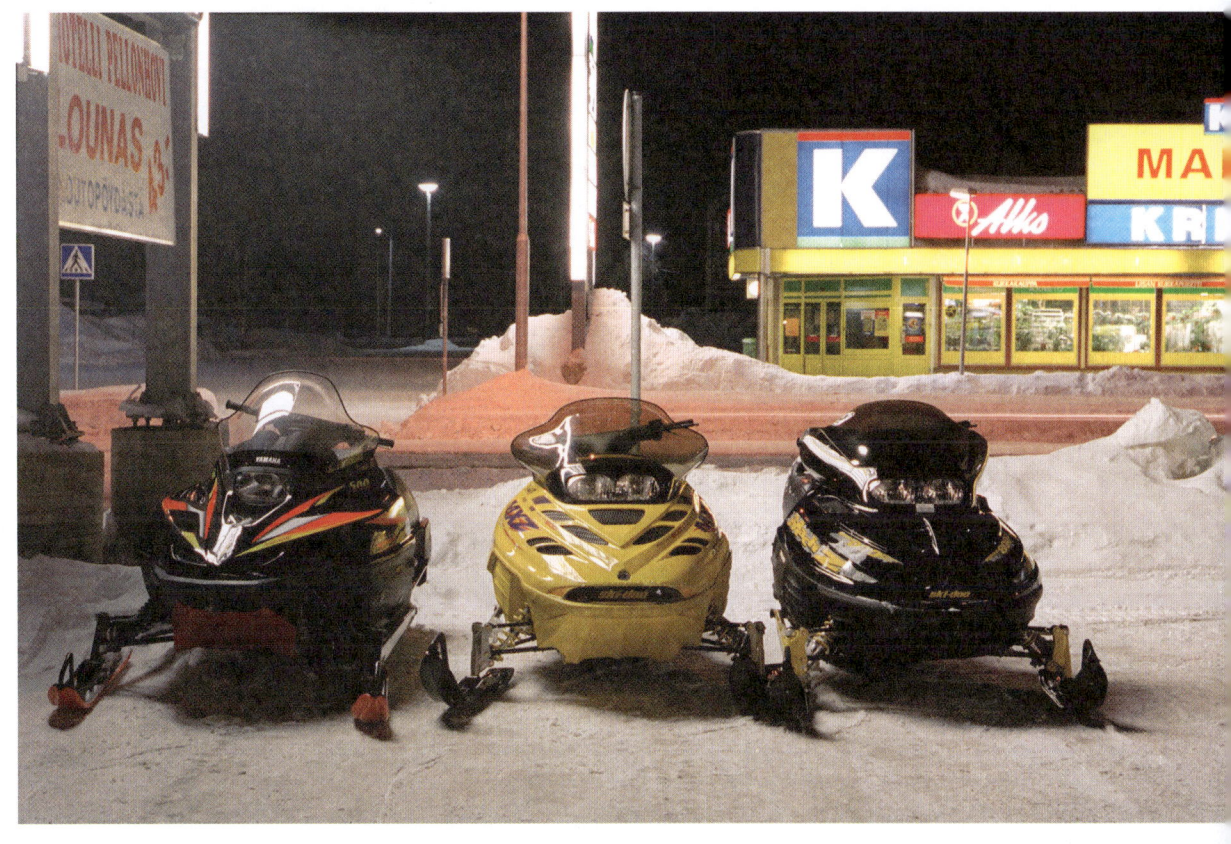

Kolari, Lapland. This was my view from our hotel room.

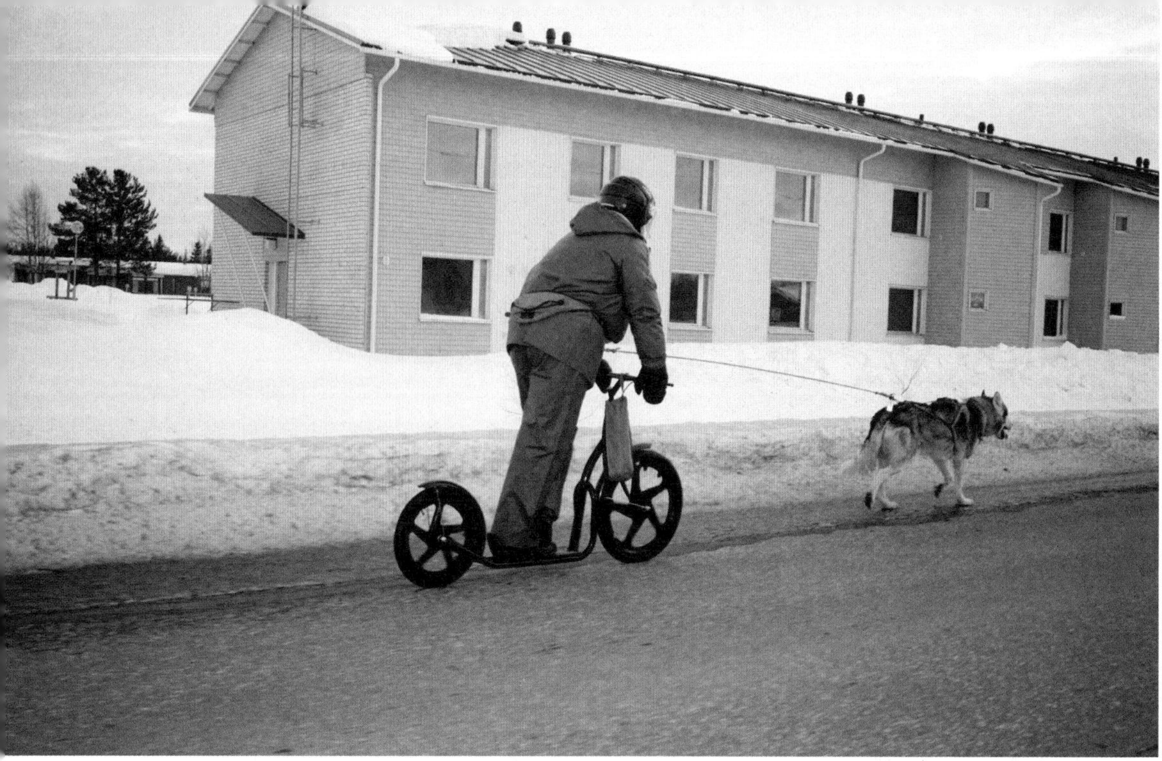

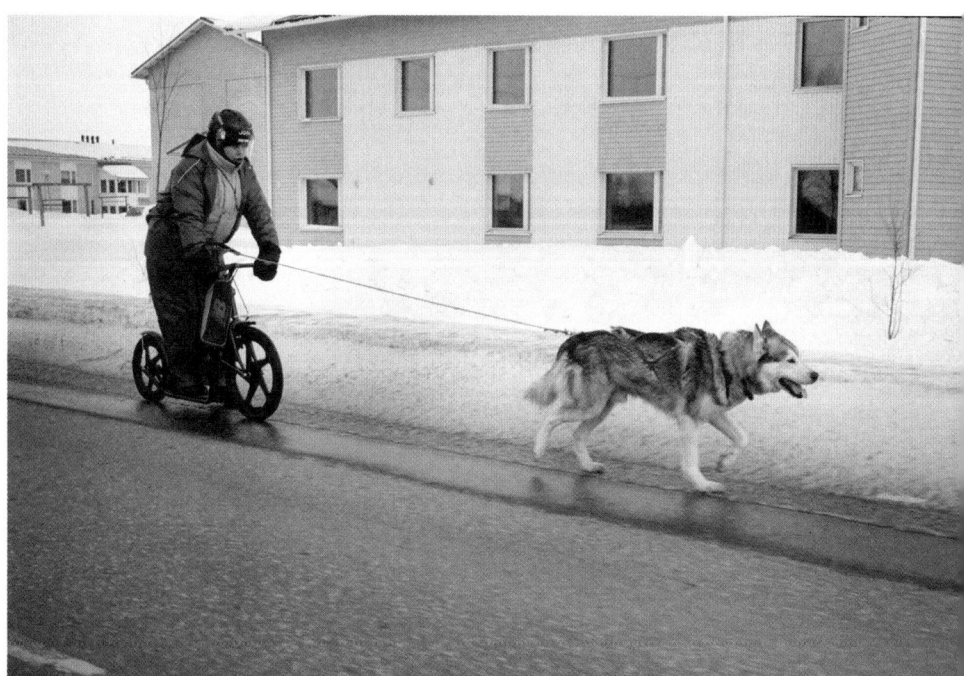

All these challenges brought me to unexpected places and situations that deeply engrain themselves into your memories. To see a person being pulled by a Husky doesn't happen in Amsterdam, not in many places for that matter. I think the world is full of beautiful places. It is always good to break out of your normal existence and see yourself in the backdrop of a totally different everyday experience. The beauty of traveling is the unexpected, unconditioned routines. This is where you see the beauty of the mind, where you get a glimpse of its beauty. You don't know how to react or act. You have to adapt. It is strange and beautiful at the same time. Wandering is beautiful.

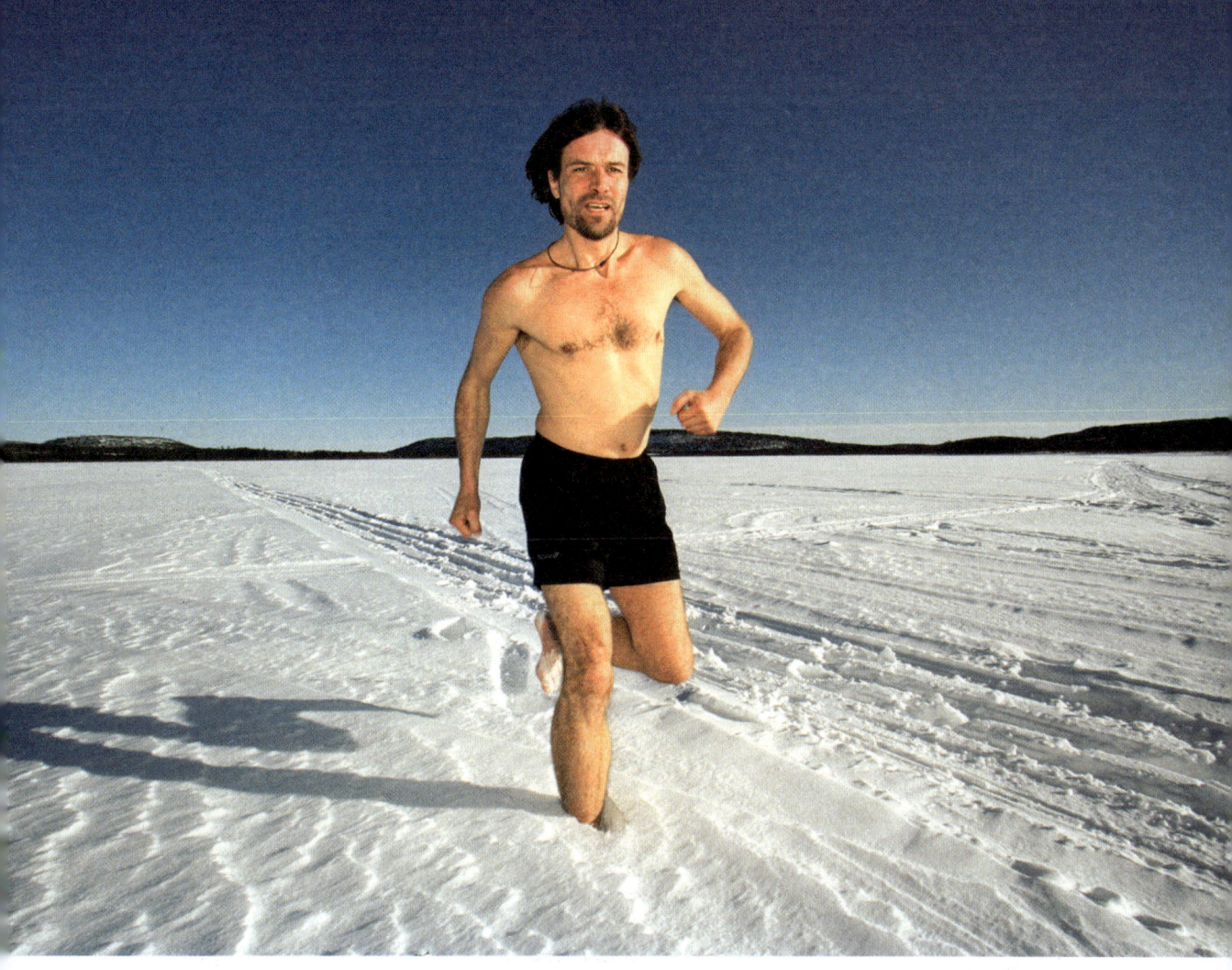

I used to, and still do, like to walk barefoot in the snow. It is amazing how the body is able to cope with this. It also makes the body feel so good. It is an extra dimension. Our feet are normally in shoes and disconnected from all that beauty. Crazy, eh?

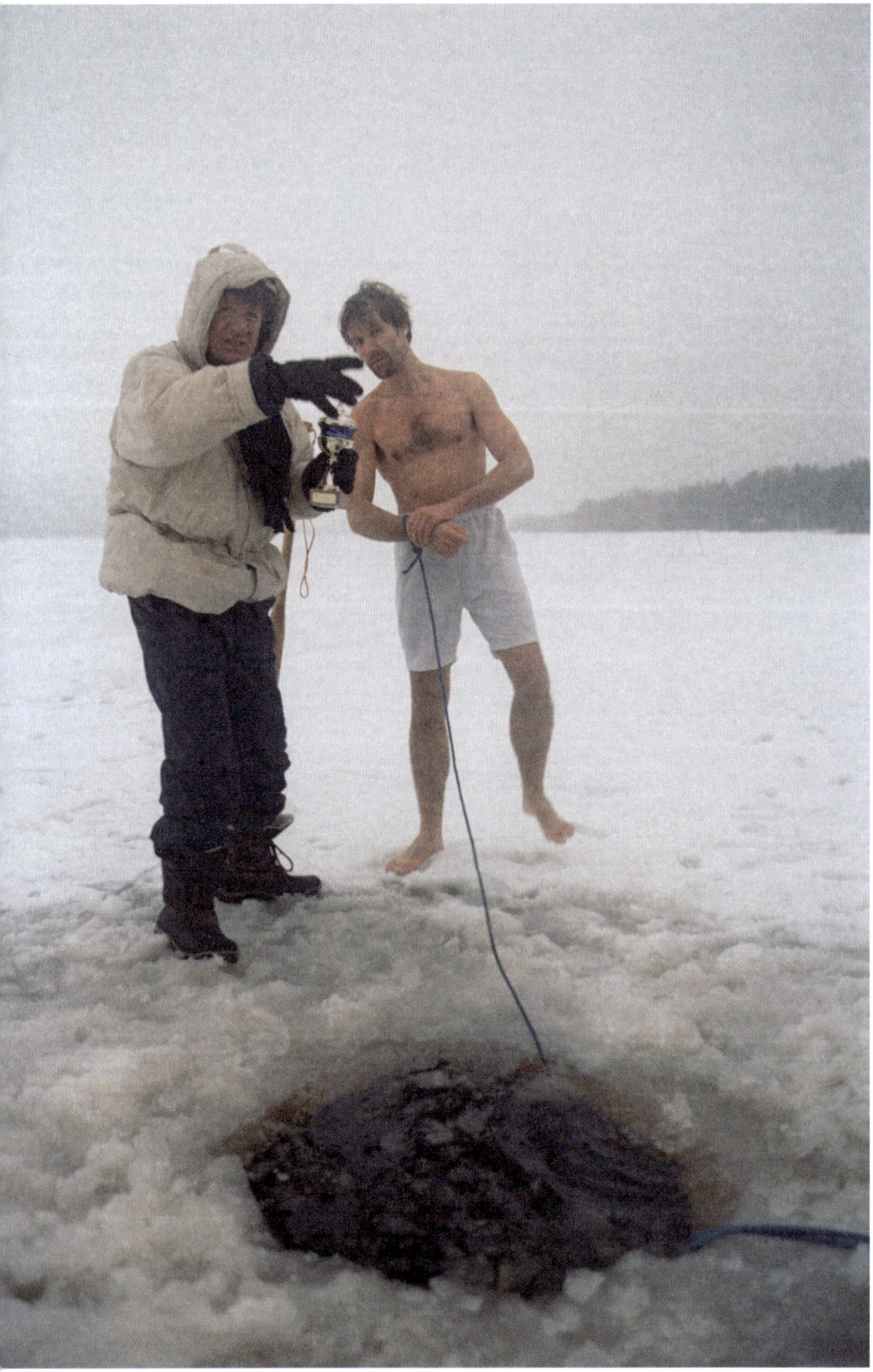

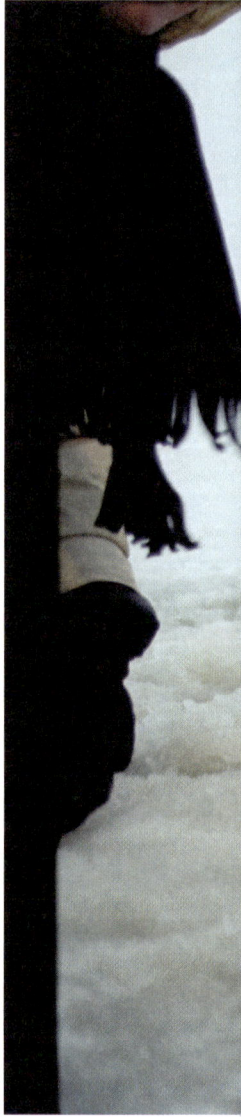

Here with a dear friend of mine, Willibrord Frequin, a Dutch journalist and television presenter. He was like my media father. He guided me and helped me with my appearances. Here we are in Lapland. It all began with just seven meters.

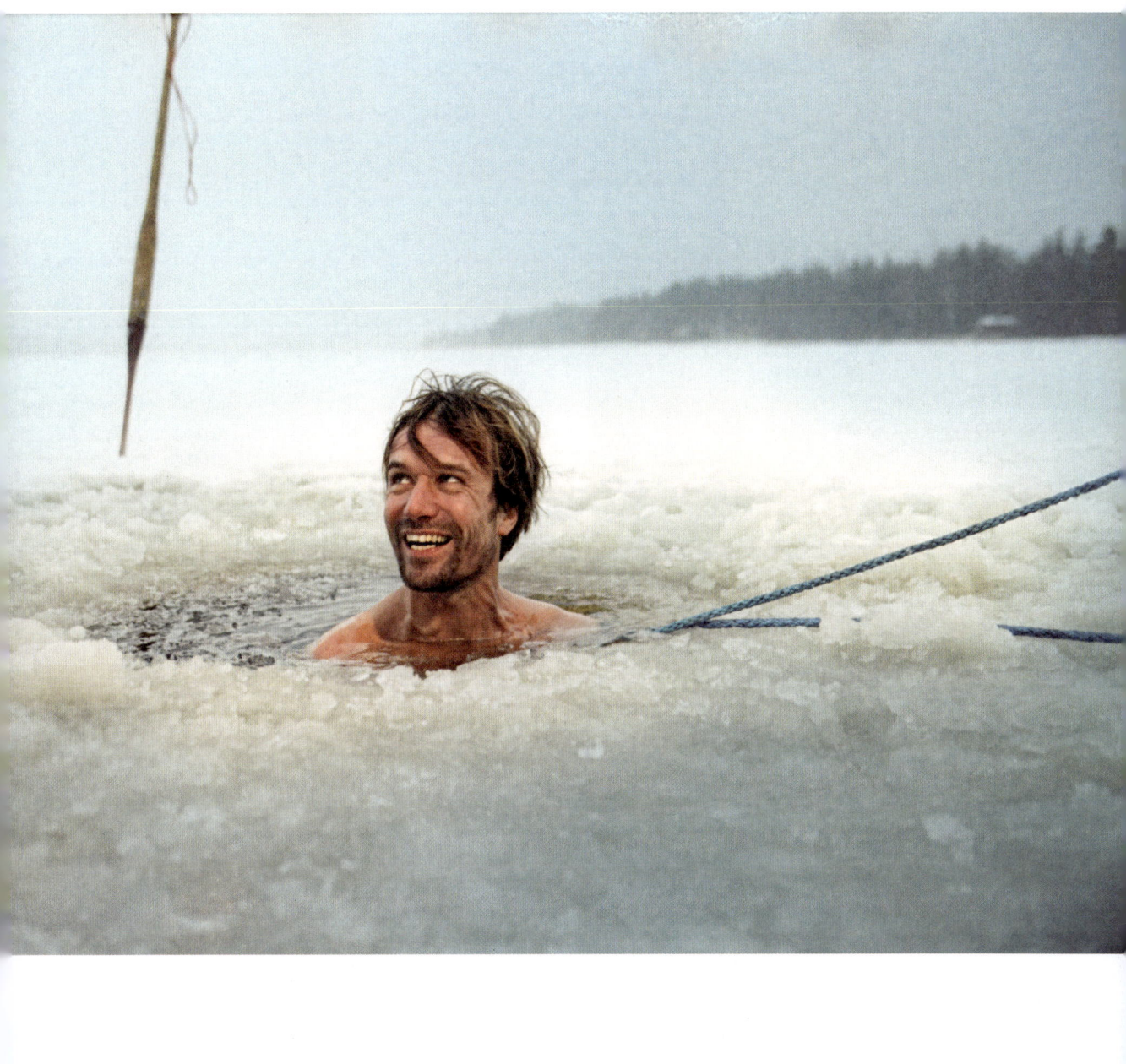

SPEED OF LIGHT

When darkness has colored the skies
Accumulating non presence of awareness, piling
Up whys
Then burdened spirits who carried their load
Finding light in the tunnel vision, the road
The path
Together we are to go far
Short cut
As the dawn of a great day of humanity arises
Entices
Minds connected to the heart, to enlighten
Where the path becomes one with all
We bring love, nature's call
The greatest of confidence, masters of
Neurology
Being free, in one's own brain
No more pain
Shaking off what is at stake
Here we are, for God's sake
To bring a powerful coup to existent paradigm
As you are the owner of your own mind
To become simply the one, kind
Ready to bring love, power, and understanding
We are kings, queens, no longer bending
The rules have changed
No longer estranged
But being your beautiful self
strong, happy, healthy
Takes a few sincere souls.

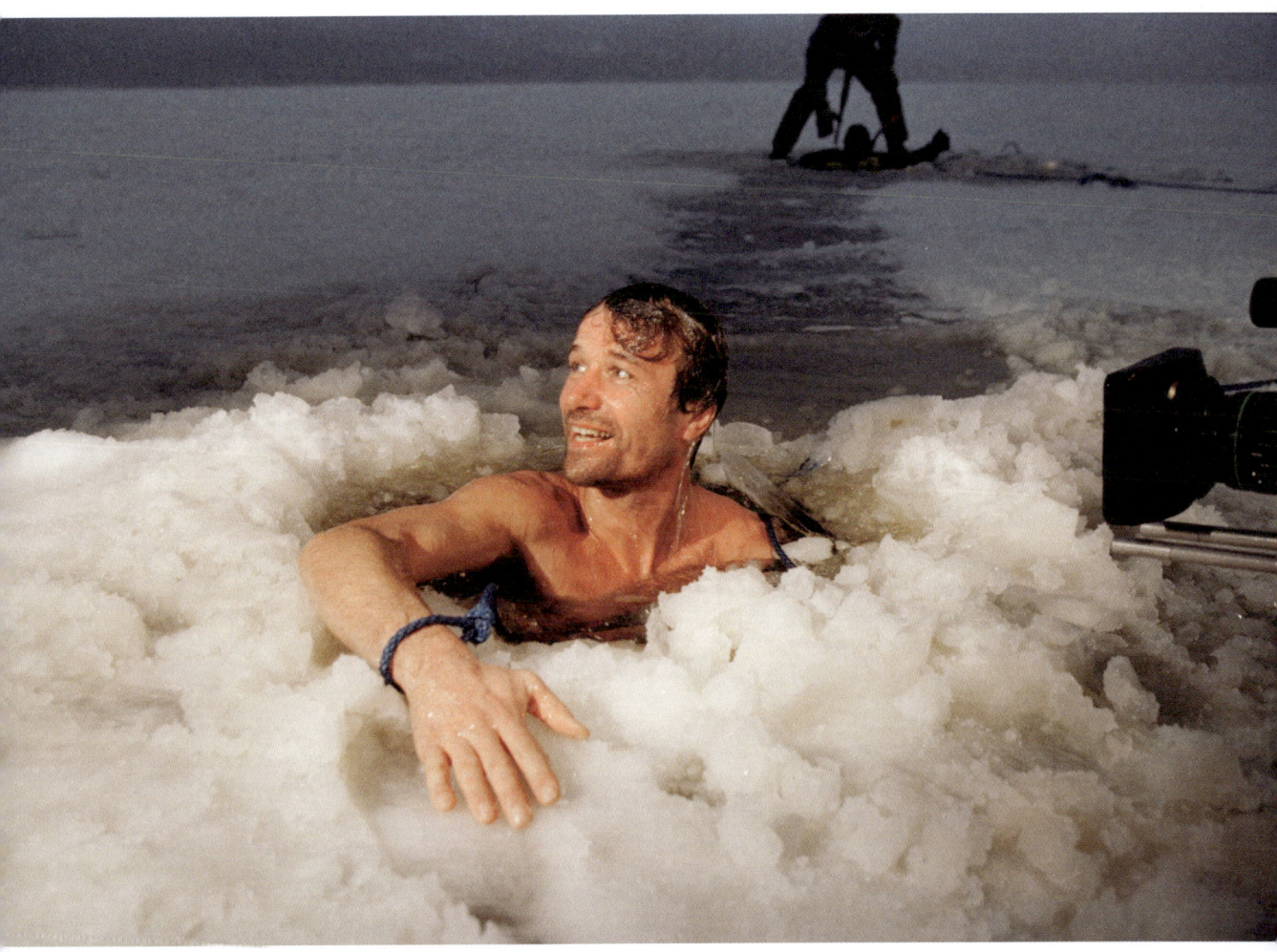

The moment the cameras were rolling, I erupted like a volcano. Suddenly all attention was
pointed to me. I had to perform. The TV world and its expectancy—you give it all and on
demand. Cut. Go. "Wim can you do this again?" "We thought of this because that looks
better." "Tomorrow at six o'clock, can we go again?" Demanding. But exciting all the same.
I was ready to go. I had done my due diligence practicing throughout the years. I could
take on the crazy demands of TV. I was not mesmerized by my exploits. To me this was
part of daily routine, but for the thrill-seeking TV world, it was a basketful of goodies.

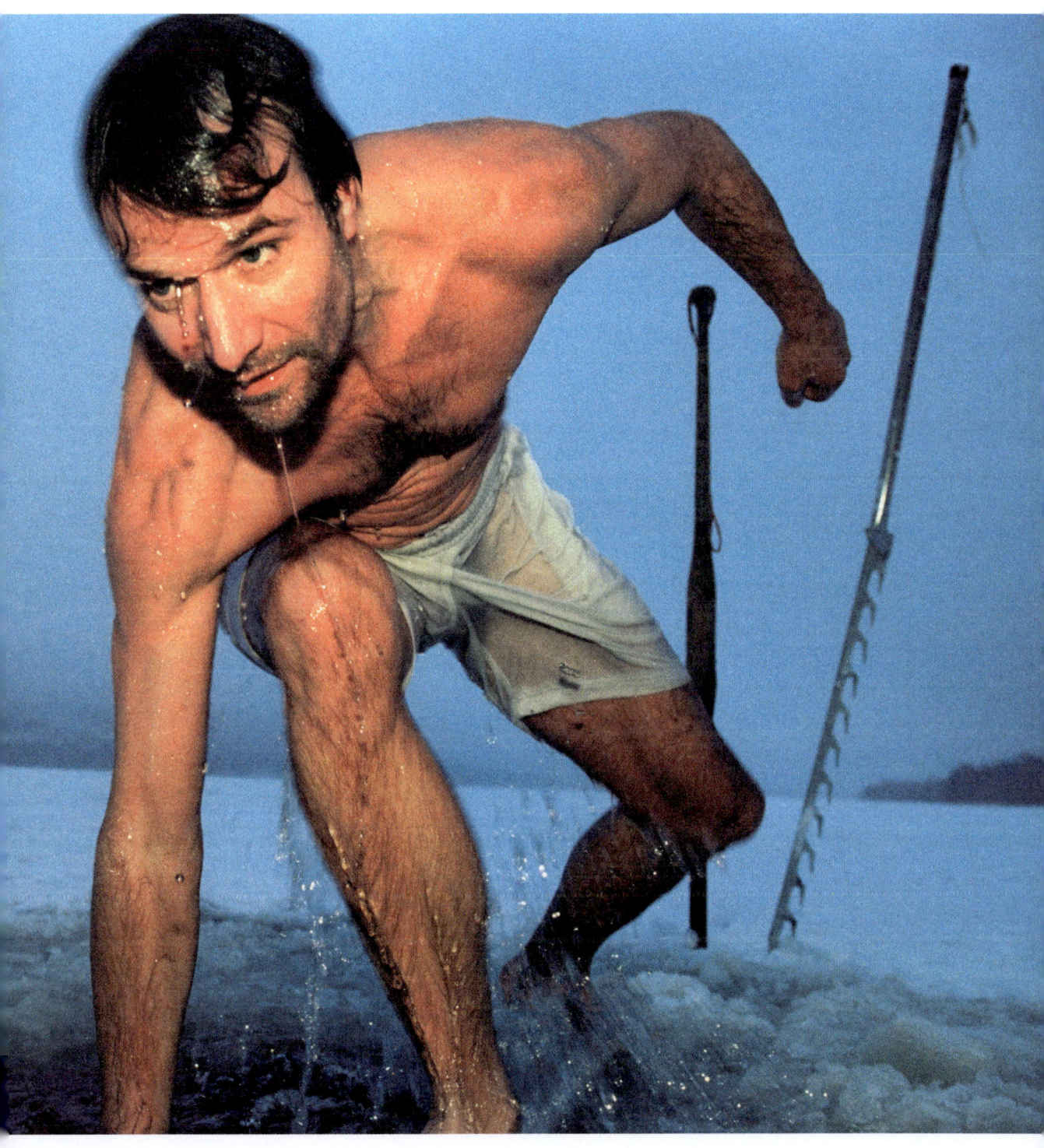

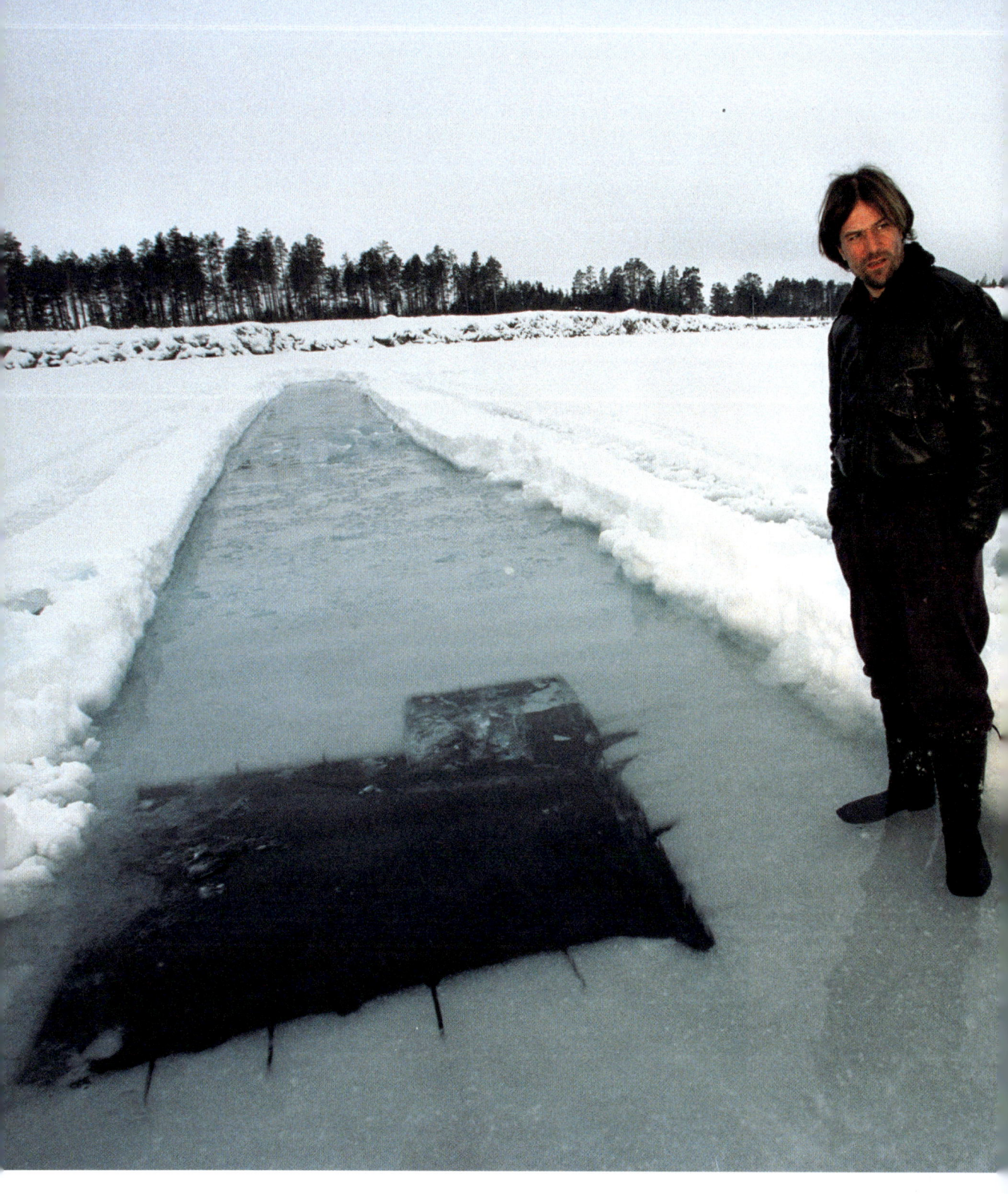

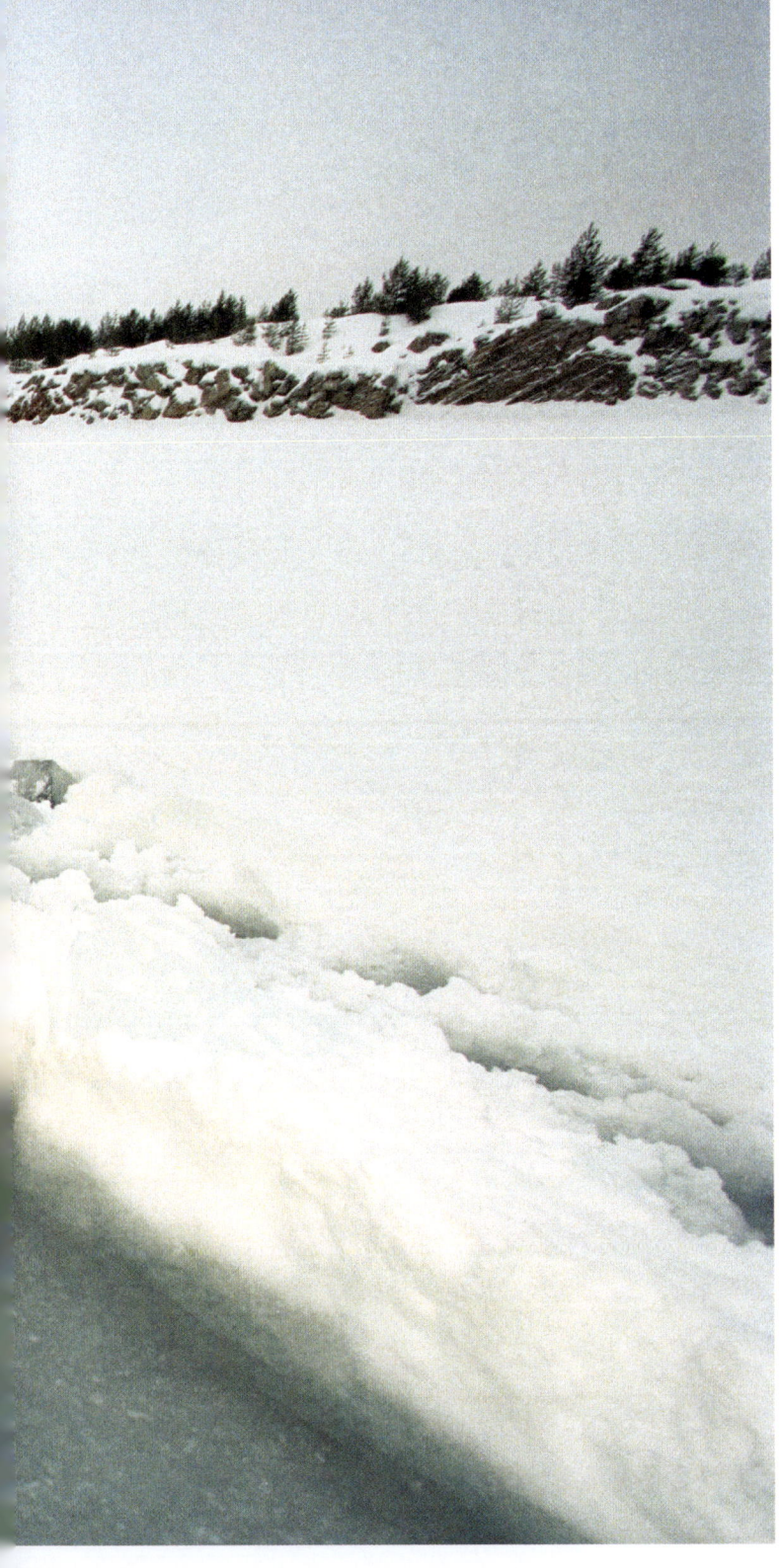

A couple of months later, Willibrord asked me if I could do 50 meters under the water, and I just said yes. His team then tried to make it an official Guinness World Record after the fact, and they did! They wanted more after that. One year later, we were back in Lapland to break my own record; this time 57.5 meters. Four European television stations were there along with an official Guinness World Record representative.

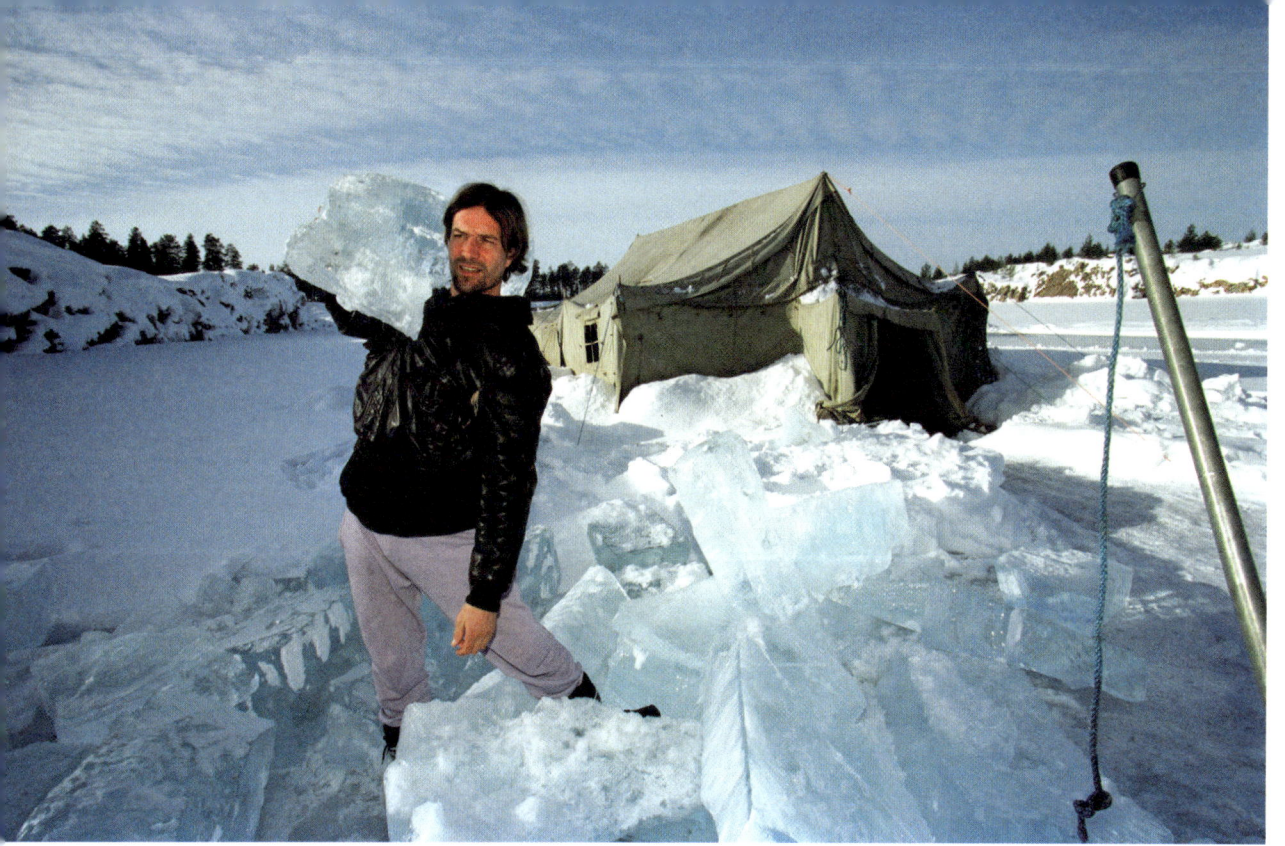

The ice that had been cut to prepare my under-ice swimming track. Soon I would be down under in my shorts, holding, losing my way.

The night before the actual Guinness World Record 50 meters under the ice, I did a rehearsal where they wanted me to do 25 meters. Since I had to do 50, I already decided I would do the whole length during the rehearsal. Once I was charged up, I got into the water, took a last gulp of air, and went down vertically until I was under the ice—and I didn't use goggles. I had never done that distance before and never thought to wear goggles. But after 26 strokes, I couldn't see and began to lose track of the straight line that's under the water to help me stay aware of the ice and distance. I knew how many strokes I needed to get to 50 meters . . . 42. So while swimming, I kept on counting and then realized I was already at 48 strokes, which meant I had to swim six strokes back. I still felt nothing. I turned my body, feeling the ice cap to see if there was a hole. Nothing. I went back and forth several times. I could only see through what was like a tube through my eyes. There was no agony of drowning, claustrophobia, or fear, just a letting go. That was when a diver grabbed me by the ankle and brought me back to the 50-meter hole. He jumped in when I had been under too long. As he pulled me, I was conscious but had no energy to move myself. My body was out of energy. Thank God he came in to grab me!

I was an extreme athlete, with a lot of experience in endangering situations, but this almost killed me. Water is a mysterious force. Seek out professional training before doing anything like this, and remember the WHM breathing technique is **not a free-diving technique. Never practice the WHM breathing in or near water!**

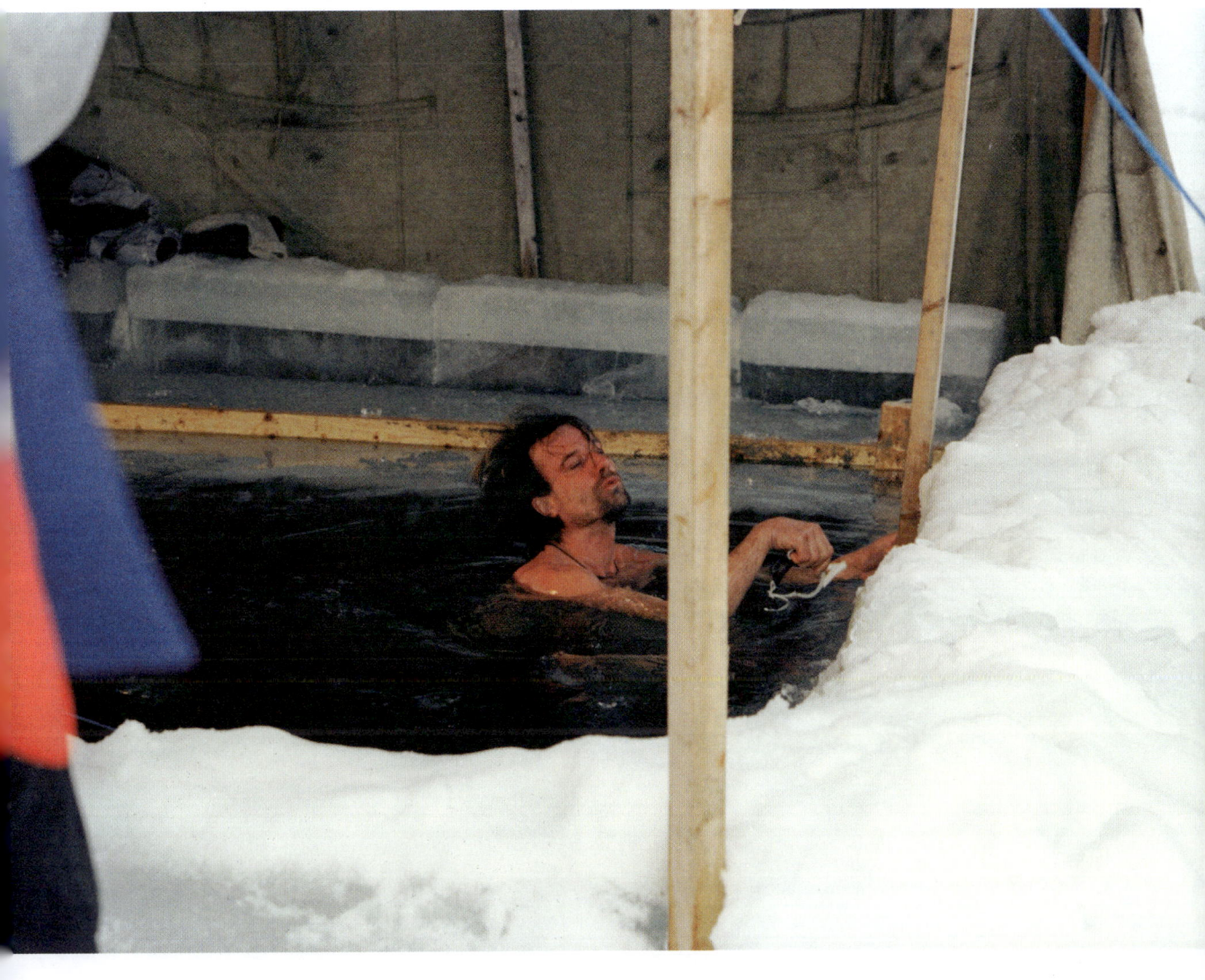

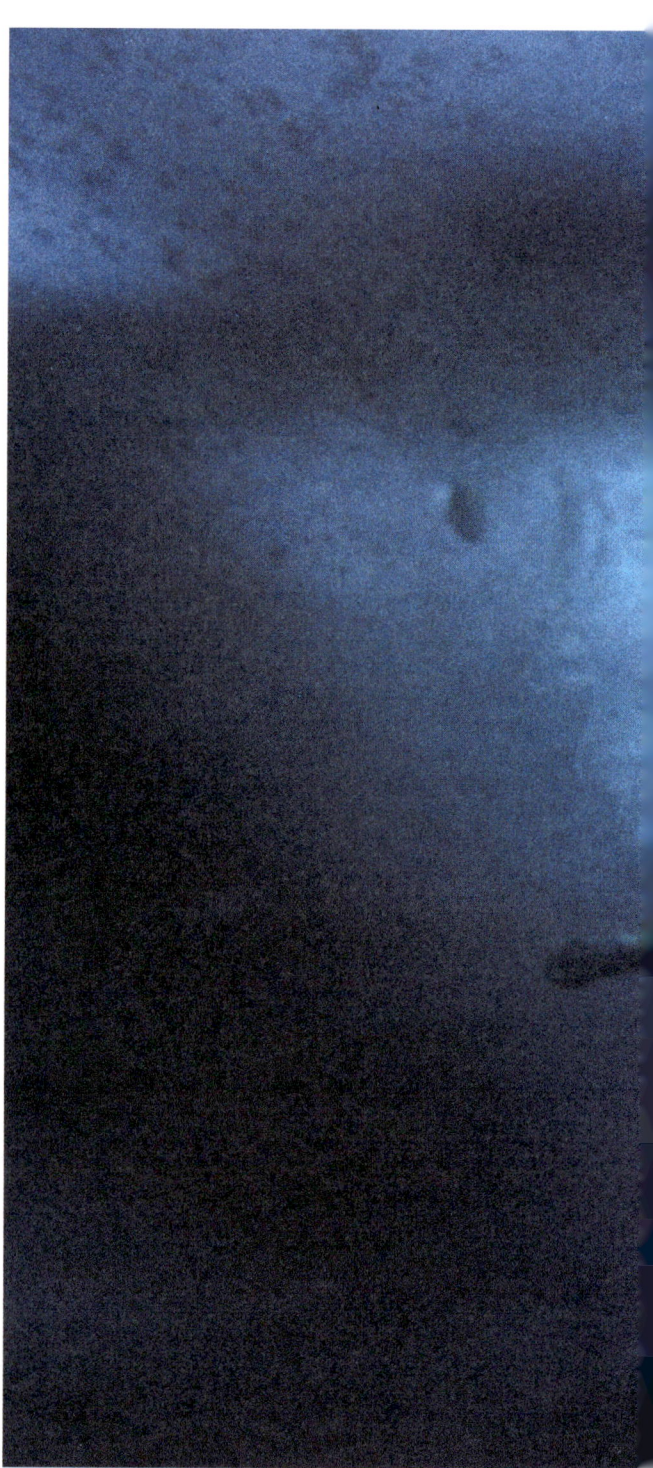

The danger of swimming under the ice is imminent. The sensation is a pressing through your body, and it exerts a deep impact on the body and mind. It is altogether a completely different dimension. It is important to remember that these were extreme feats. Absolutely not to be taken lightly. That is the beauty of the method as it is. That there is no need to go to the extremes to get extreme benefits.

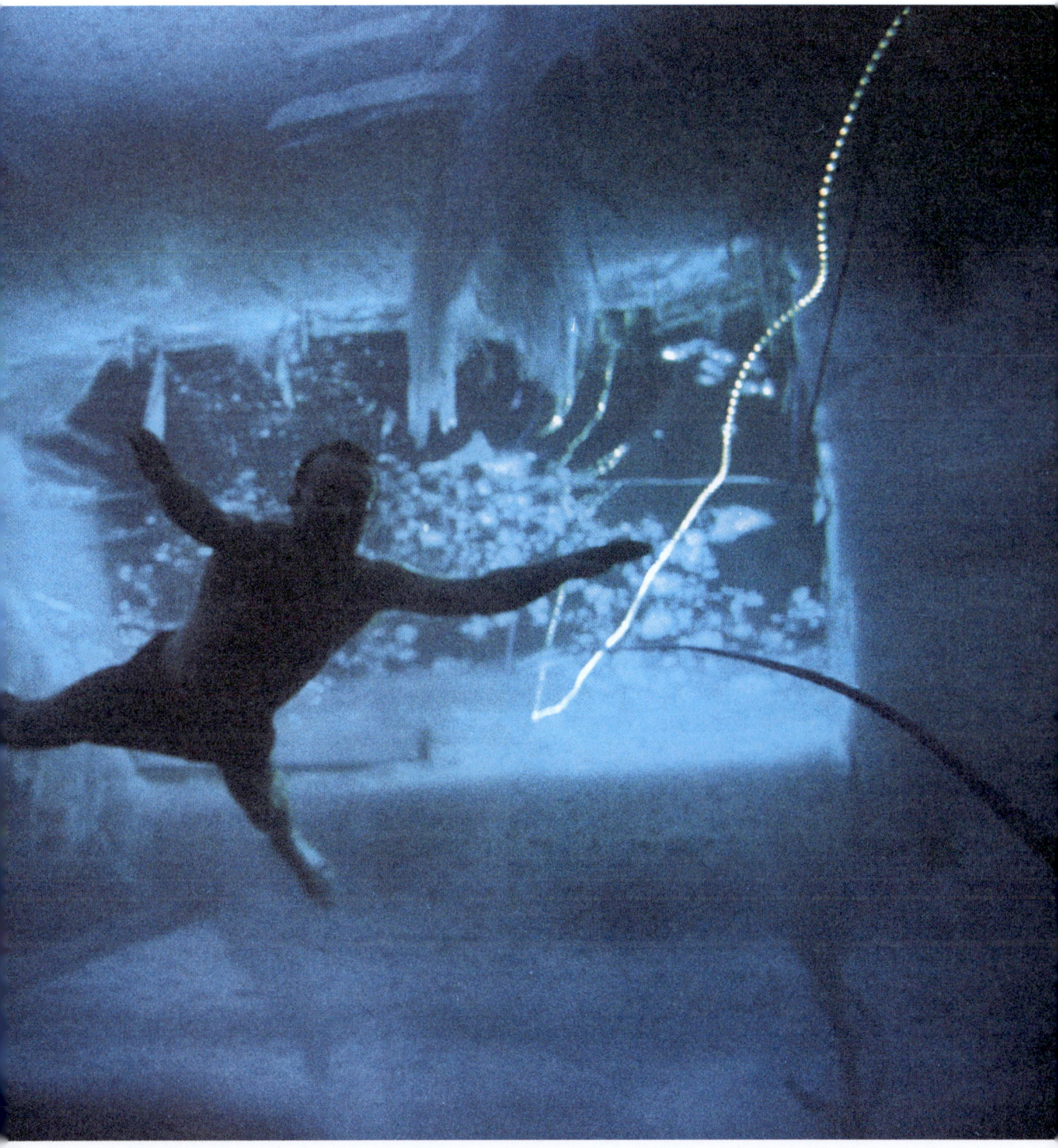

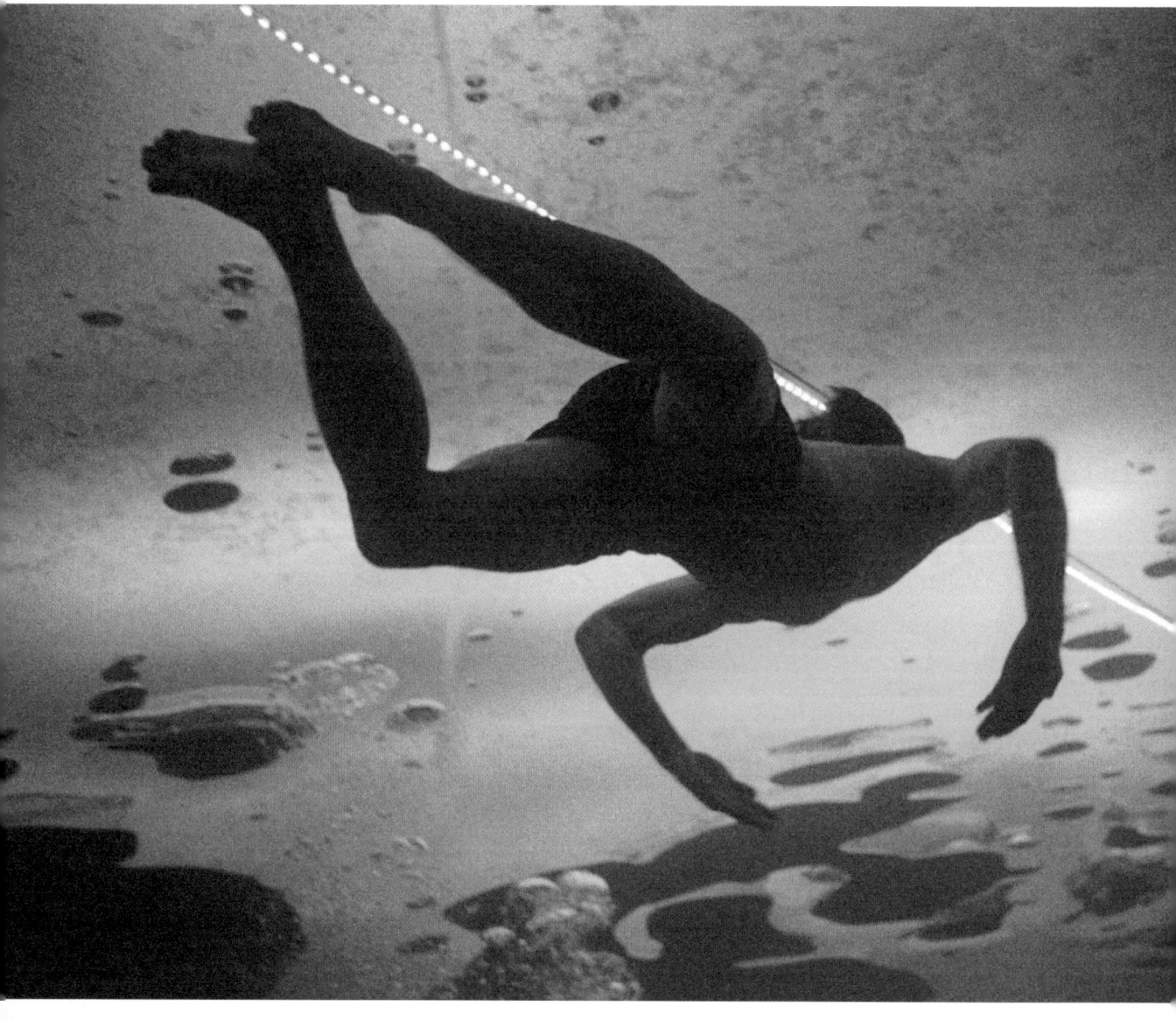

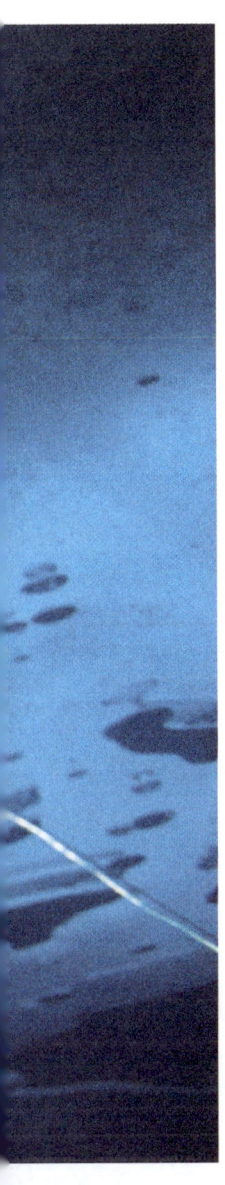

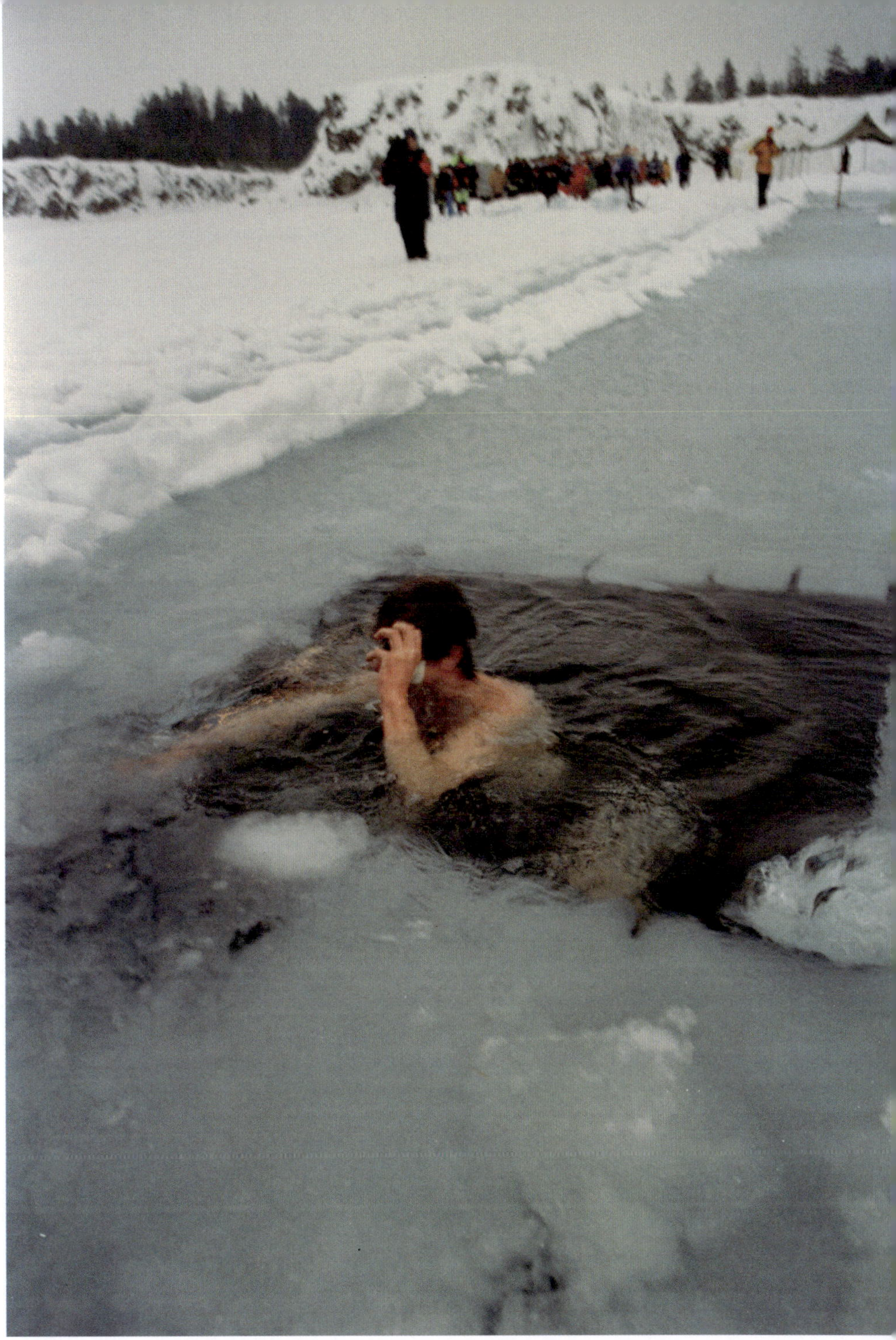

Did it! Fifty meters! What I felt was
astonishment—nothing more, nothing less.

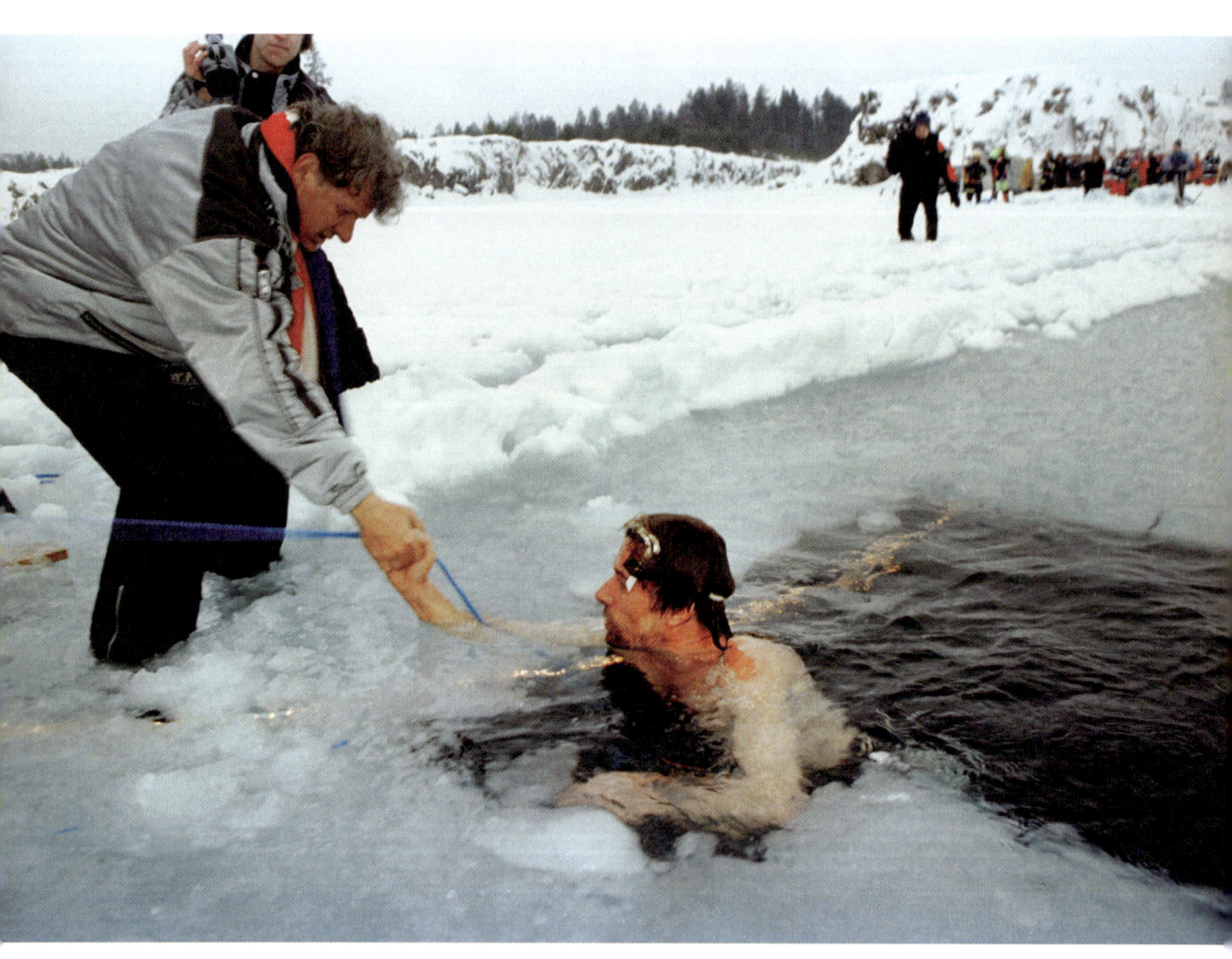

OH SUN

You

You

Always there, relentless rays of life

Dressing all beings with a warm drape

Nowhere to hide

Even in the shadows I see your presence

Coloring it all with this golden brush

All what fires becomes so lush

That falling in love when you rise

Taking the light into new heights

Or missing in the northern hemisphere

Short days, long nights

Awaiting for the turning

Thoughts are churning

To see burning desire

From a slumber wire

Coming to a halt, shoots bullets

Everywhere

Out of a triggered soil

It's a shoot out

Shout out

Sun wins

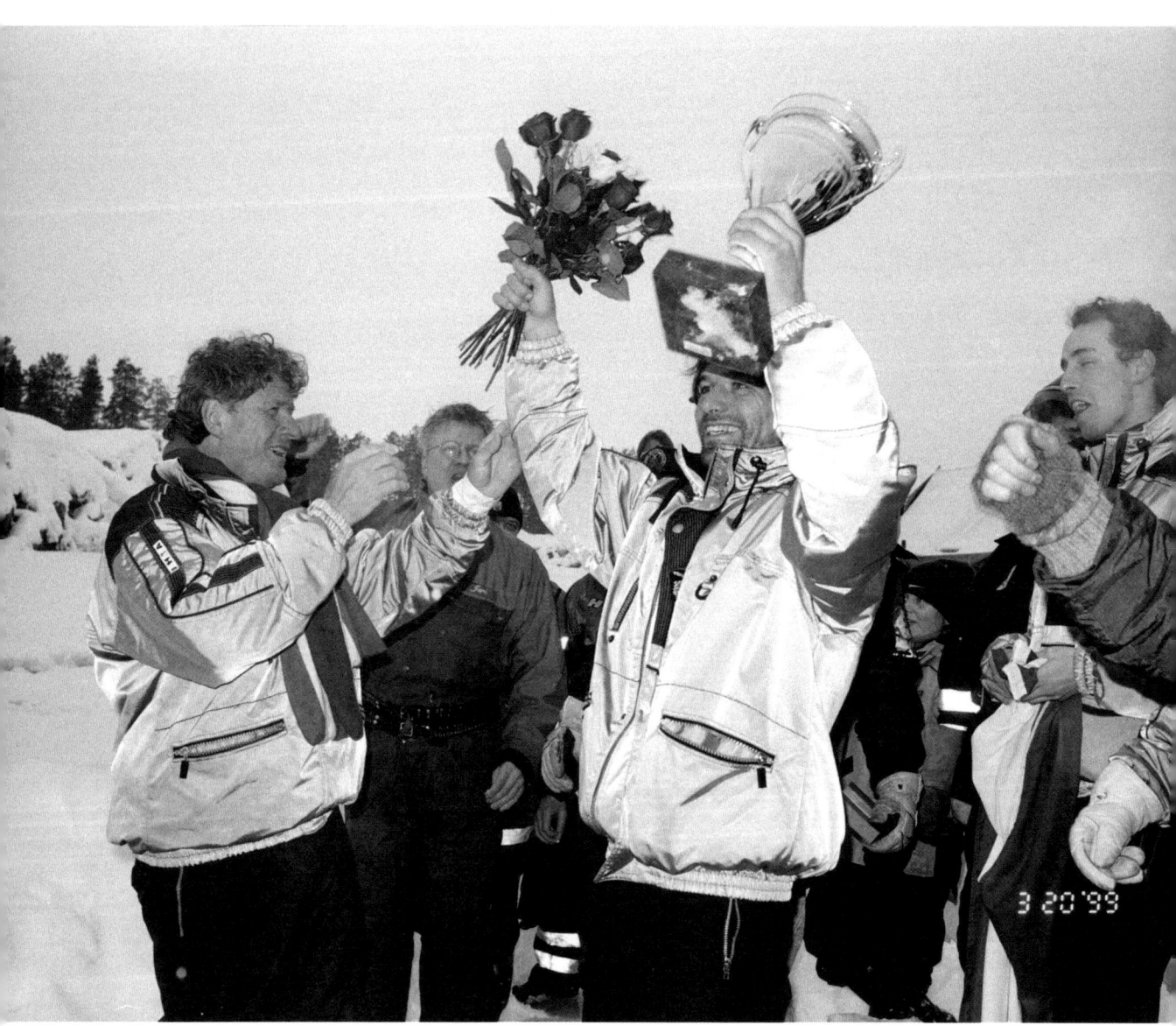

Celebration of my second Guinness World Record.
Crazy, beautiful stuff.

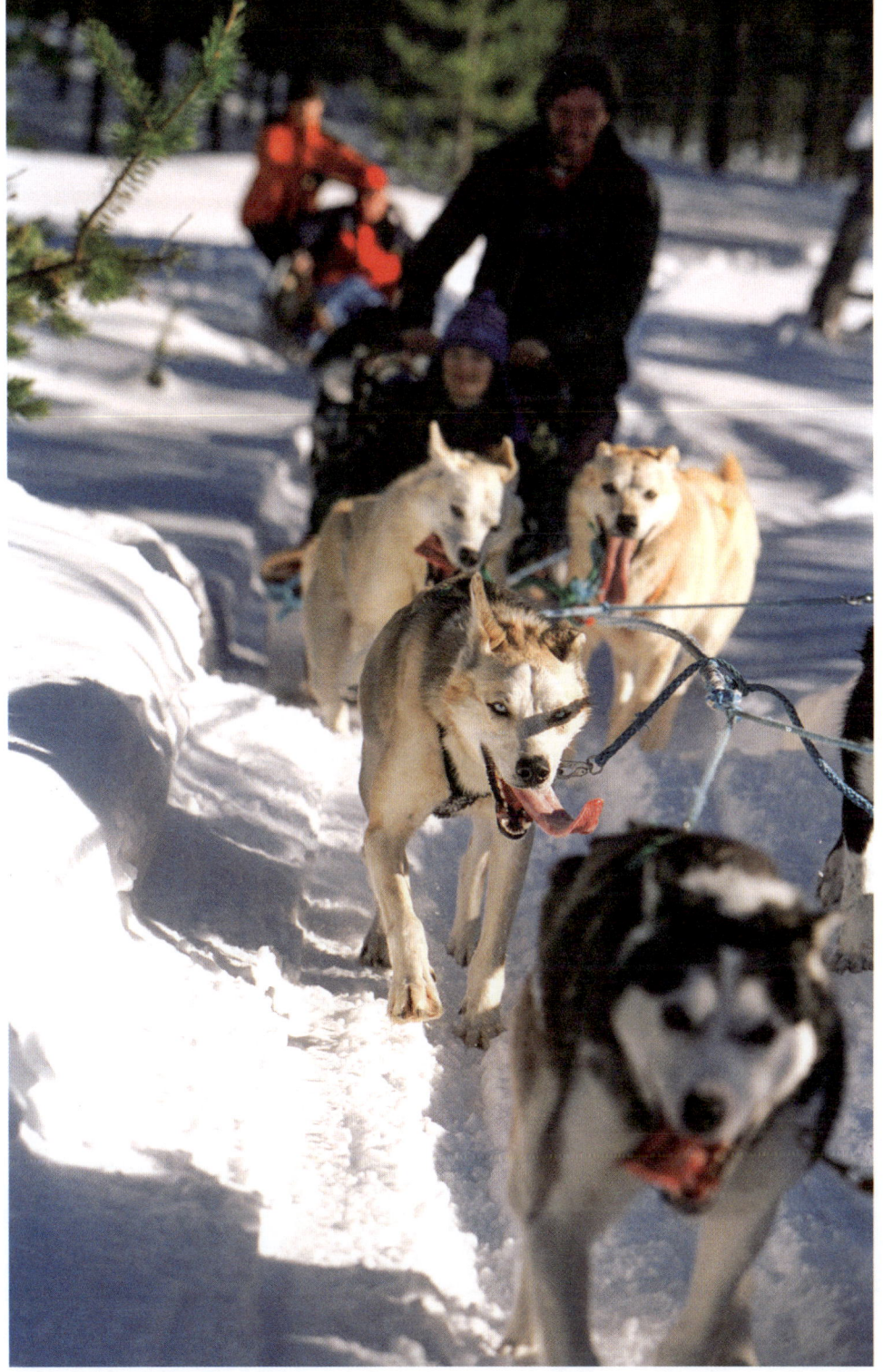

Some downtime after the celebration.

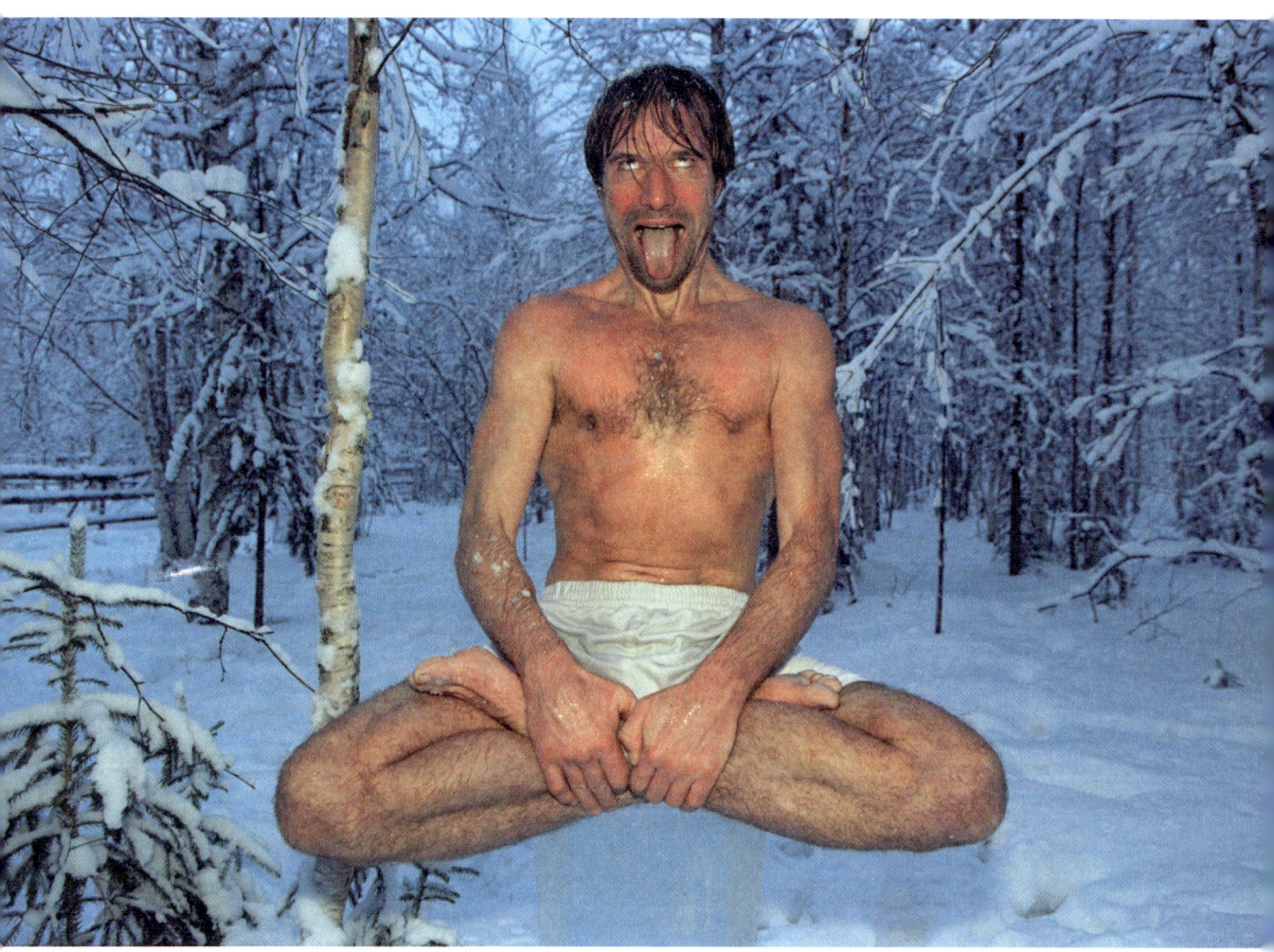

Simhasana—the Lion Pose in the cold. I loved to practice these yogic postures. They became part of my life, like an extra limb. The cold practice, however, goes straight to the depth of the body. Depth and power become yours through regular practice.

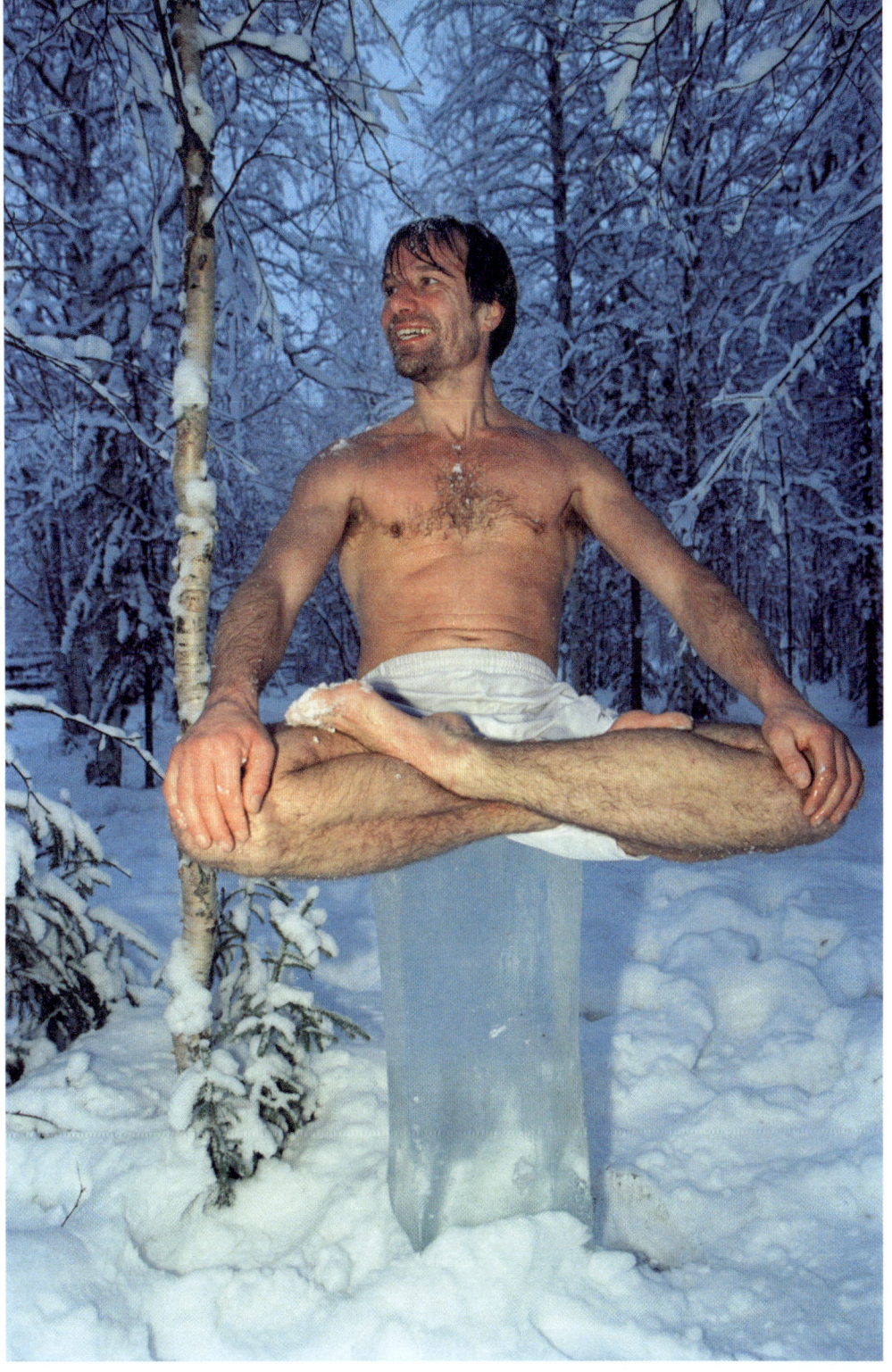

Lust for life in the cold and fun.

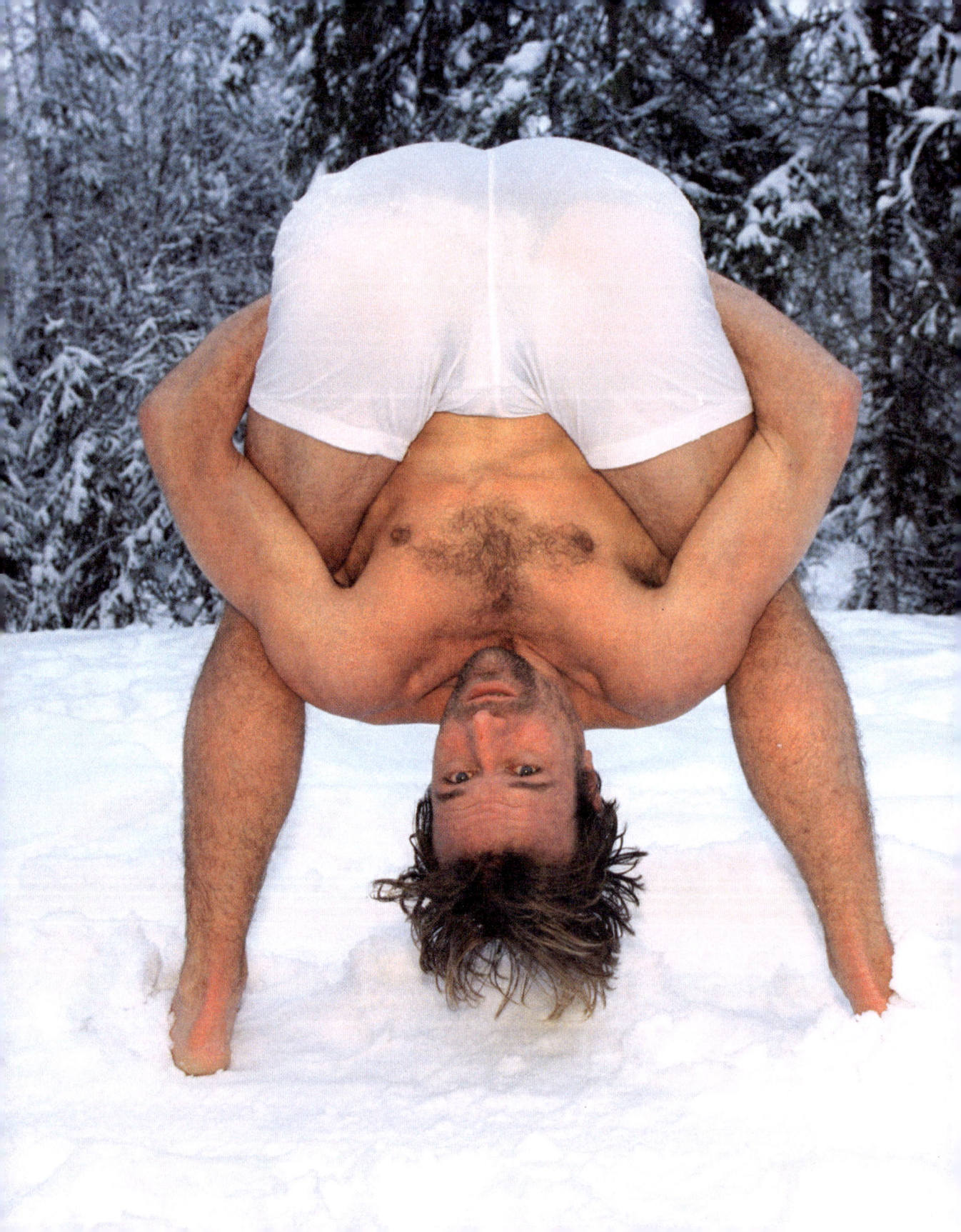

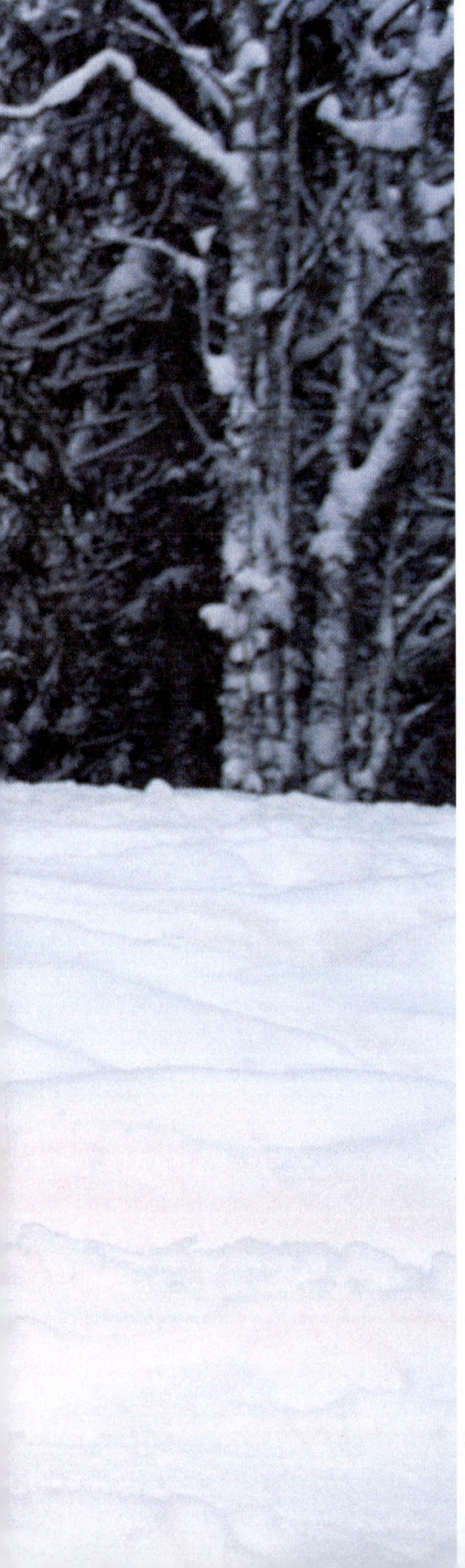

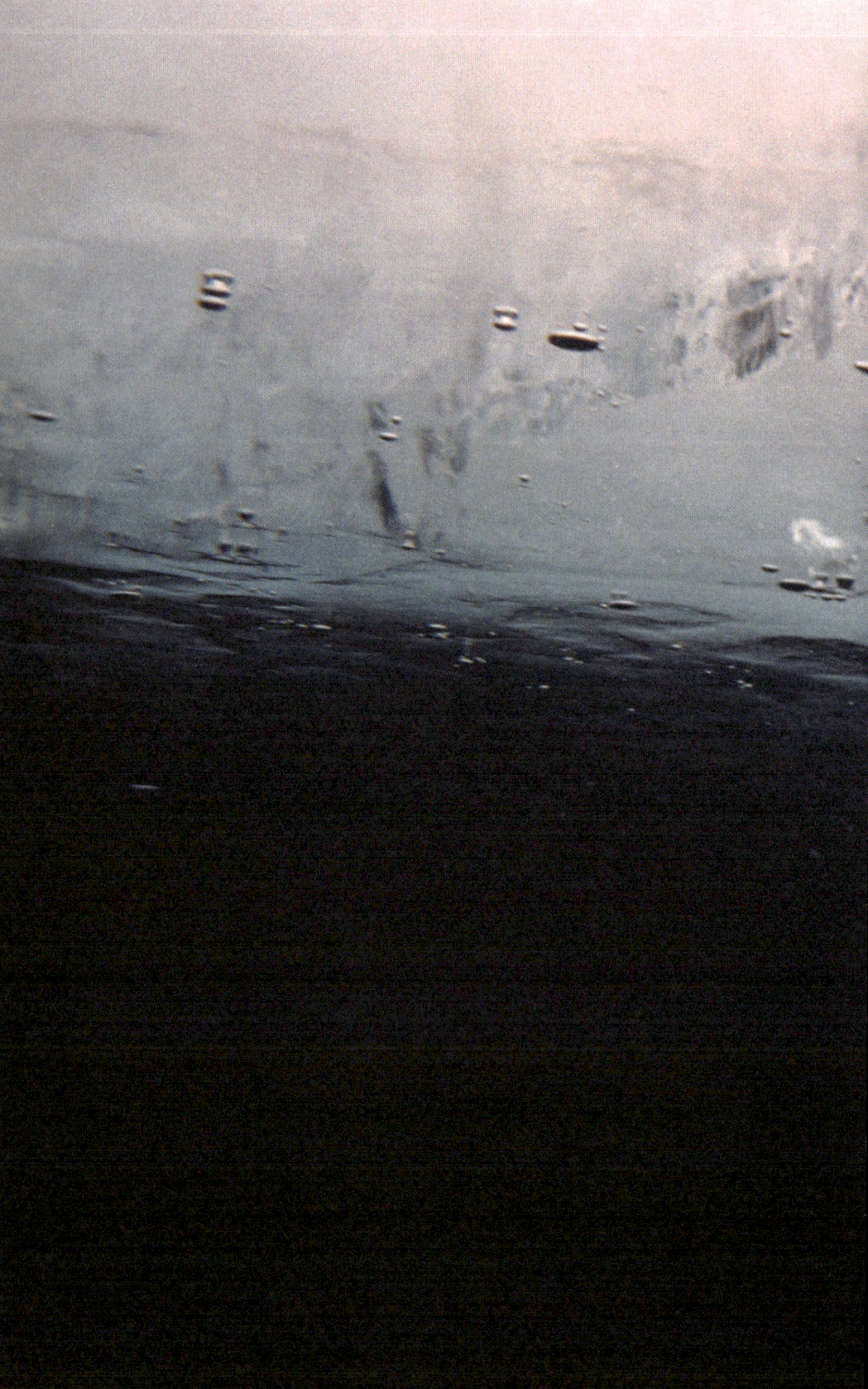

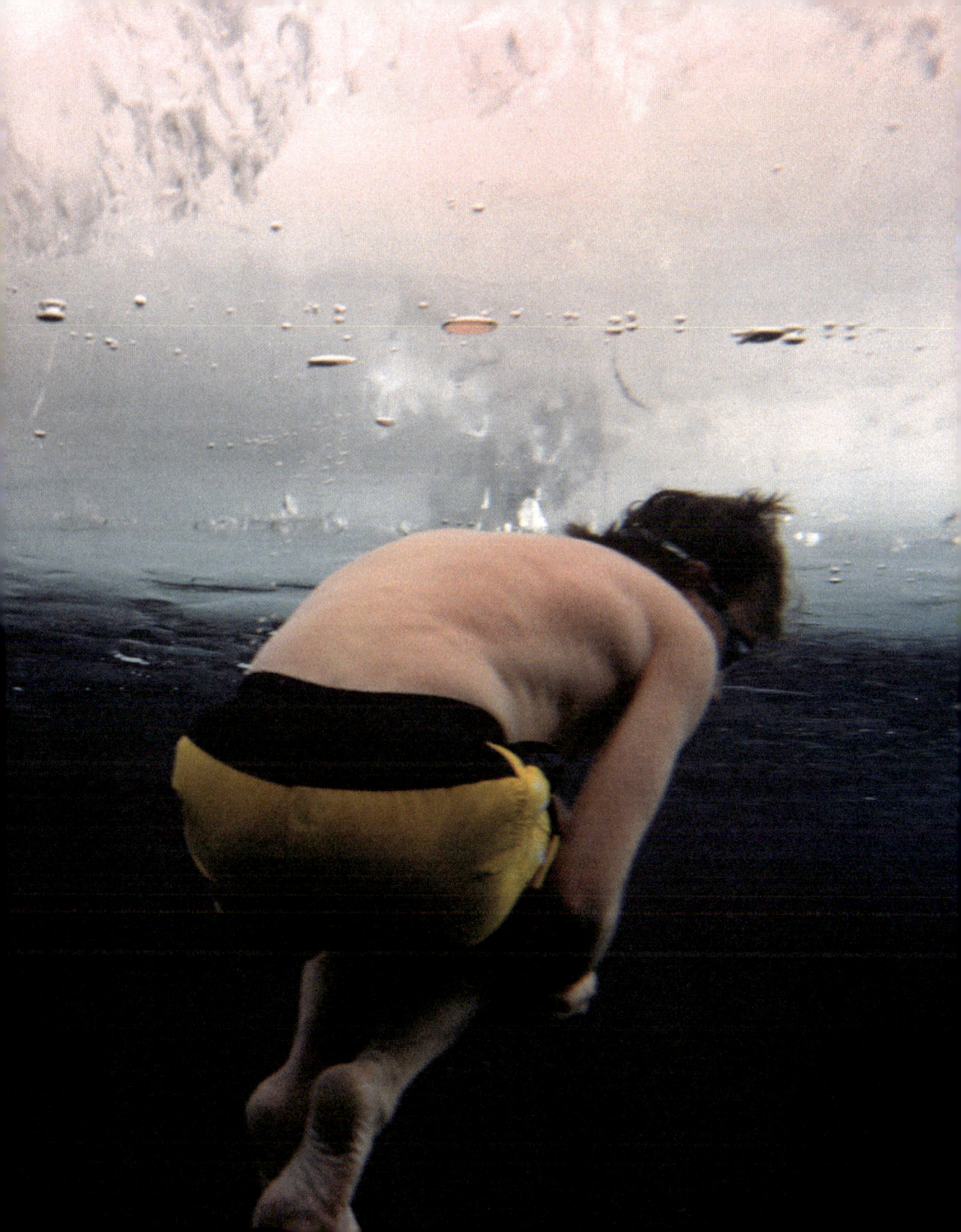

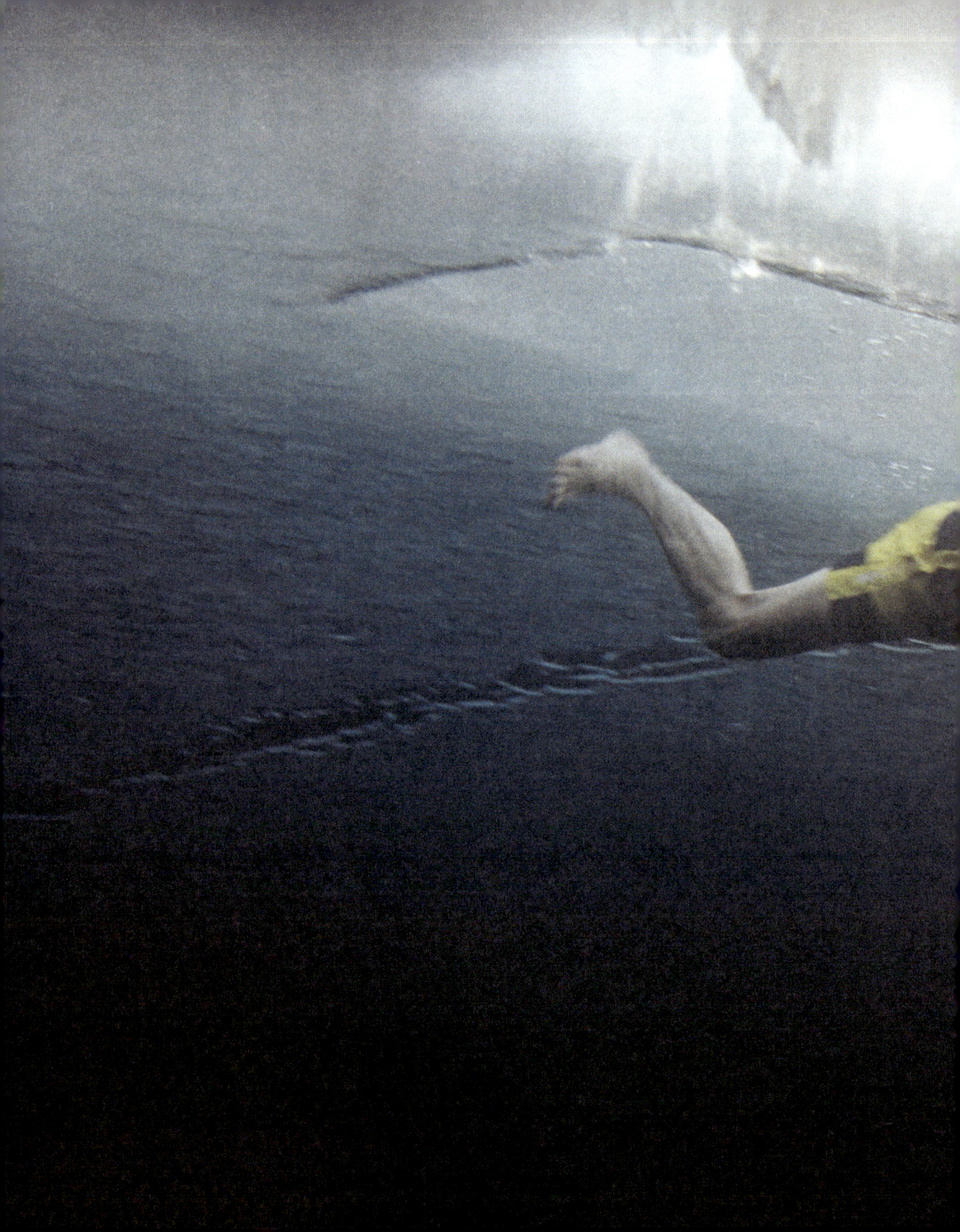

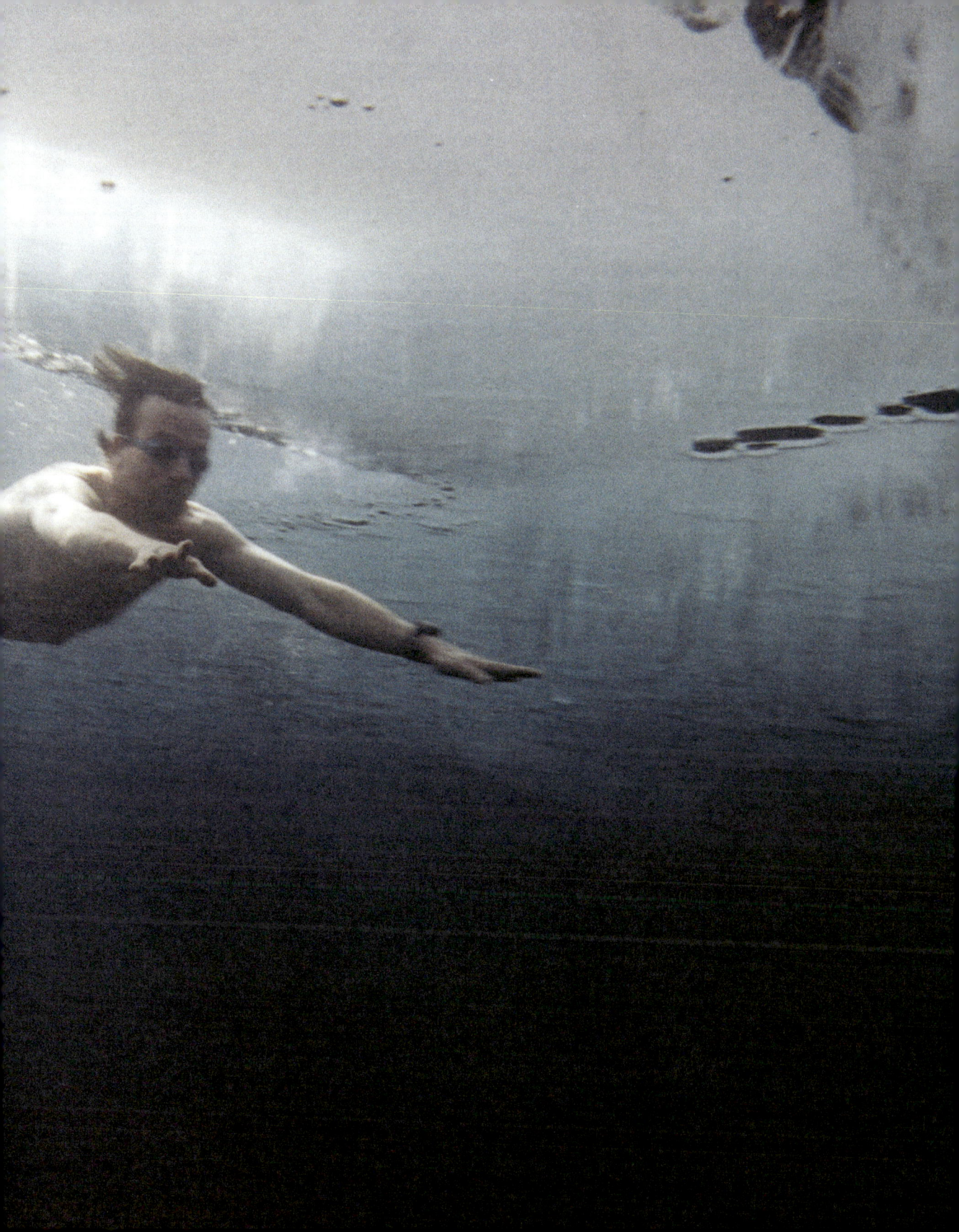

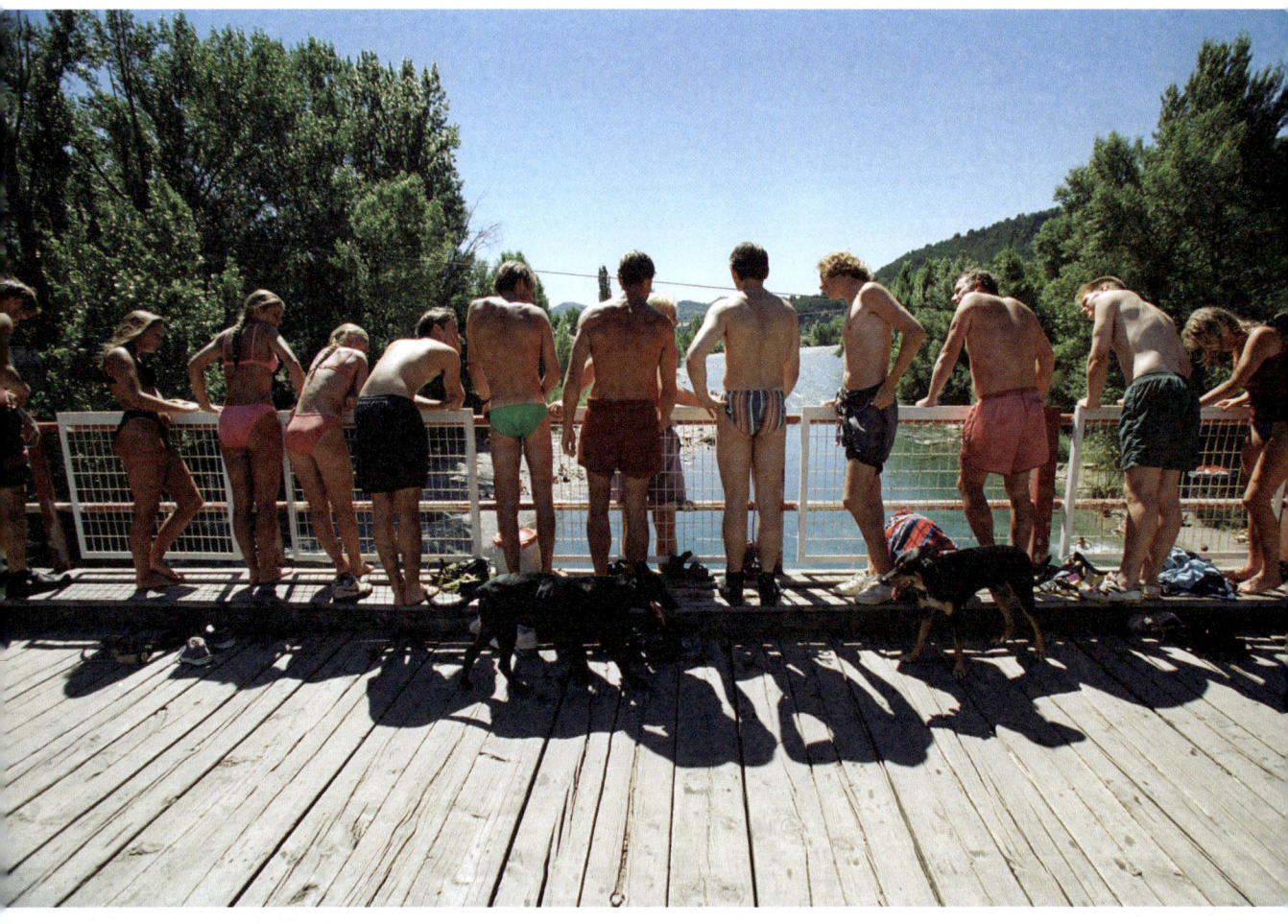

From the ice to the sun—Boltana, Spanish Pyrenees.

Before going into the canyons in the Spanish Pyrenees, we bond as a group, jump from bridges, and learn to rappel down. I loved coming together and seeing the emotions open up. People from all walks of life. You get to know them before going into unpredictable challenges in nature.

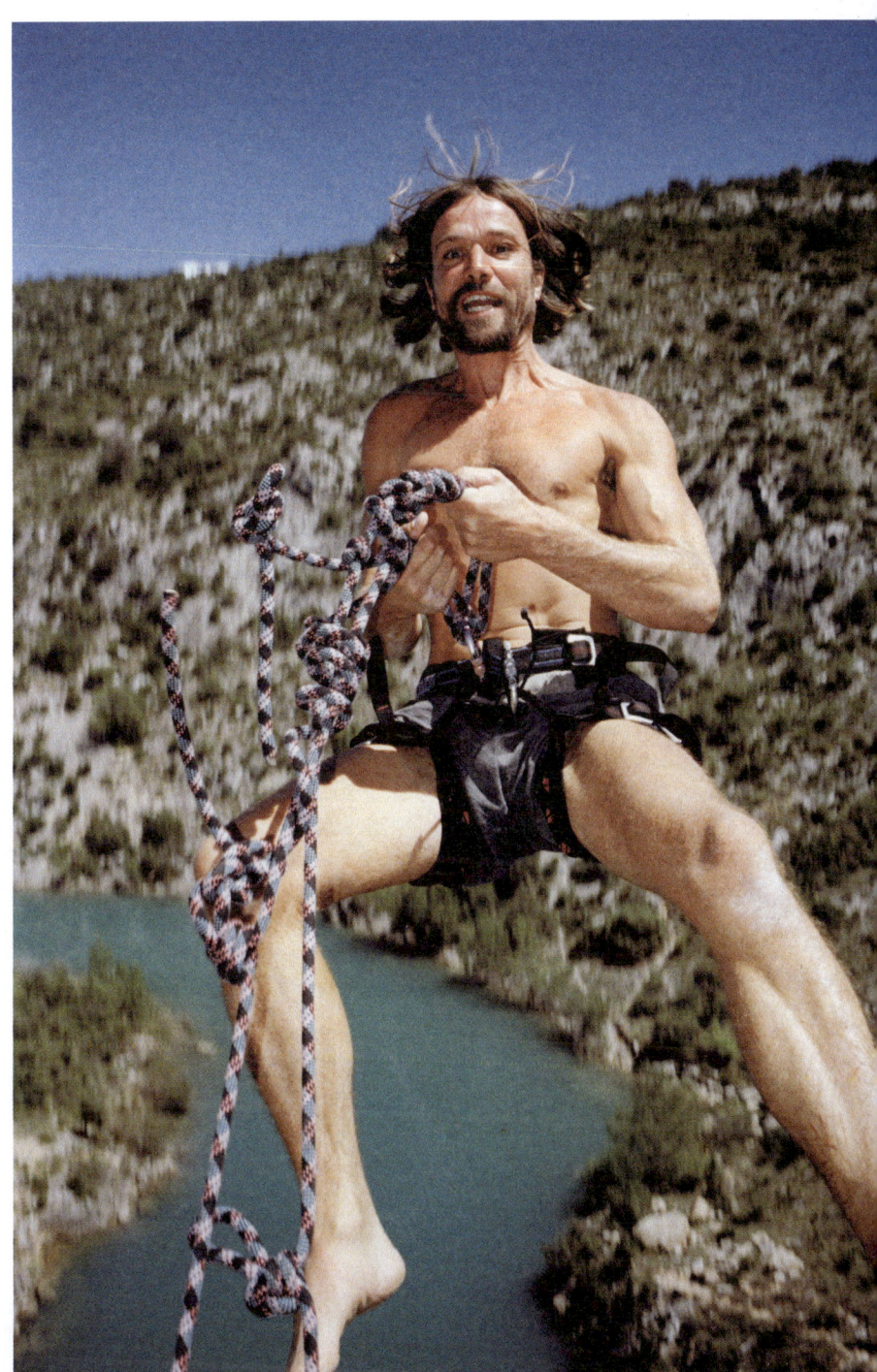

Puenting—to tie your dynamic ropes in a triangle to the side of a bridge.

I look like an adrenaline junkie! I learned to get out of my conditions, the conditioned state of my mind and body, through things like bridging. It felt like an explosion of freedom. But if you do this same thing ten times, then the tenth time it really is less than half. It's different from going into icy water. The body and mind adapt to these adrenal kinds of stunts, but never do you get habituated to icy water.

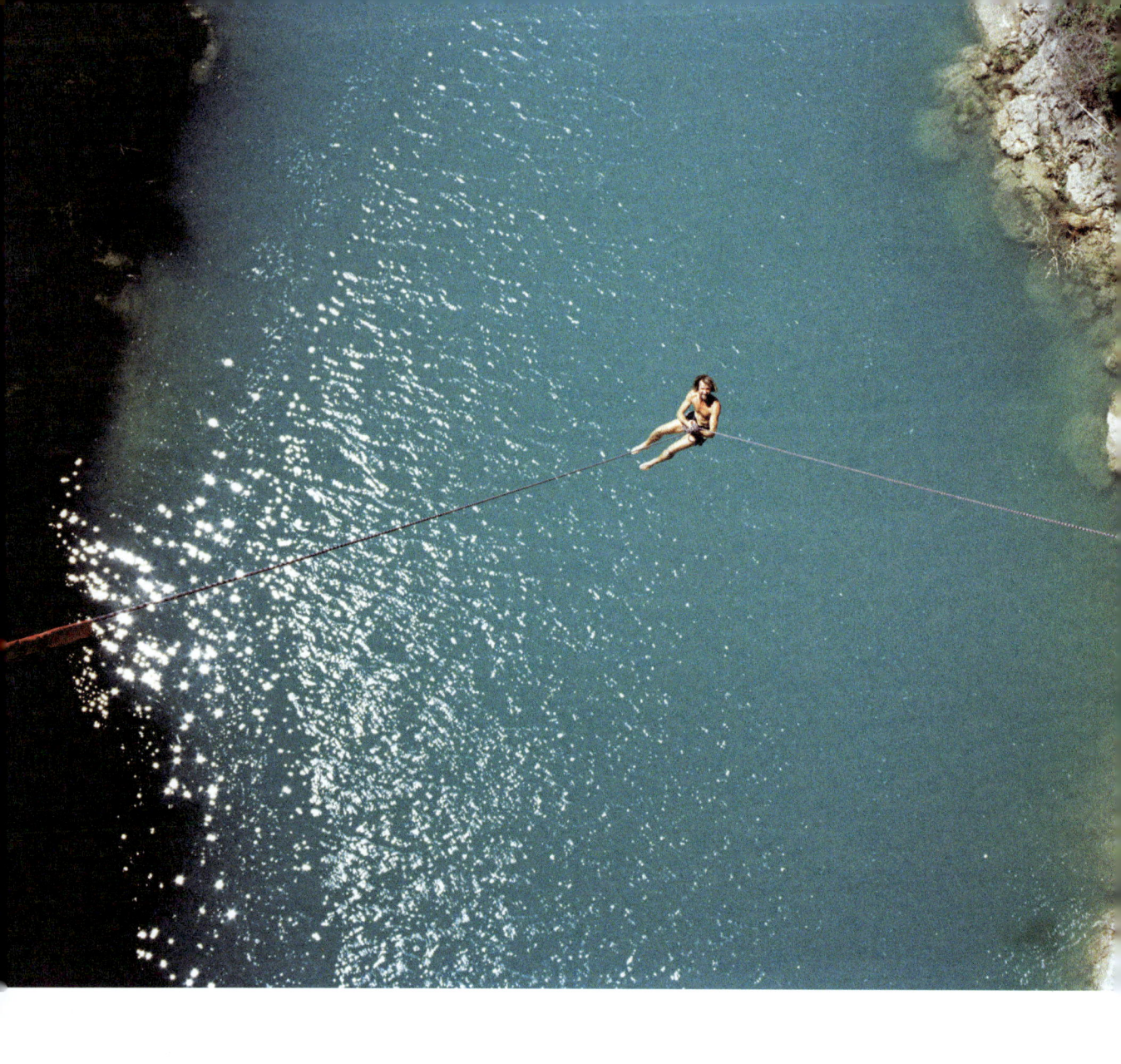

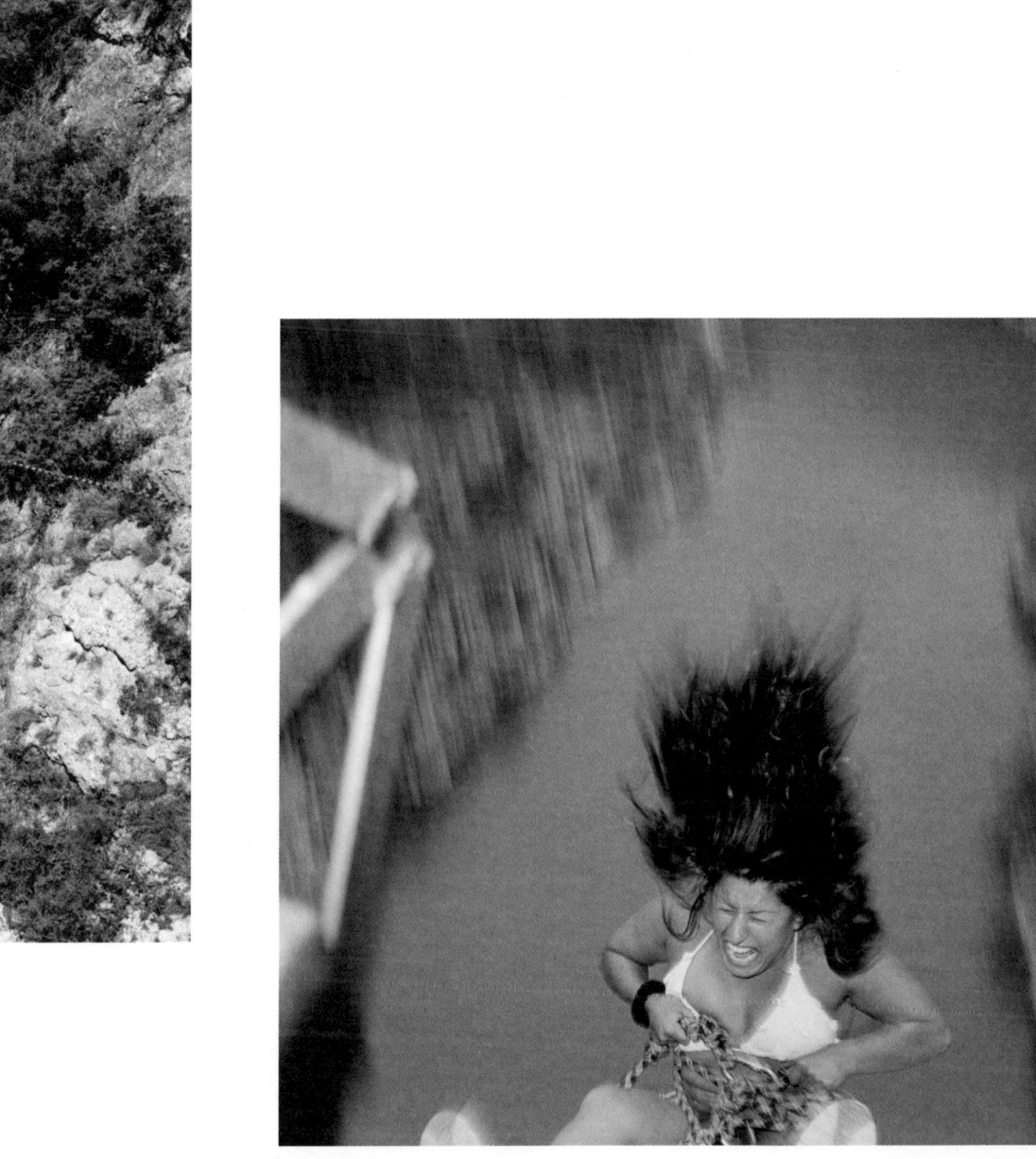

This was a travel activity to overcome your
fears. It's amazing to do. To stand there and
to jump backward, you will be confronted
with the deepest fear within yourself.

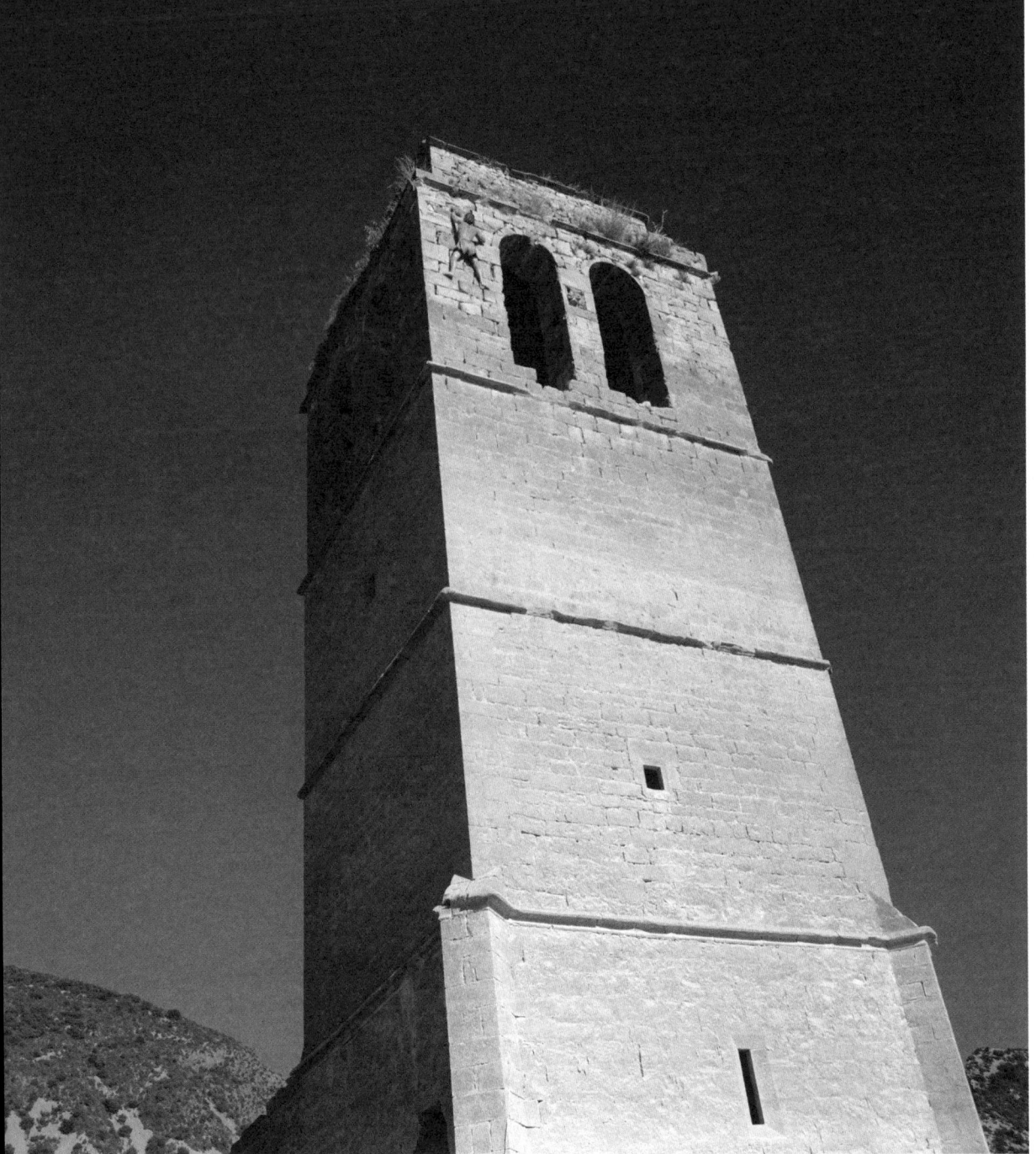

The church symbolizes sacredness. My sacredness is
in my body. Flowing through my body and challenging
it past the fear of death, saying, "Be alive, feel alive,
where there is no death!" Everybody has their own
way. Trust your gut and find your own way.

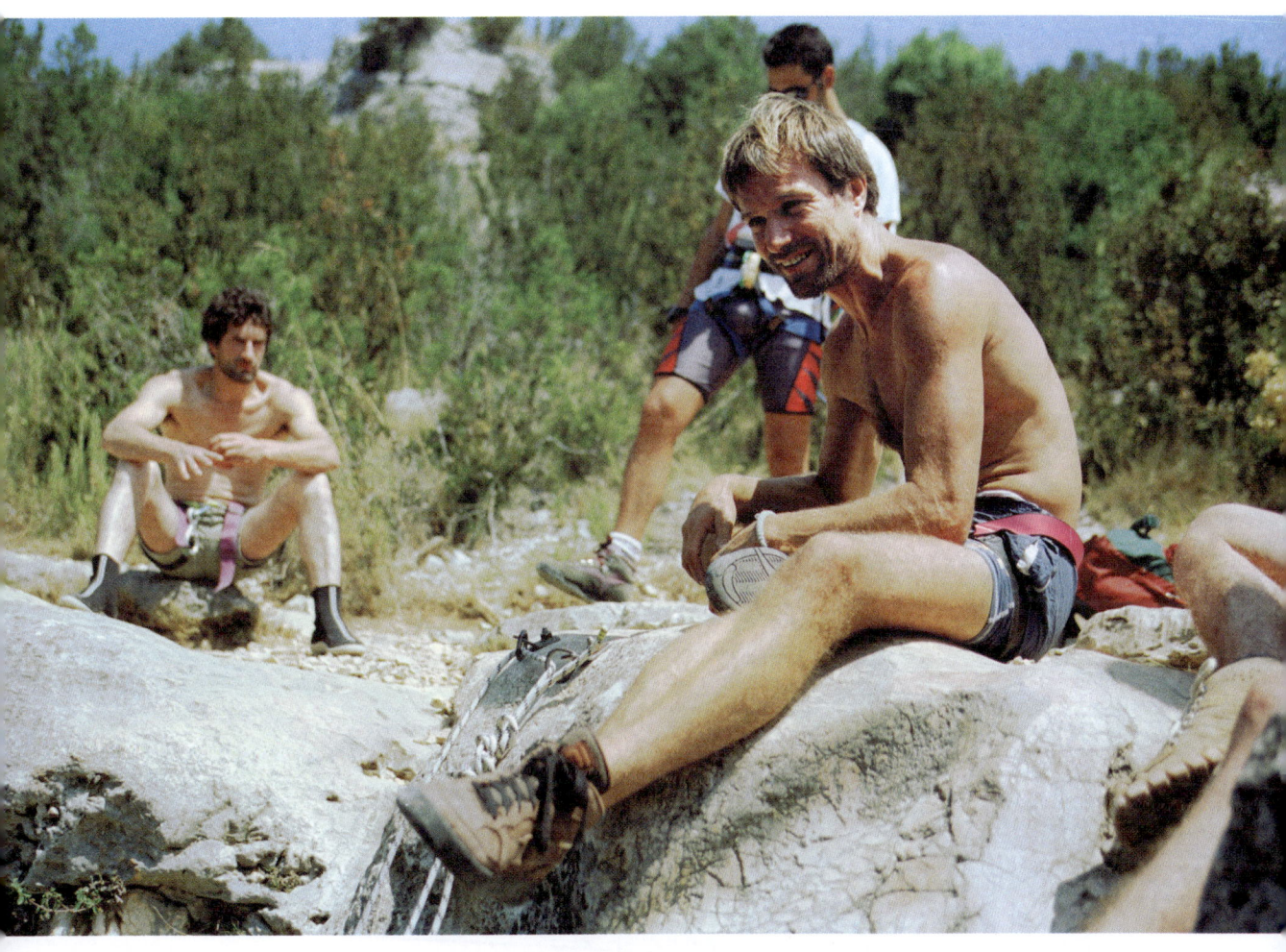

Waiting before the descent; rappelling.
If you are peaceful and restful at the
brink of an abyss, then people with fear
feel safe. When we feel safe, we have
much more control over ourselves.

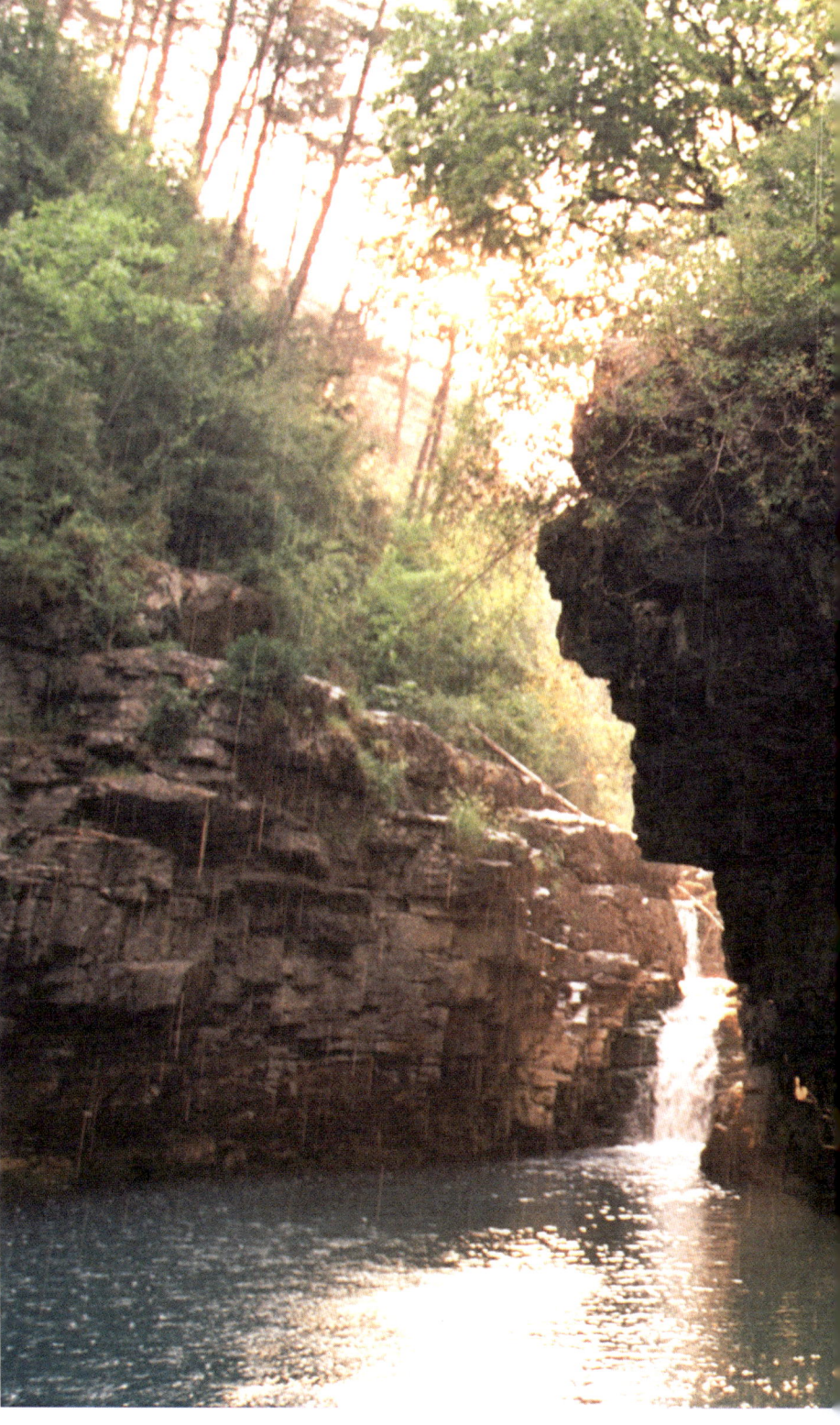

Monkeying around.
Bouldering in the
Barranco de Anisclo
in the Pyrenees
after we did the
cave La Cueva de
los Moros. Or just
a beautiful pic.

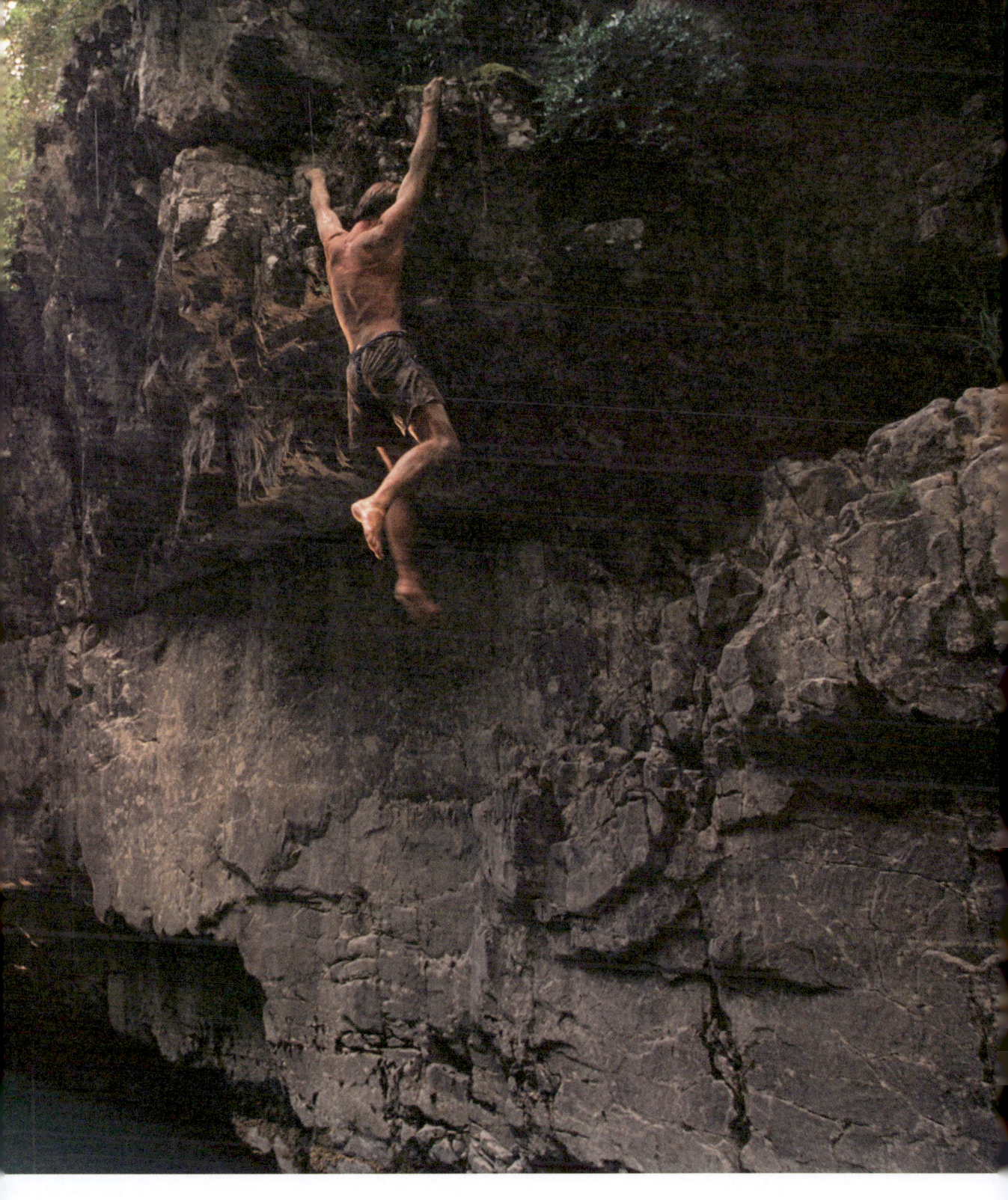

LOUNGE

The space between the days is ever

Meditation in the waiting room is

Just relax, sit back, and launch

Breathe deep and lounge

Let the mind go into the heaven sphere

The feeling of being in love, anywhere

Matter serves what does not matter

What you are then will only get better

Let go attachments as birds set free

That's where they belong you see

Frivolous, circling around

Innocent, beautiful sounds

Like a water stream reminding eternity

A voice of droplets bringing clarity

No words, just lounge

Amazing state of mind

Kind, all there

No more searching, just find

Awareness, fairness, light like a breeze

Clear like drops, before they freeze

Are you ready, steady, beautiful as you are

Any moment now, and you become a star.

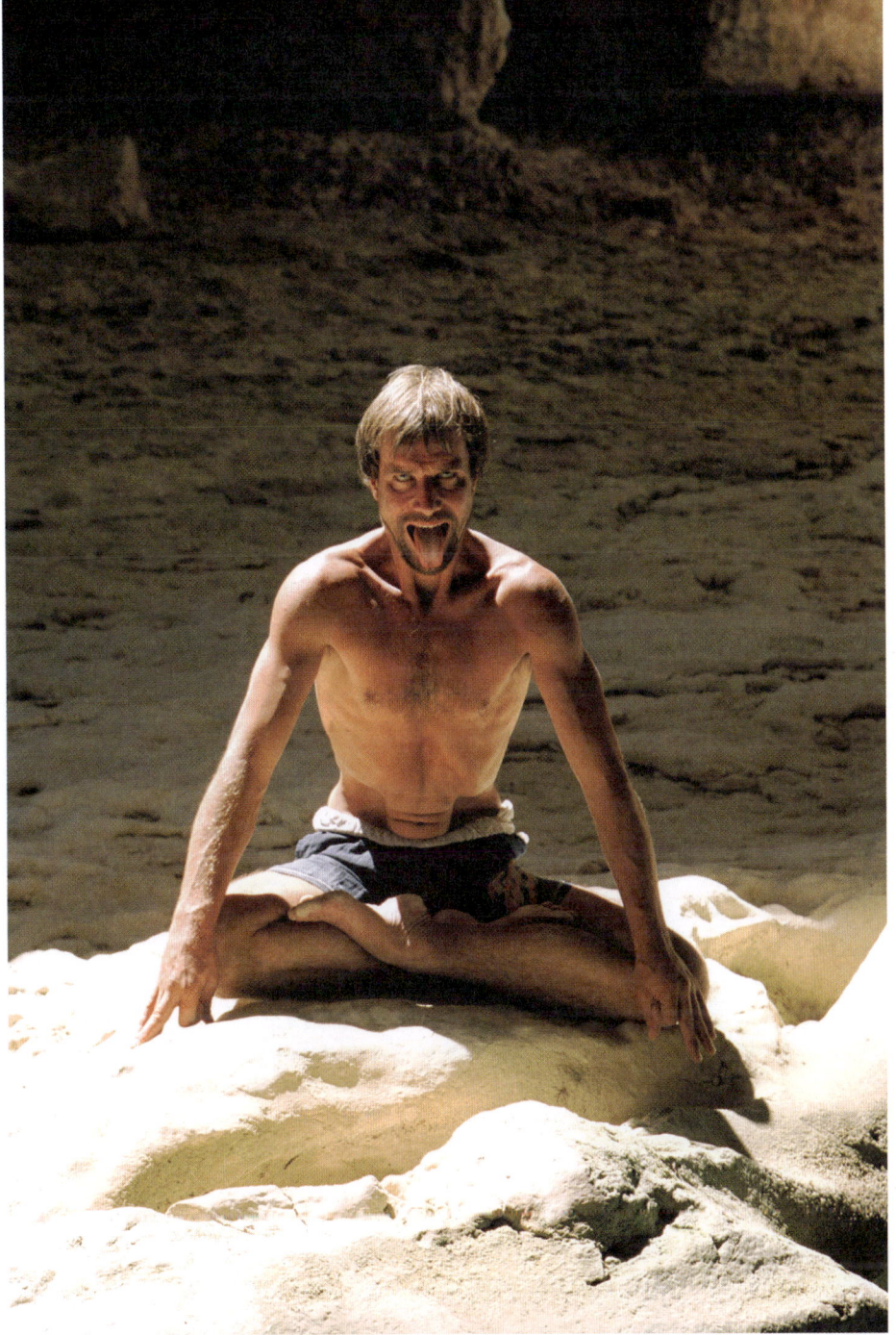

Anytime, anywhere Simhasana—the Lion Pose in the Rio Vero Canyon. It takes about six hours walking, strolling, swimming, diving, jumping, to get to the other end. Marvelous journeys in the canyons. I remember my friend Javier bringing me to this canyon for the first time. It is where the world opened up to me again. Deeply moved by it all. Nature.

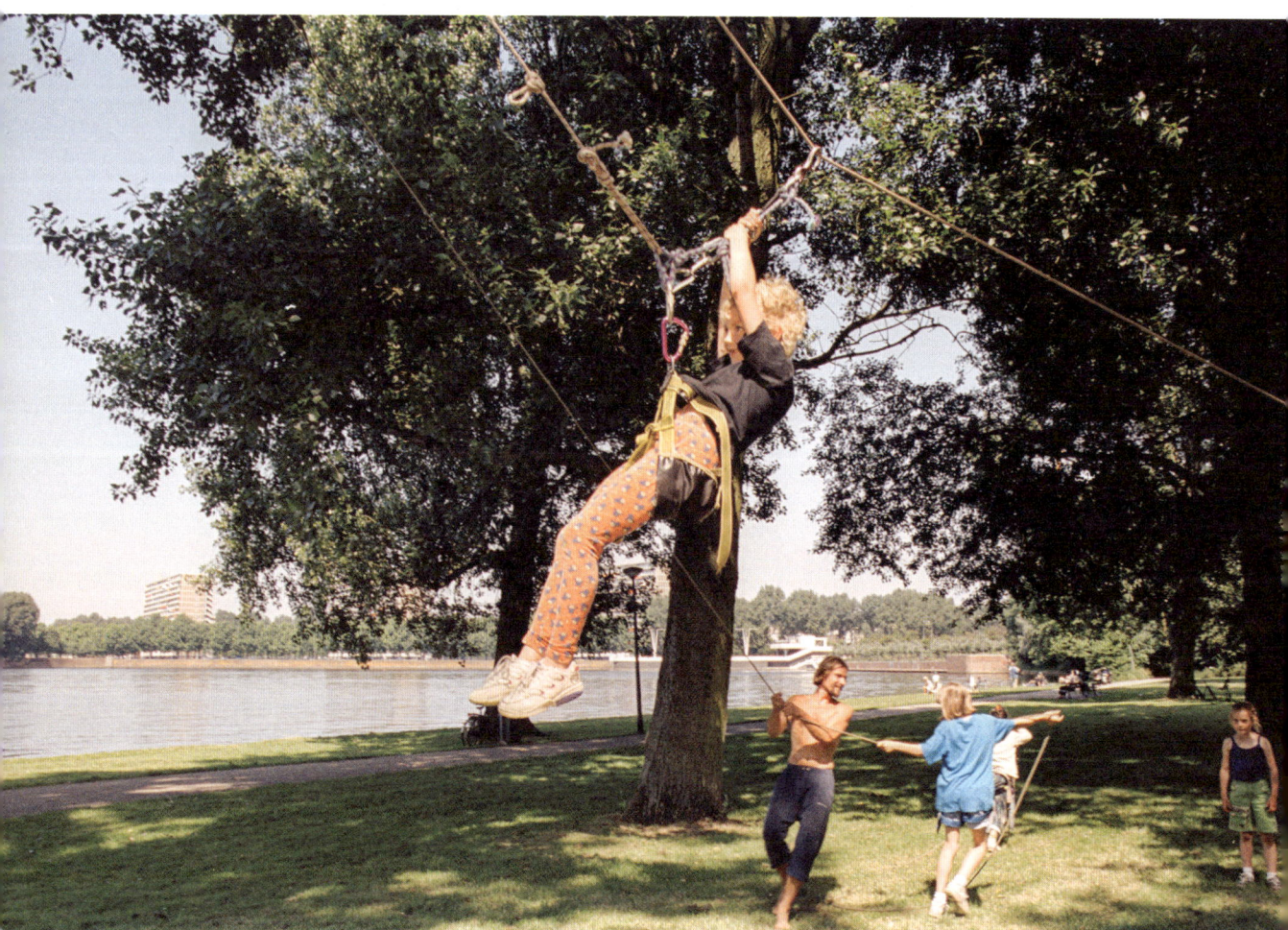

Back in Amsterdam. Six years doing tree-climbing birthday parties. Children have a natural drive to learn, to be in nature. They loved it! They go faster and are more focused and controlled. After it all, they are positively silenced. Serene. Parents are the most astounded as they see their children so different! So much fun and power.

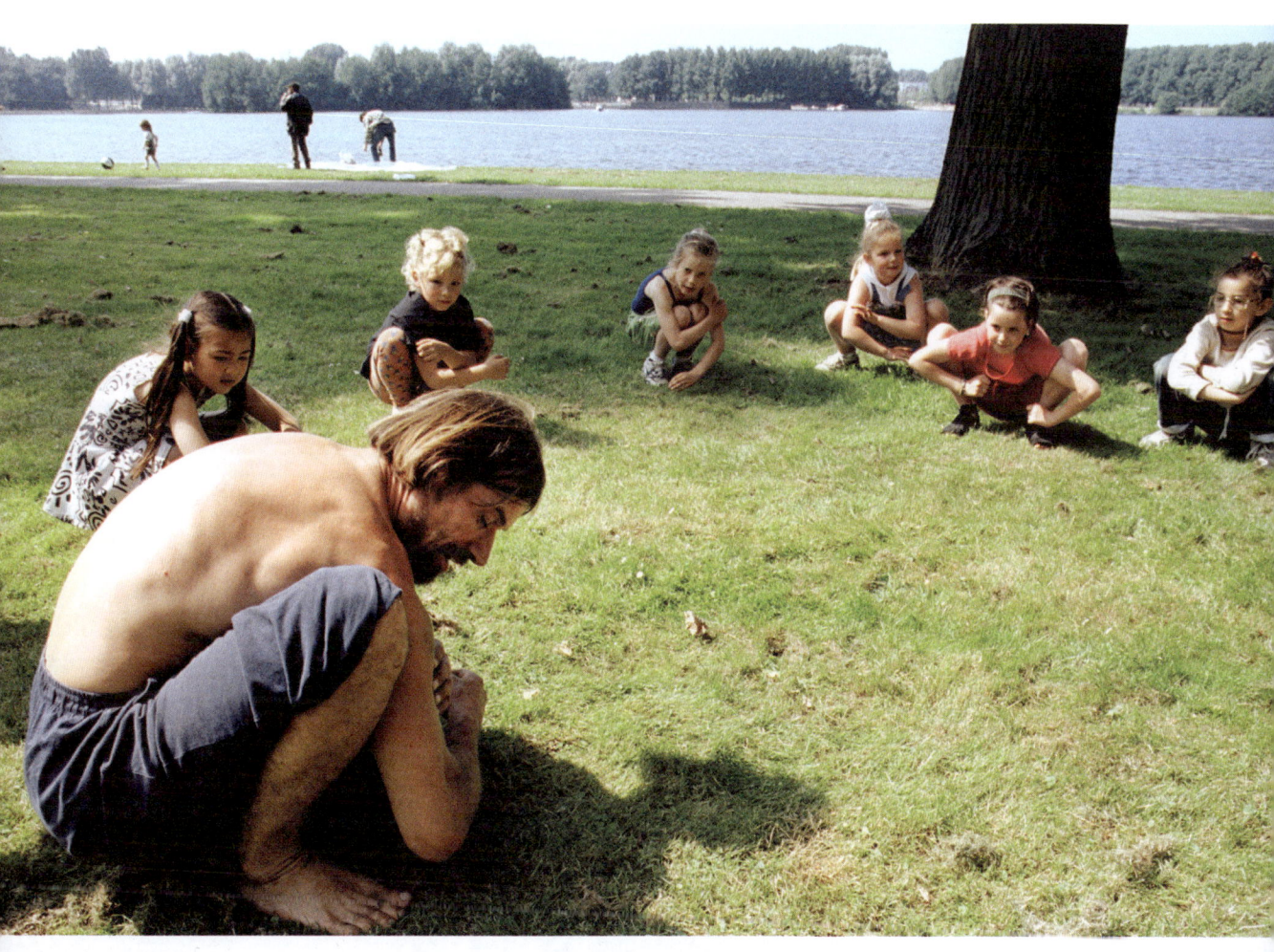

Once you capture their attention, they follow. Here, teaching yoga postures, Crow Pose, Headstand, Frog Pose. Children love enthusiasm; they are heightened beings themselves. Learning to connect with themselves and with nature is of utmost importance.

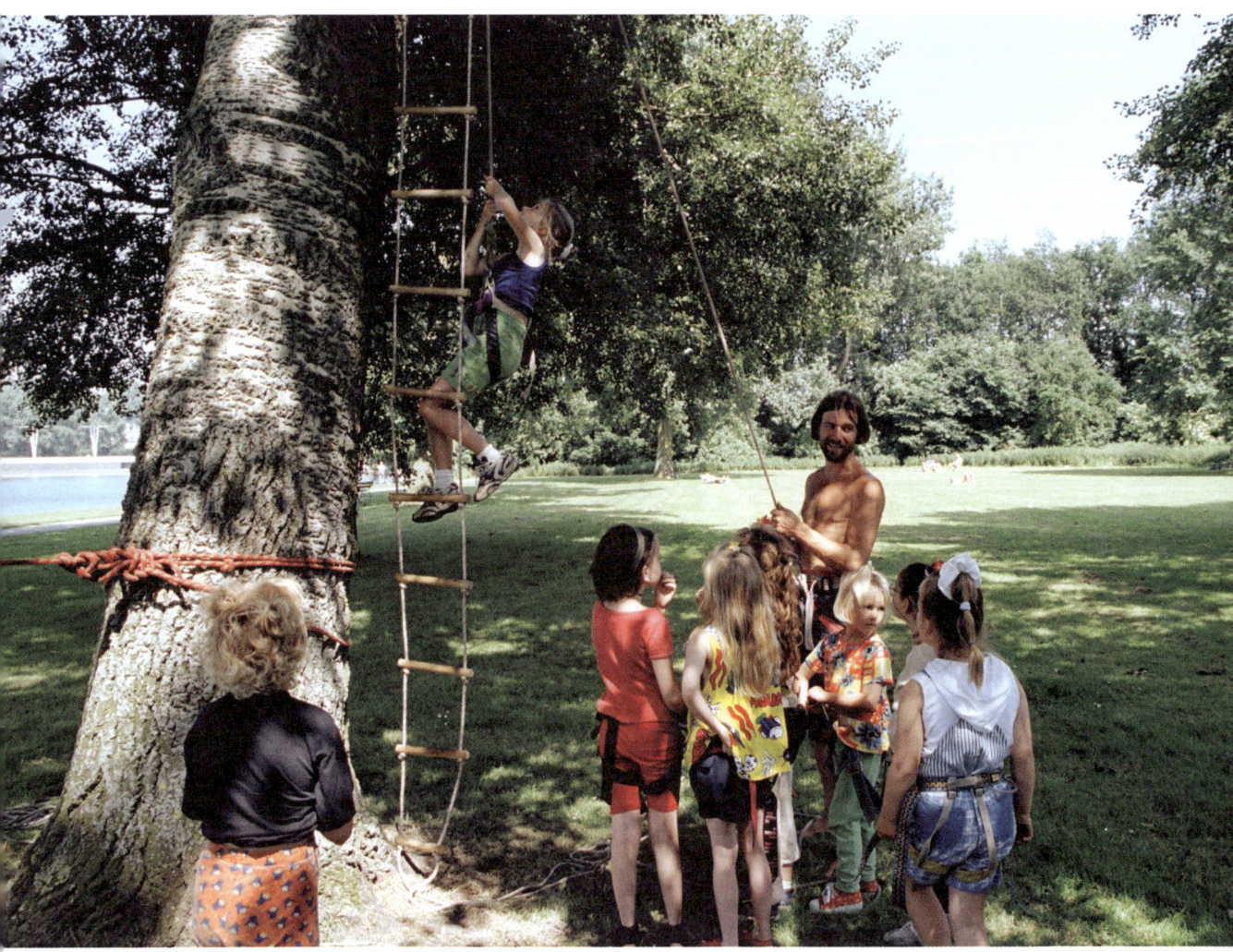

Instructions are part of the focus.
Excitement stalled pays off.

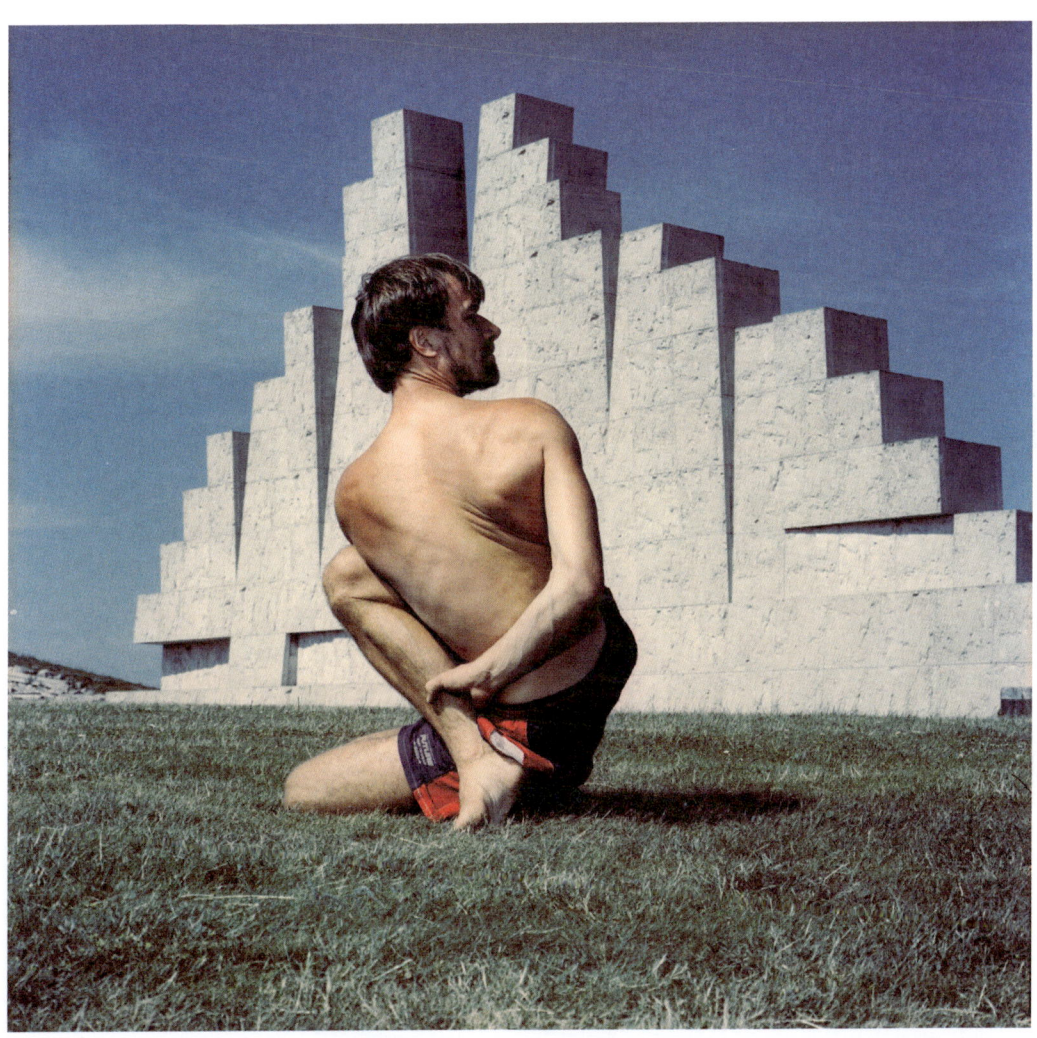

Ardha Matsyendrasana—the Full Lateral Twist. Great feeling to lock yourself half a minute into more and more twisting. Good for the kidneys as the blood flow is coerced to flush that area.

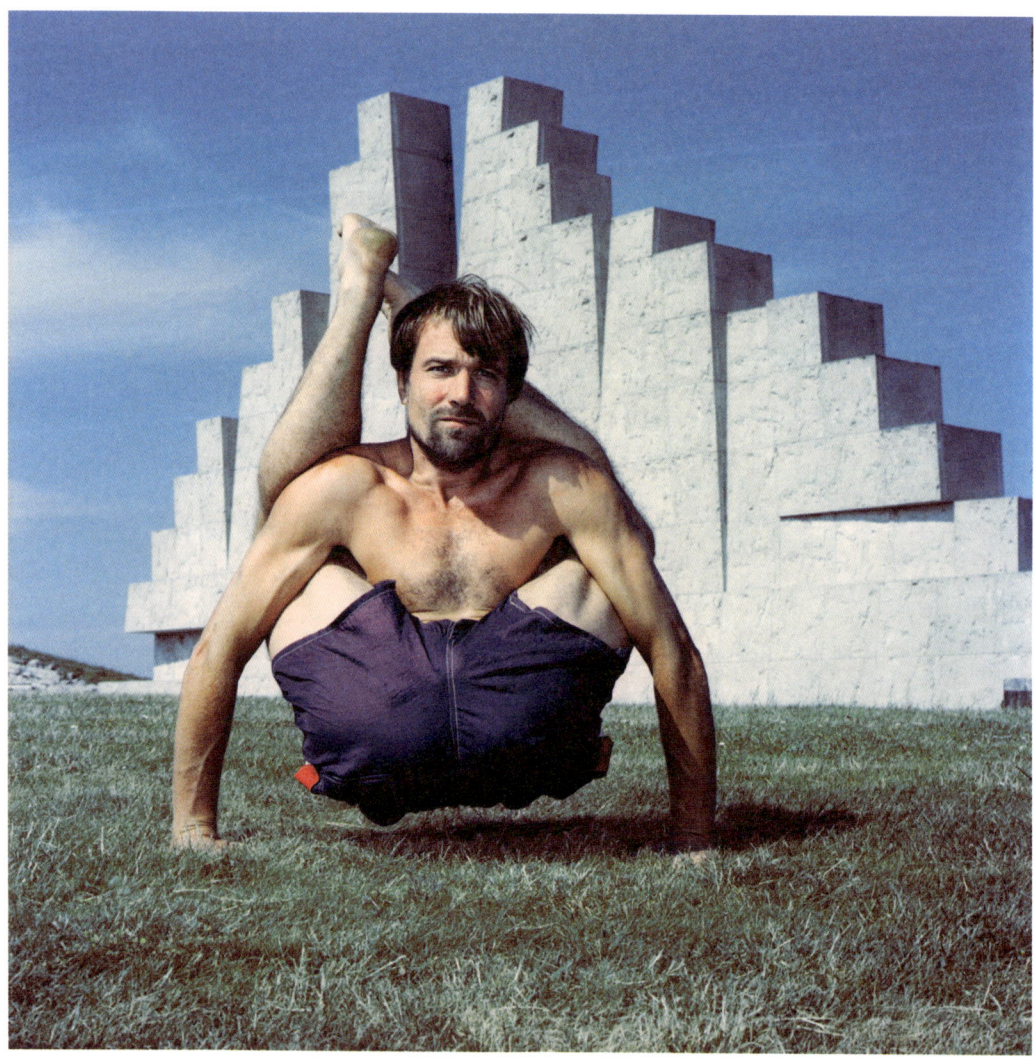

Yes, love this one. Looks ridiculous but
feels amazing. It's the full contraction of
the abdominals and forward bending.

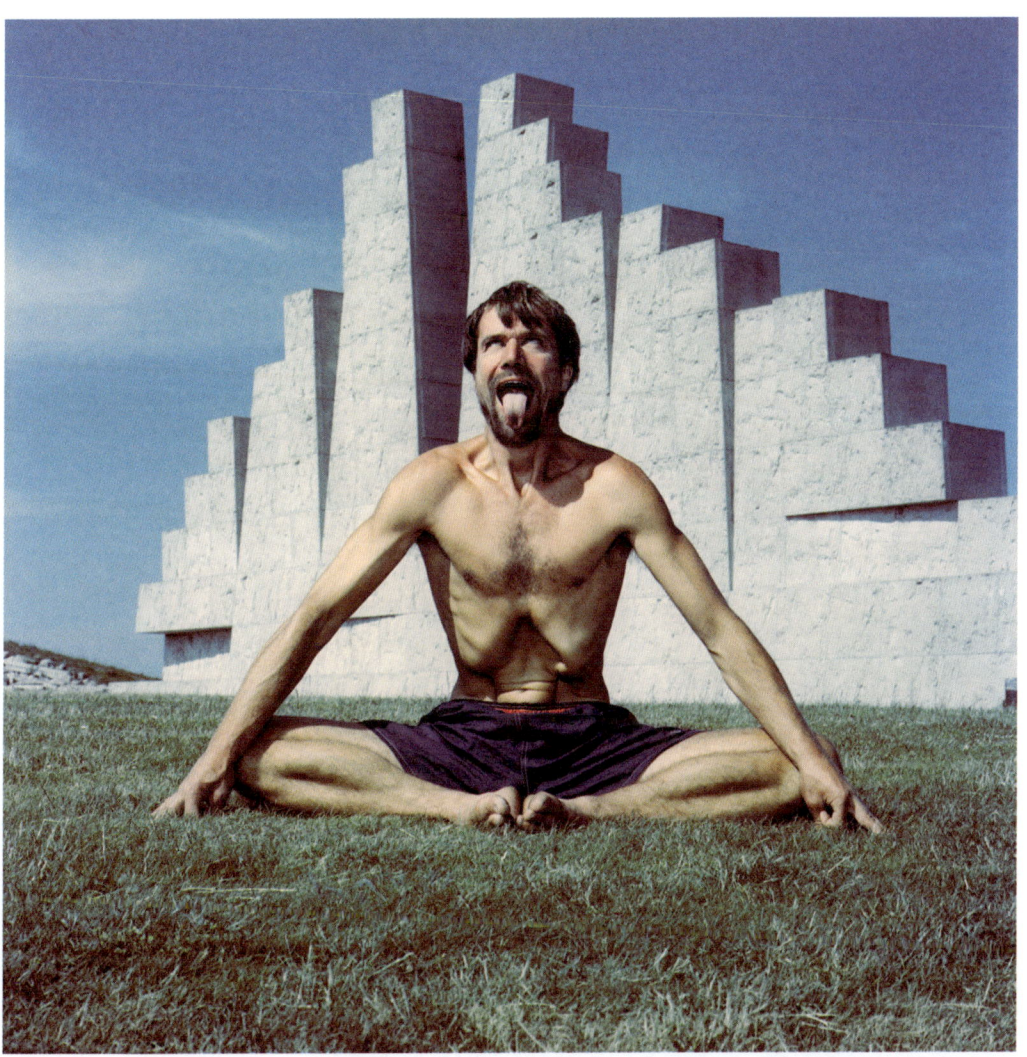

Simhasana (Lion Pose) and Nauli (the Wave). This pose
opens the kundalini (subliminal nervous system currents)
through the spine (sushumna) so it has an uninhibited
flow reaching the full brain (seat of the mind).

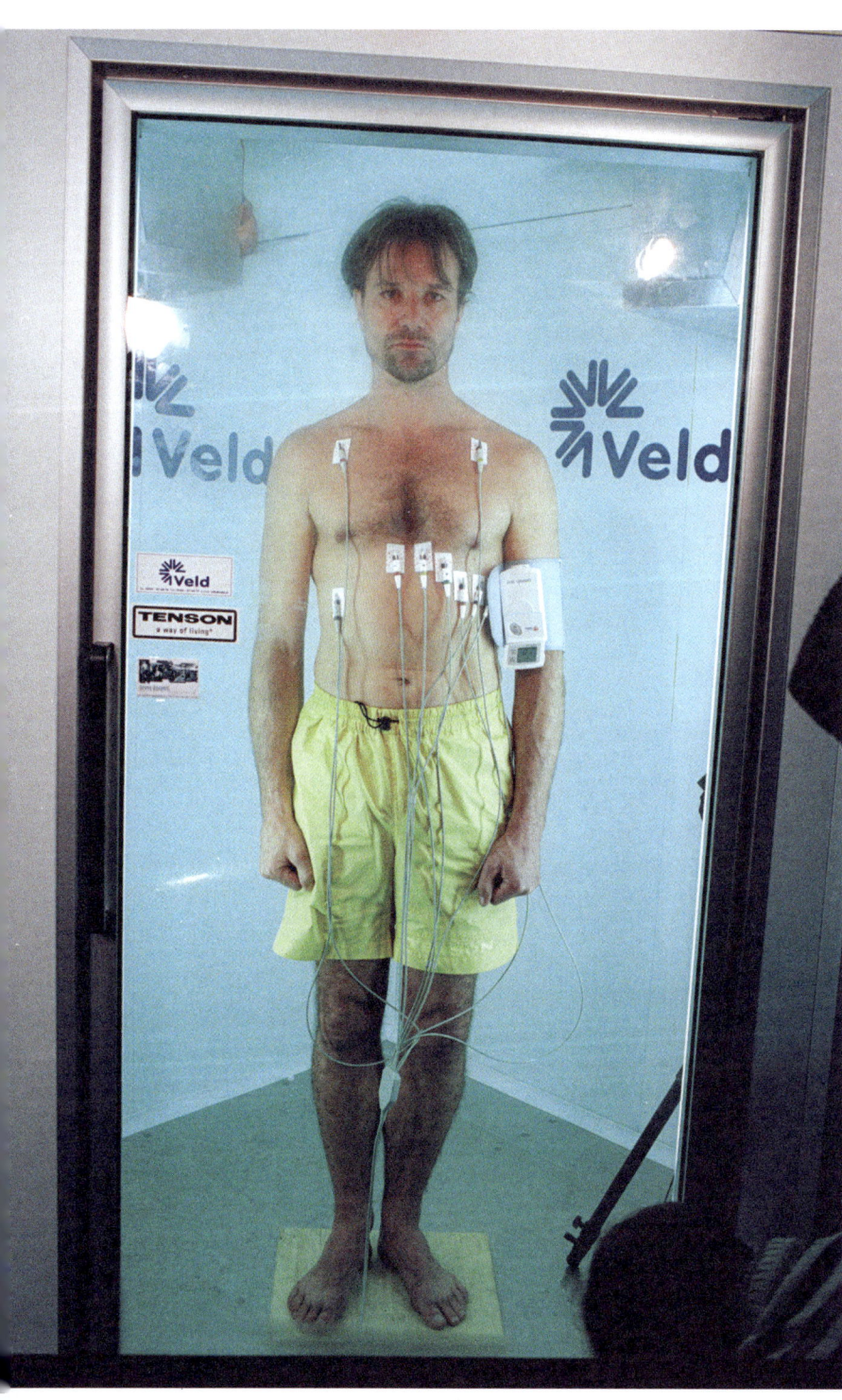

Rotterdam at an expo on thermodynamics. Standing for an hour in -30 degrees Celsius was a piece of cake (ice-cake) for me. I ingested temperature pills measuring my core body temperature, which almost never dropped!

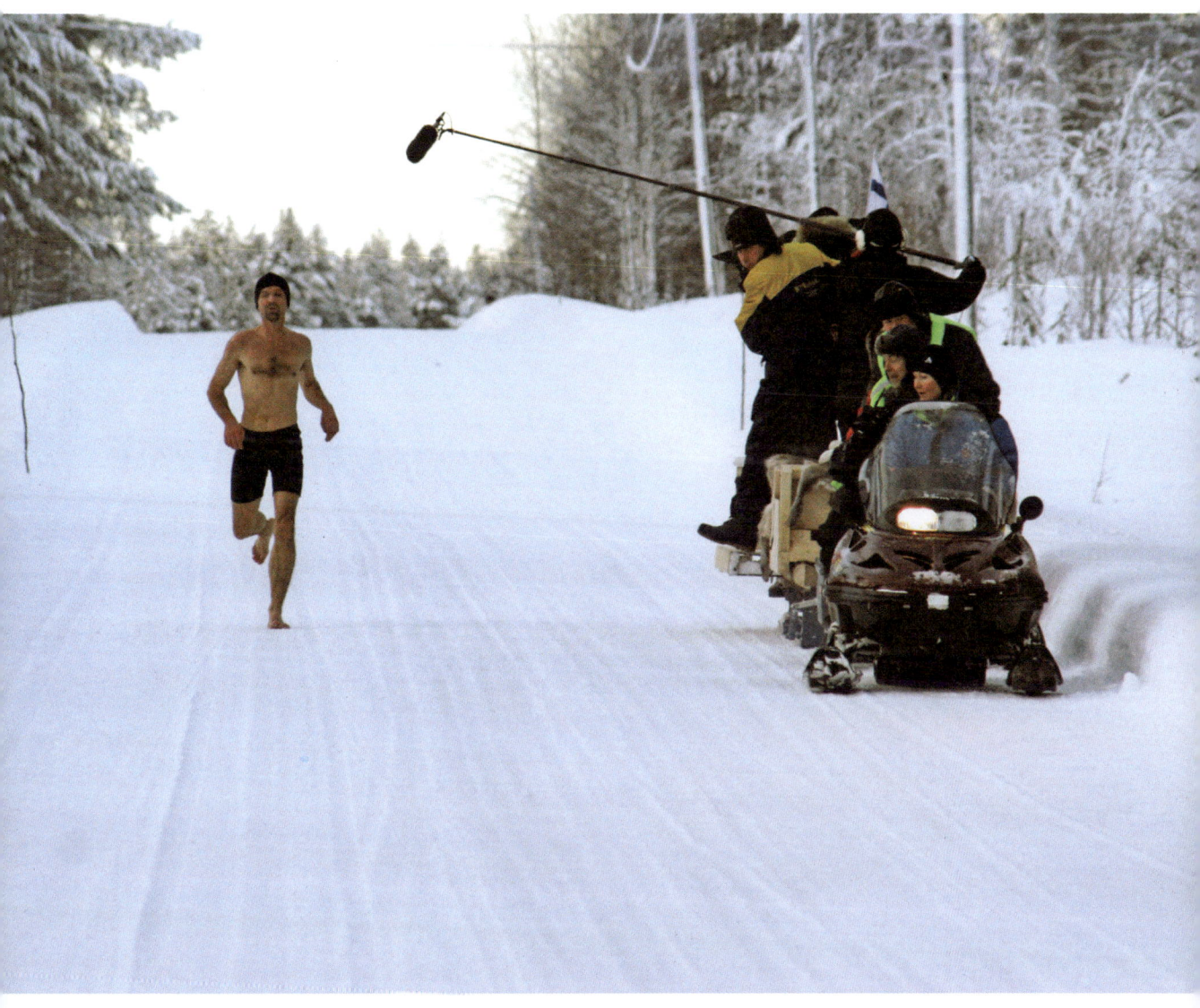

Running beyond the polar circle in deep freezing temperatures. The night before I had some doubt. I thought, *Am I going to be able to do this barefoot?* Imagine then, when you start, and the doubt disappears. You feel great. I even started making jokes! Yet, at 18 kilometers my left foot, actually my whole left leg, felt like wood. I couldn't feel anything anymore. I ran on and completed the half marathon. Normally I would have stopped. I listen to my body, but this time there was television and this abstract number, 21 kilometers. In a high-performance situation, you can make mistakes. The body gives clear signals. But I overruled it in this case, and the damage was done.

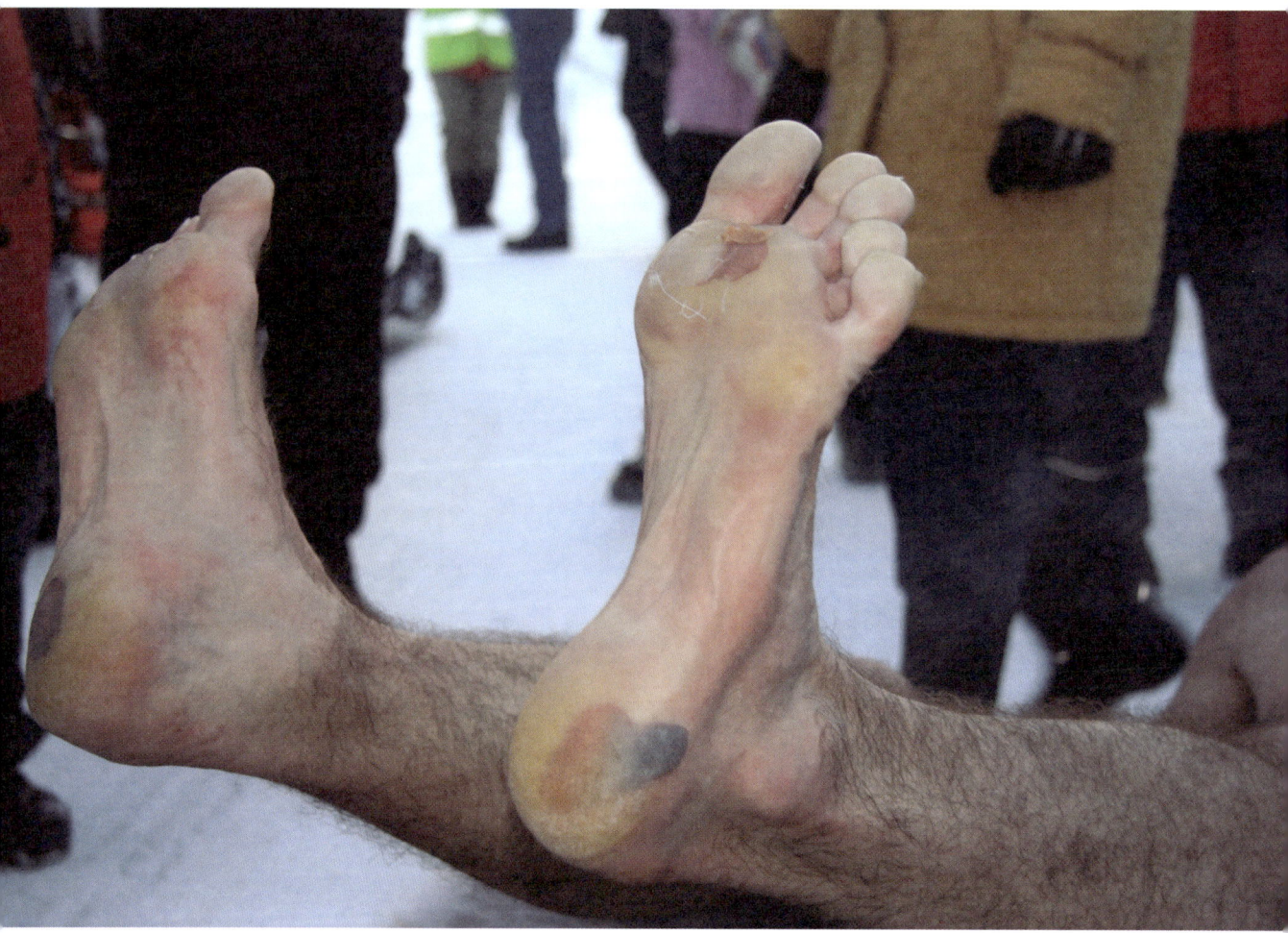

The mind may be stronger than the body, but my feet took the blow. Look at the blisters! The worst part was that I could not feel my feet anymore. That means my blood flow had stopped, which can cause irreparable cell damage. A dermatologist warned that it may be impossible to heal from this, but three months later, I was on Mt. Everest. It was quite a healing process, though. Don't just think the mind can overrule the body because you want it to. It is a back-and-forth communication. There is a stretch you can take in overruling, but with risk, so always be aware.

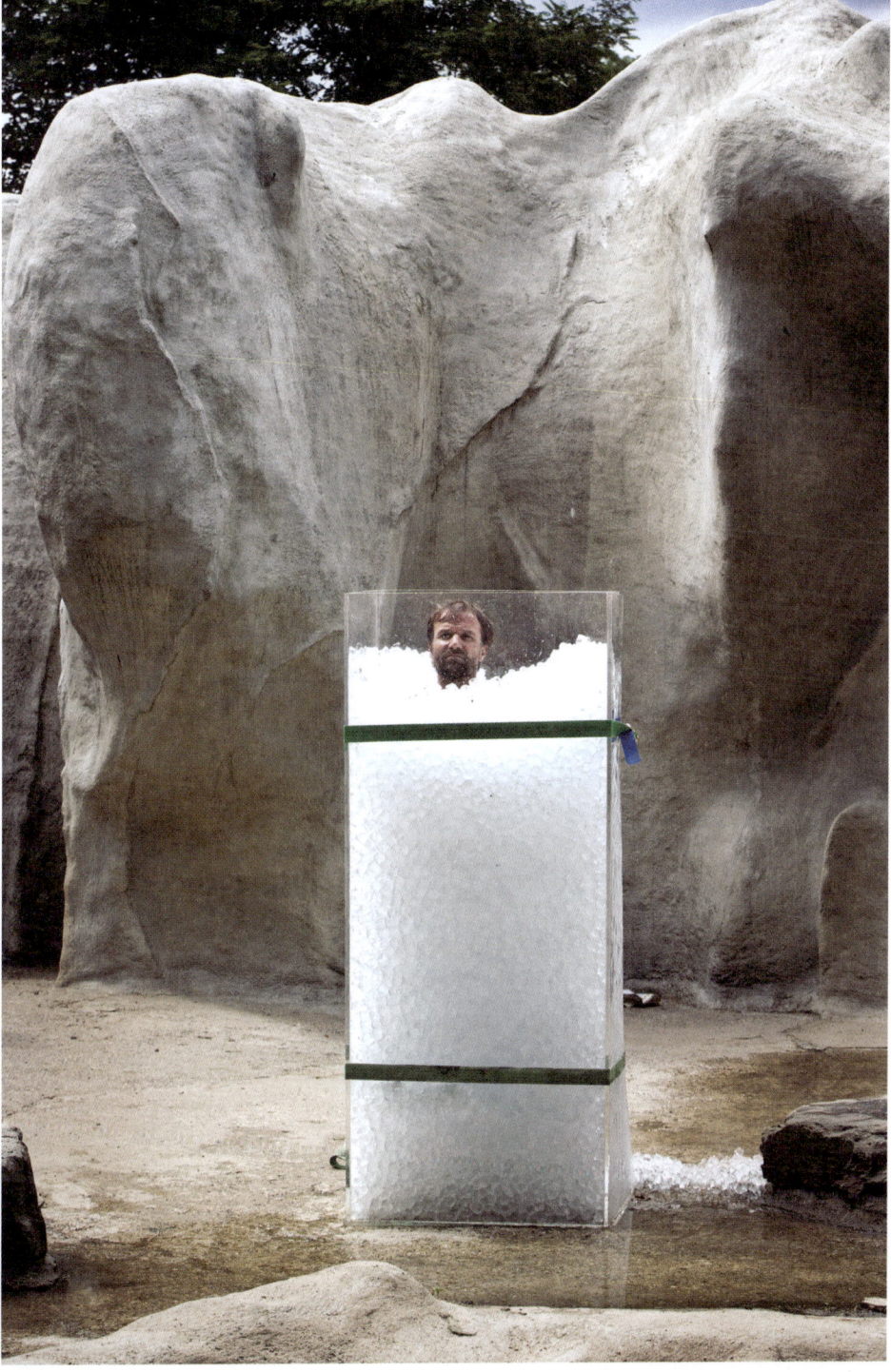

A world record in the polar bear compound at the zoo. I invaded his territory and thought he would have eaten me if he had not been brought to an adjacent compound. Polar bears are huge when you see them up close.

BREAKTHROUGH

Though

Existent paradigm, cementing the presence of a

Wall

That kept our freedom at bay, as if something

Utopian, fallopian

Tube, you have a rebirth coming to you

A key of the universe, passing through

Ovarian wisdom to grow into magic

New light, away from being tragic

Feeling your way simply great

No longer held back, just wait

A minute, a moment, a flash

You are here, gone the trash

Unconditional love settling down

You might notice, the weight of a crown

The you are as it is

When left alone, leading to bliss

Every moment just let it be

Like all flowers do, just see

When all the compensatory temptations fade

Astray

Then the cozy temperature of all is here to stay

Where faith listens to you well

The source, the heart, out of hell

Hell yeah, into heaven

Break through!

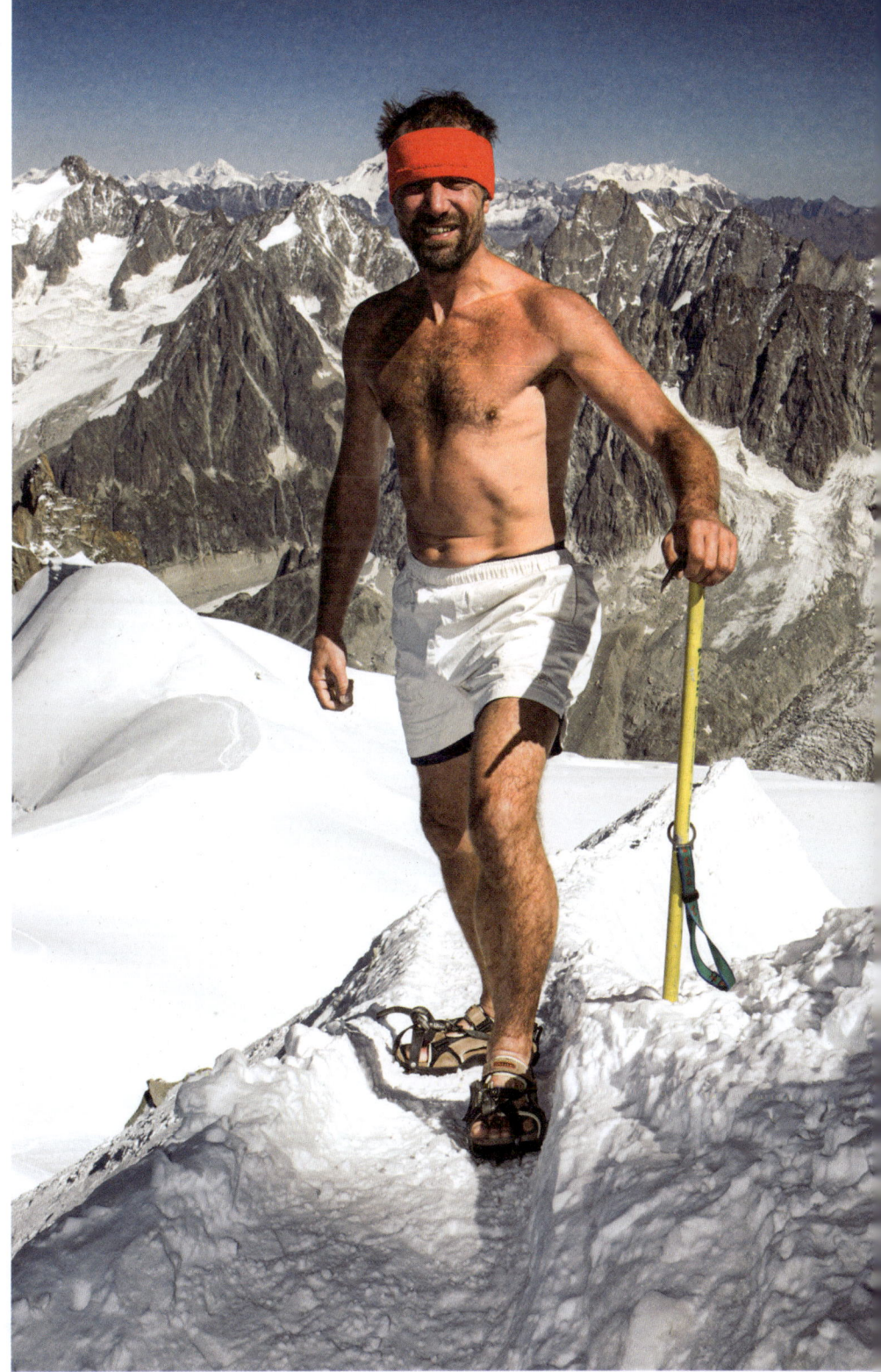

High in the mountains. I challenged myself so many times. You feel pure confidence when you are naked within the hostility of nature, and because of that, it becomes your friend.

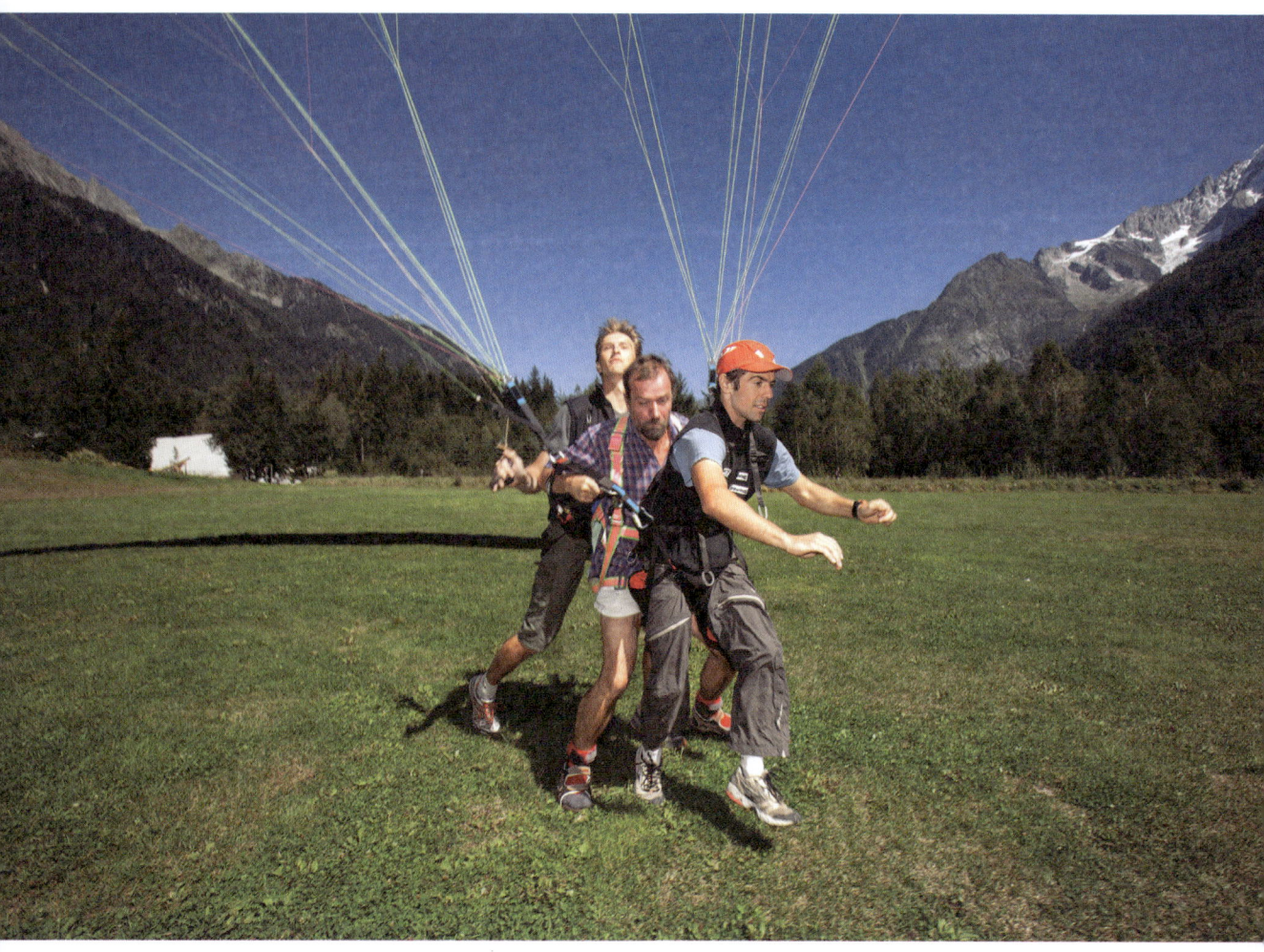

I met these two French guys on Mt. Everest in the advanced base camp. They planned to go parachuting down from the summit area. It did not work out, but our friendship did. Here the three of us got ready to jump from the slopes of Mt. Blanc together, something that is normally done with two (in tandem).

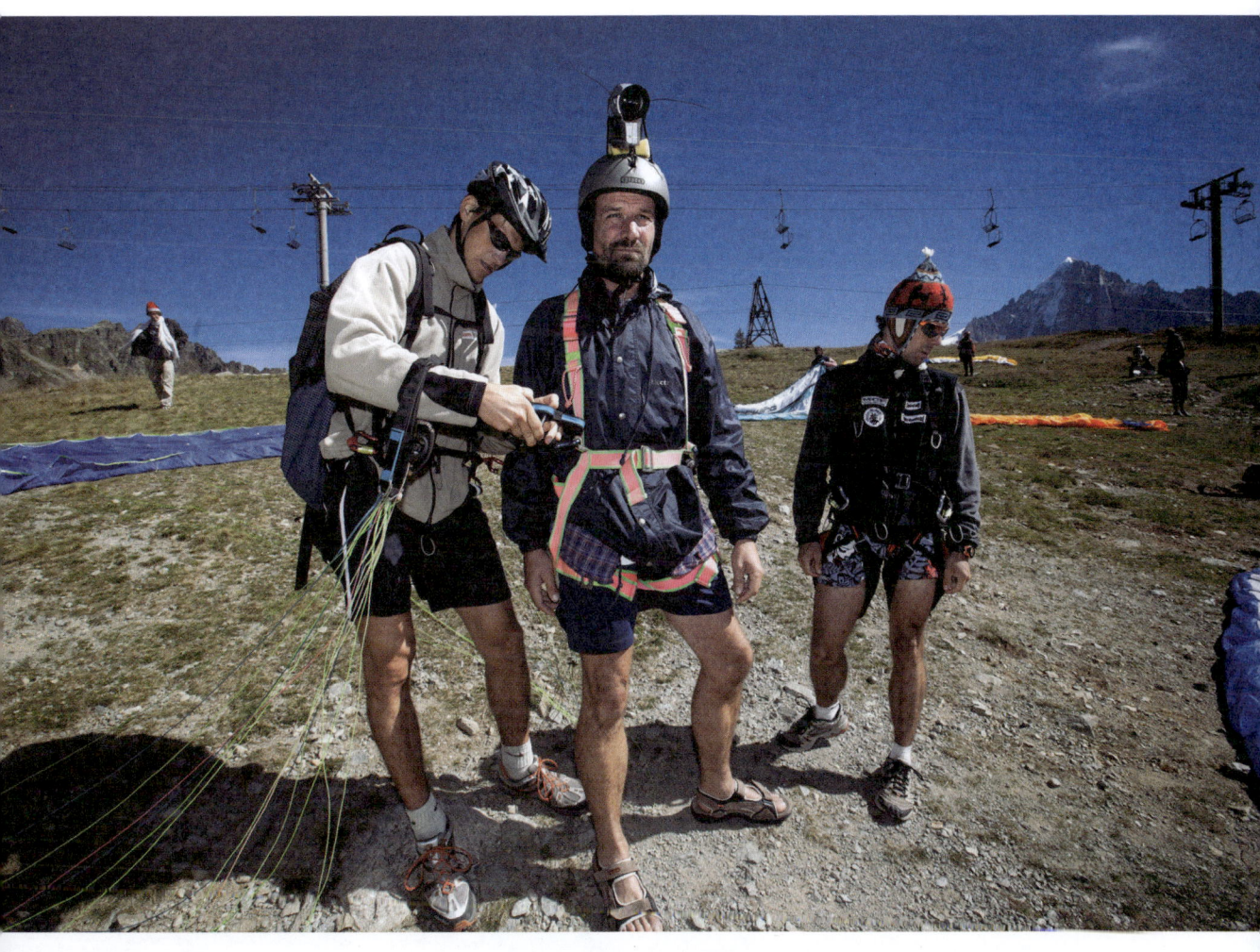

With my friends from Everest, just before the jump. Just the three of us. Excitement and trust because three is more than two!

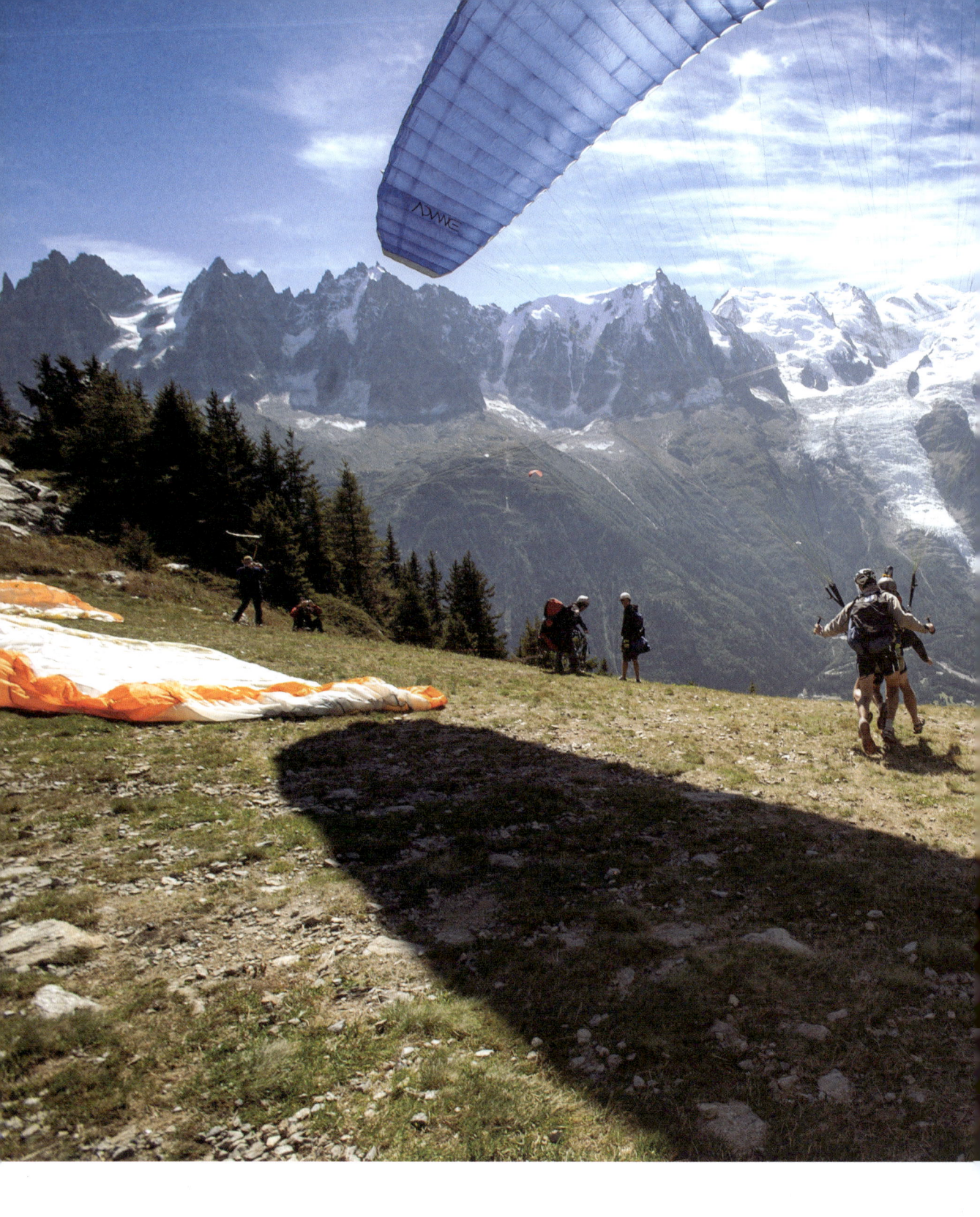

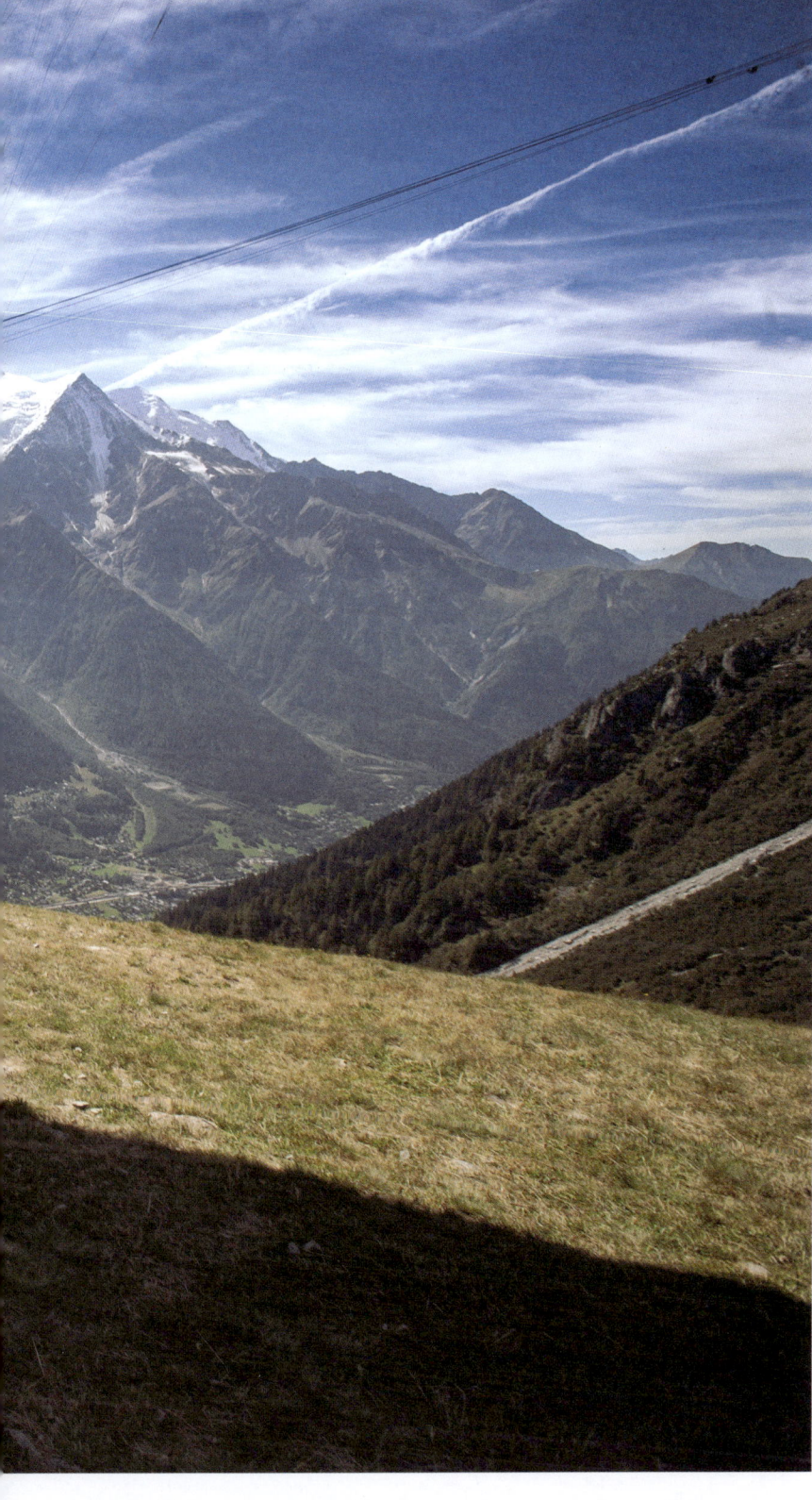

On the runway out into
the blue. Quite amazing
going down and making
these big circles and
even somersaults.
Imagine . . . the three of
us. Wooooooooooaaaaaa!

130

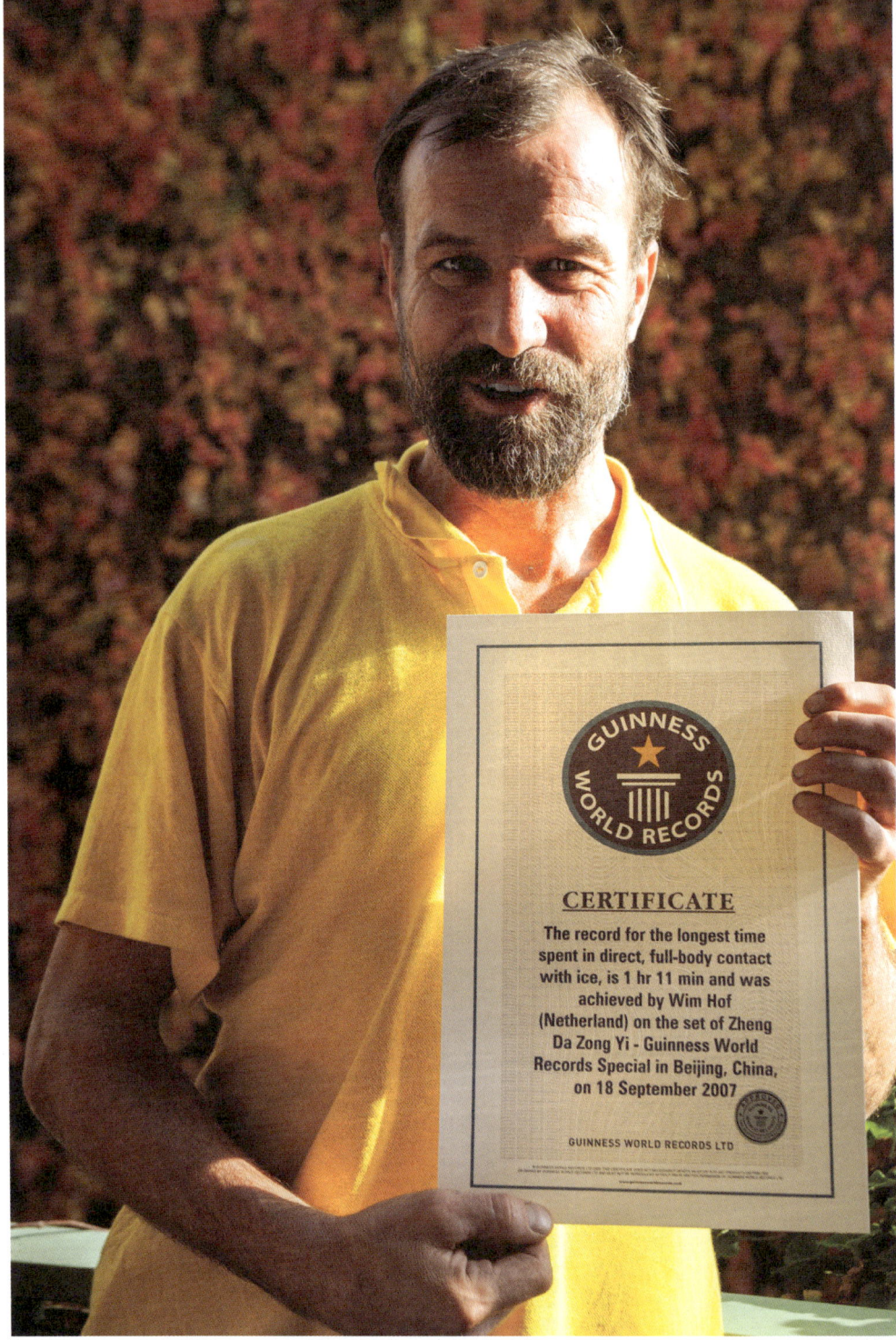

One of my Guinness World Record
certificates. I was invited all over the world.

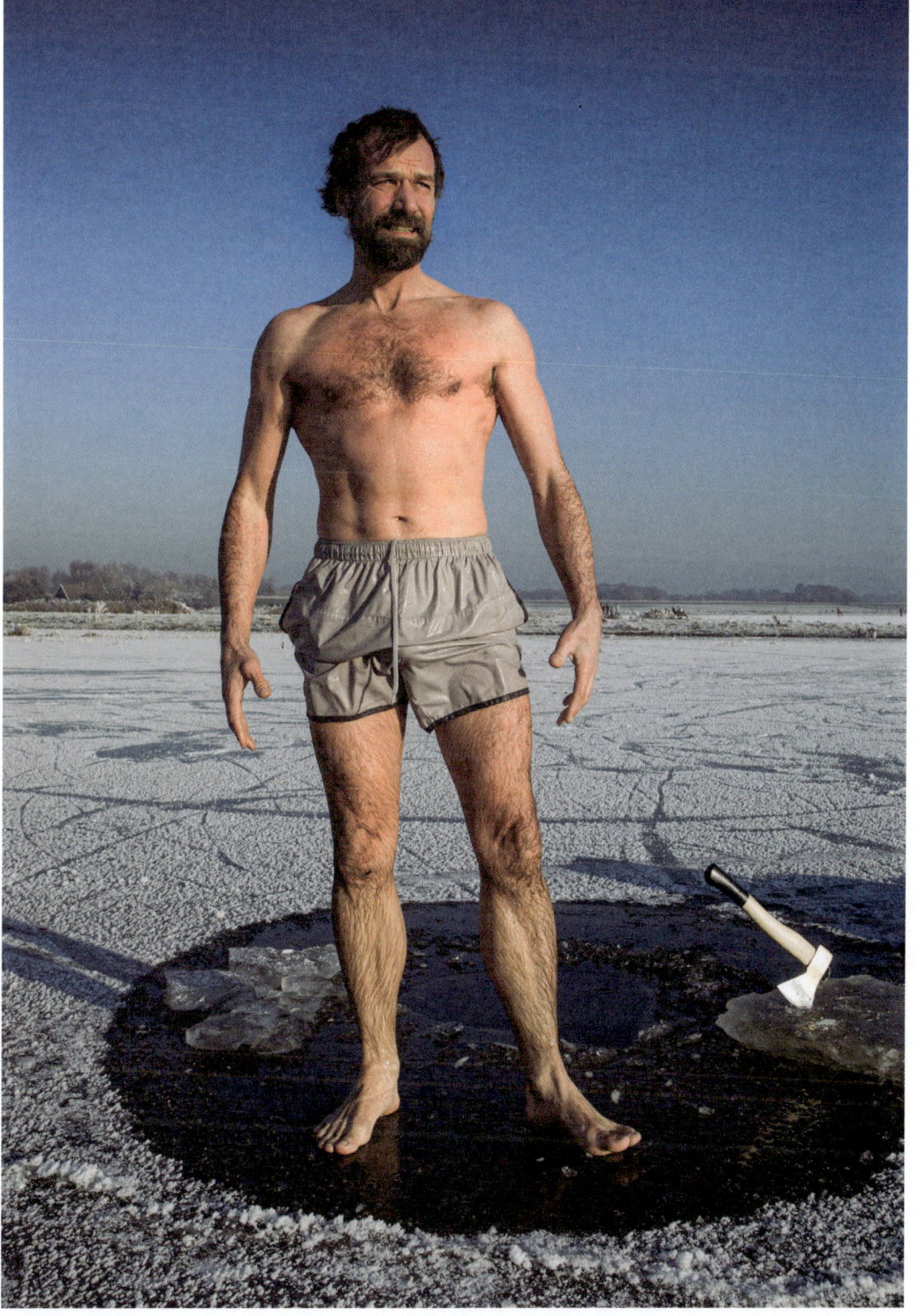

The cold trains the body's functionality best. It looks like you are
doing nothing in the water, yet the body is working like hell.

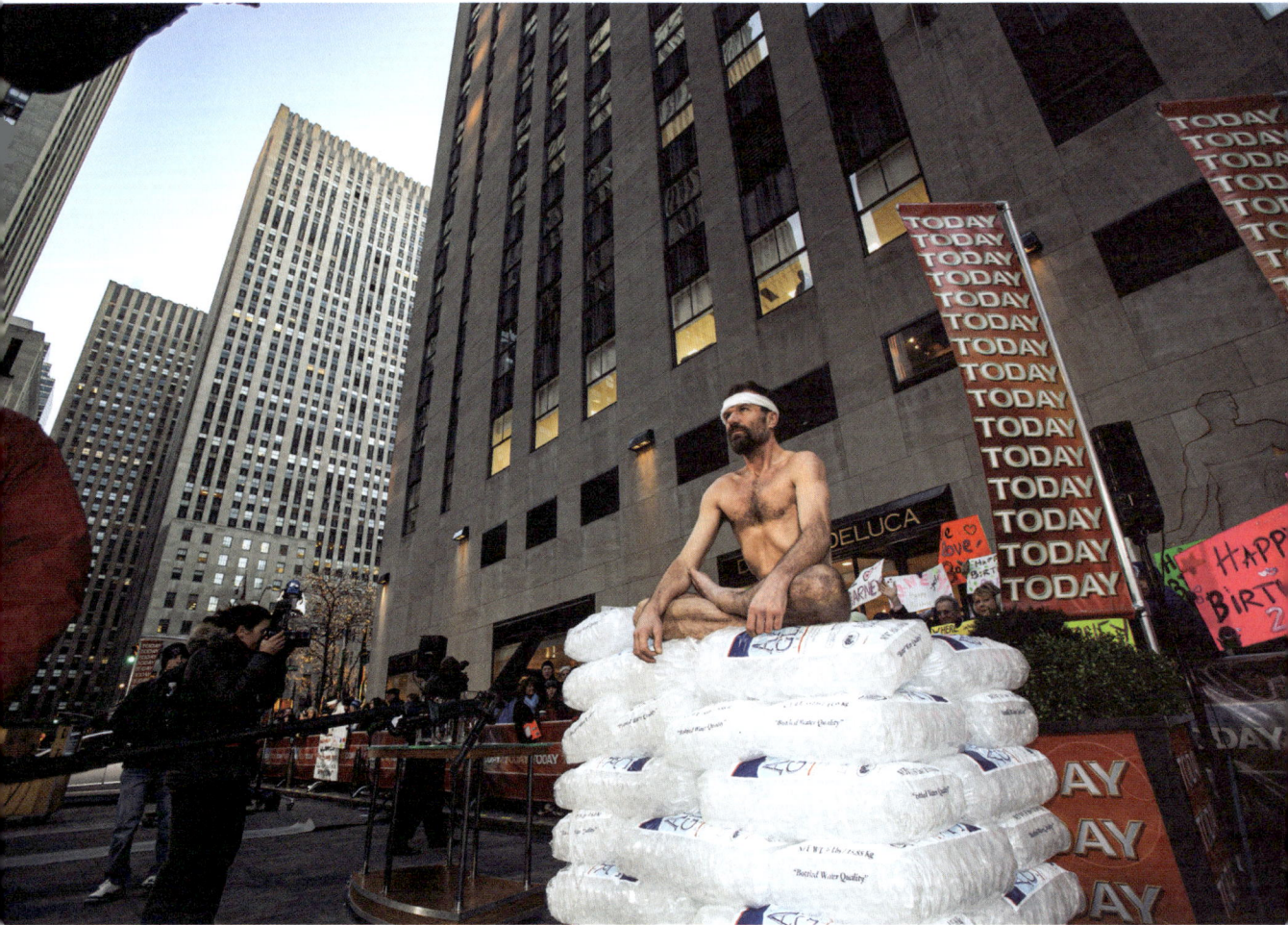

A chilly January morning on *The Today Show*. New York, 2008.

It was a spectacle for everyone there. The thing is I actually did those exhibitions to show we can do more than we think. This trip would also prove to be a crucial turning point in my life.

Fifty minutes in the ice.

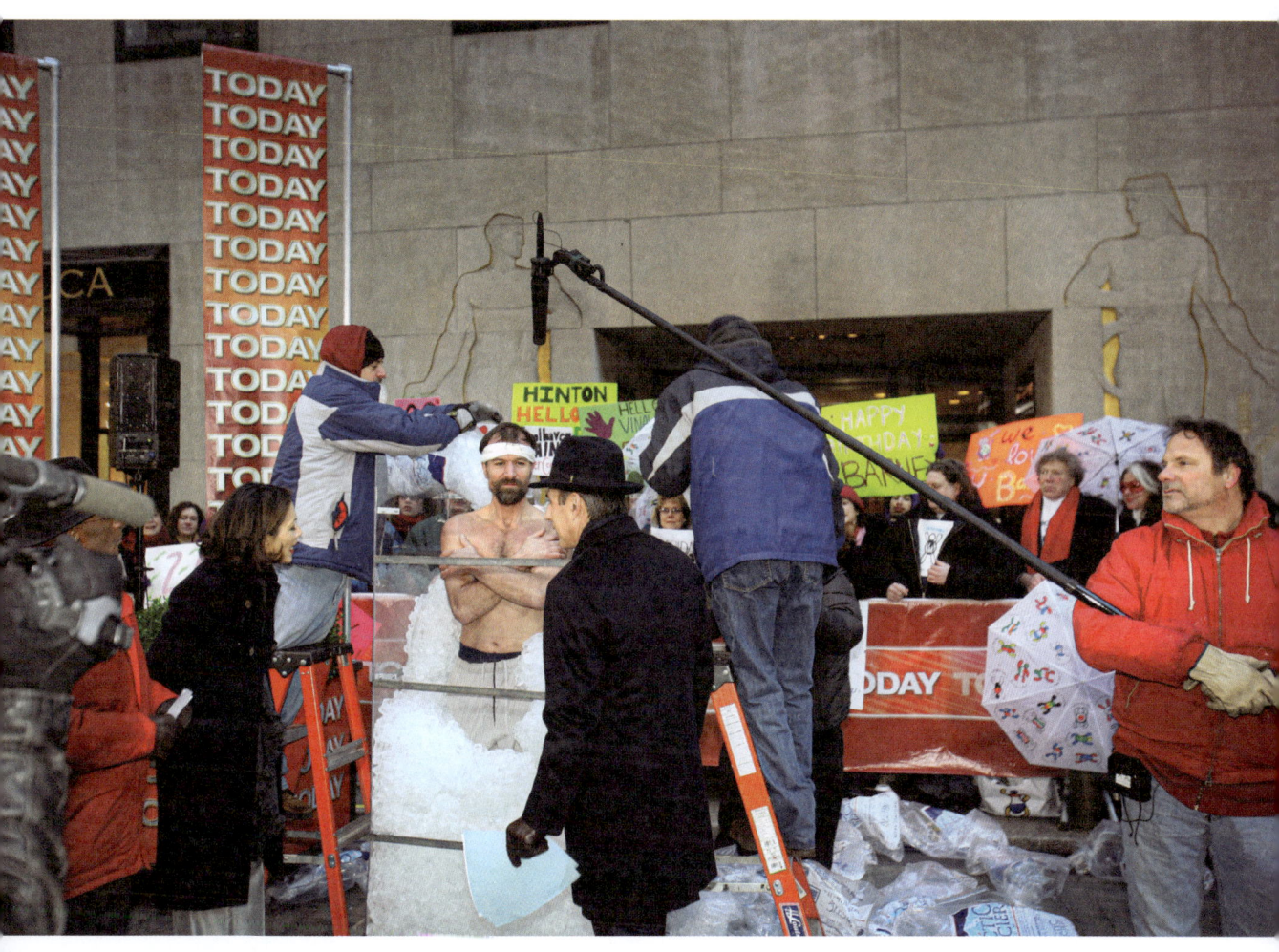

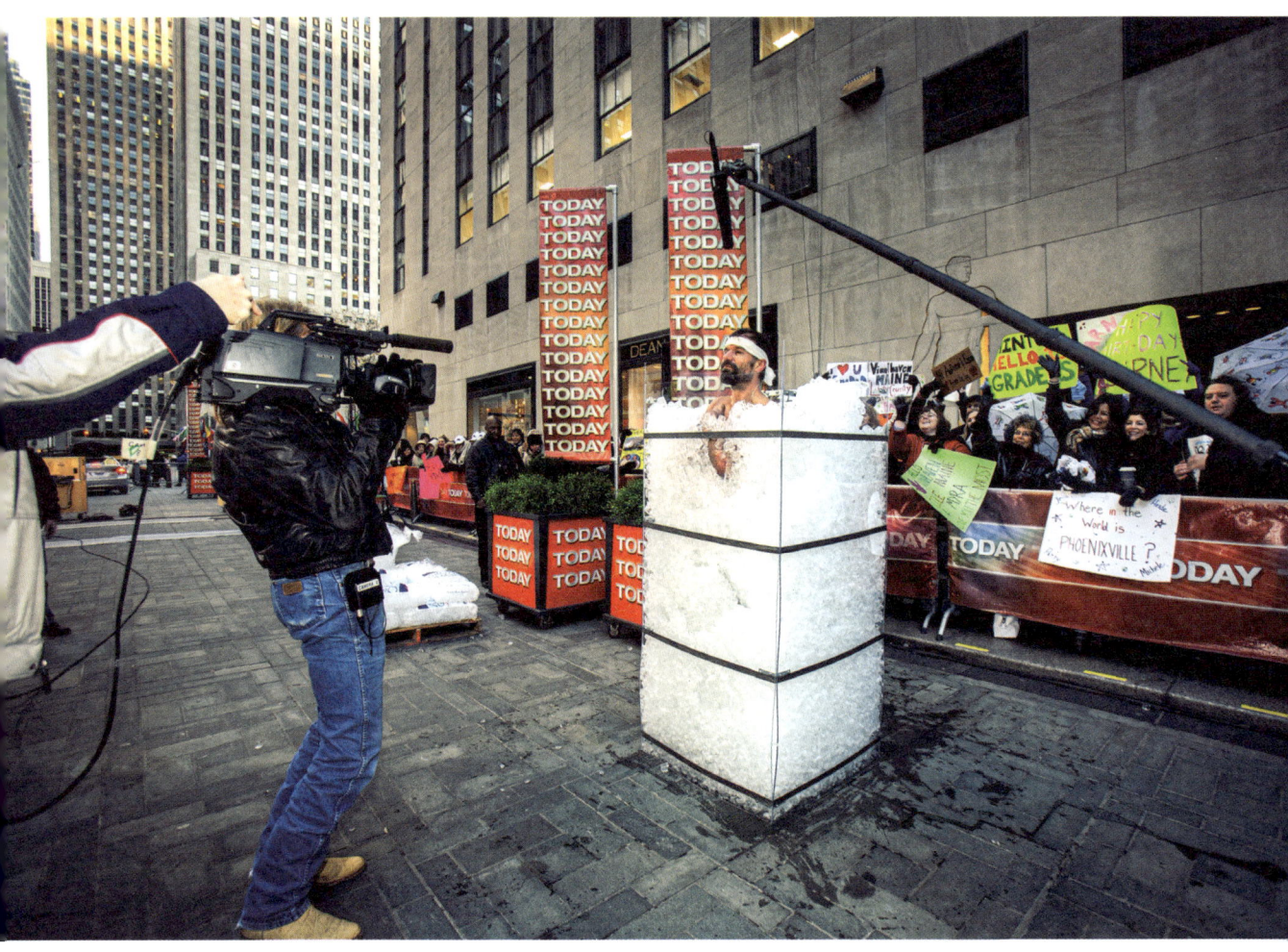

Times Square, the evening
after *The Today Show*,
moments before I saw myself

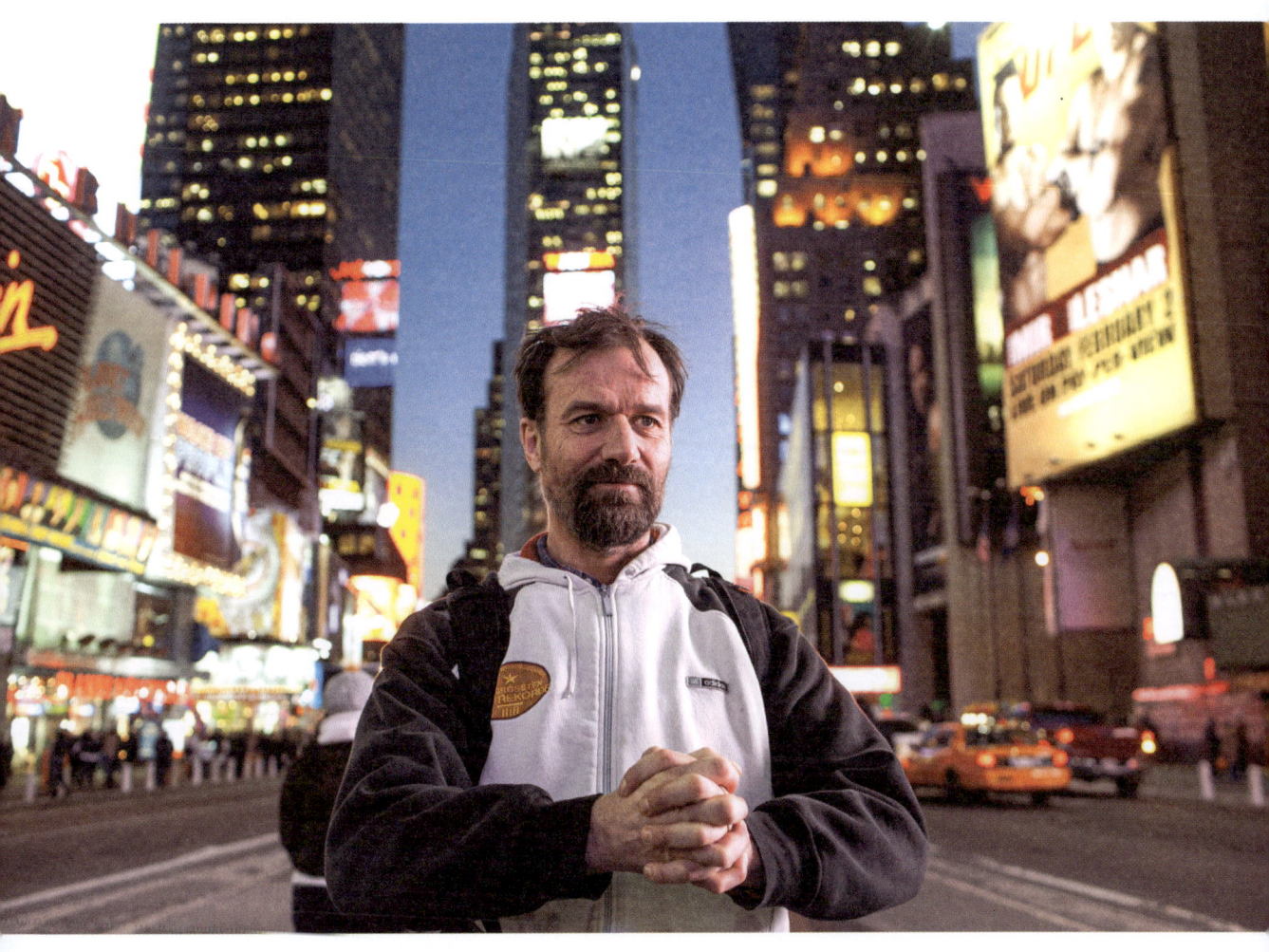

on those screens. All of a sudden,
I was right there! I was flabbergasted. Directly after, I
went for a hot chocolate, and there I was. Once again,
what a contrast it all was with my normal daily life.

BREATHE

Leave
Your thoughts behind
Just breath, being kind
Like a leaf falling
Beautifully
So light
Bright
Like being left with nothing but
In, out, in, out
A silence falling in
Beautifully
So light
Yet like a flower
Tangible fragrance
Great power
An angel whispers in my ear
I now can hear
They talk through the heart
Making me part
Of their celestial songs
Inspiration that belongs
To no body
No mind
Just being
Your thought behind
A whole new world
Where babies are being birthed
Breathe, its innocence
What only remains
Angels bliss

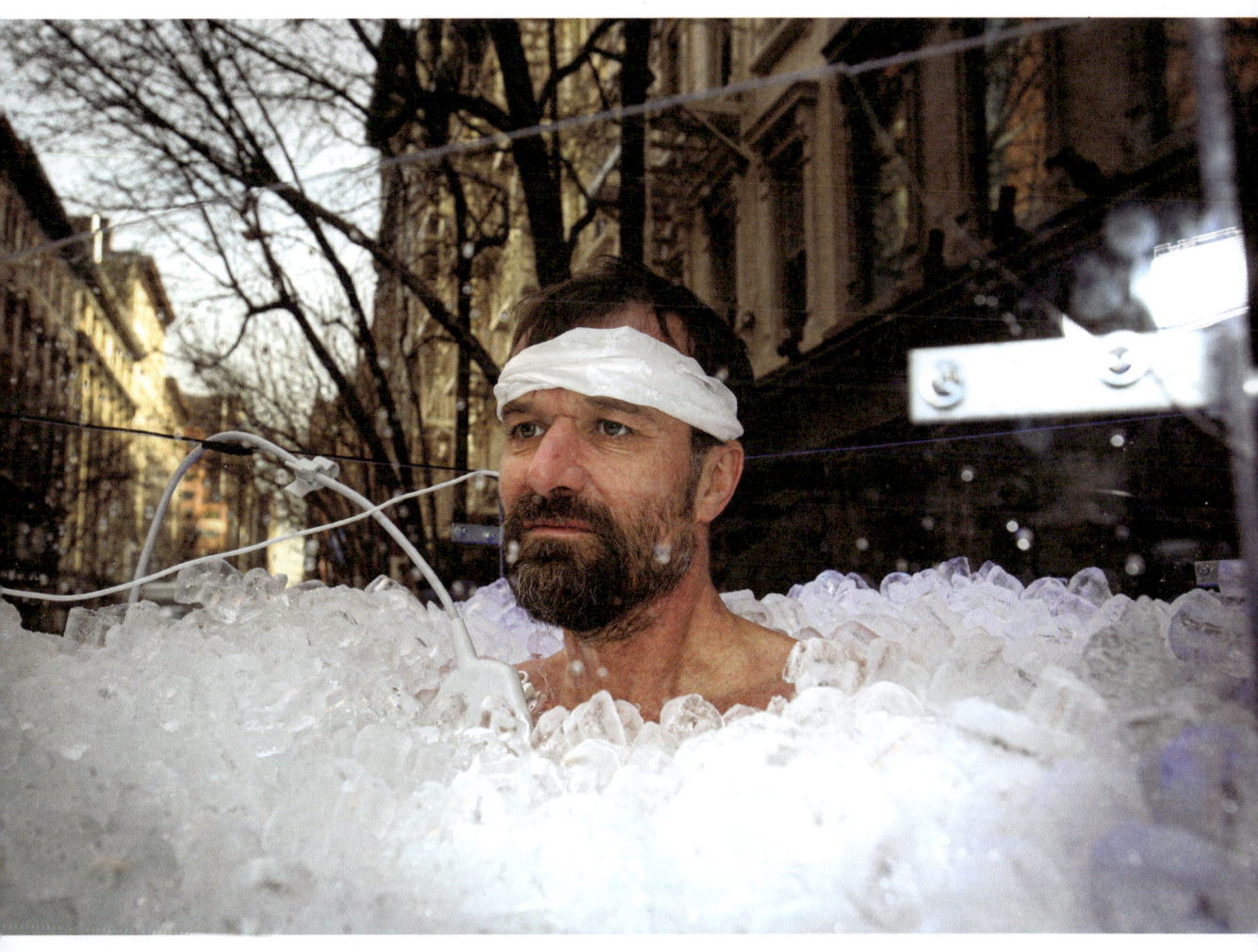

The day after *The Today Show*, in front of the Rubin Museum of Art.

I was in the ice for 72 minutes. This was different. I performed under the supervision of Dr. Ken Kamler and Nurse Granis.

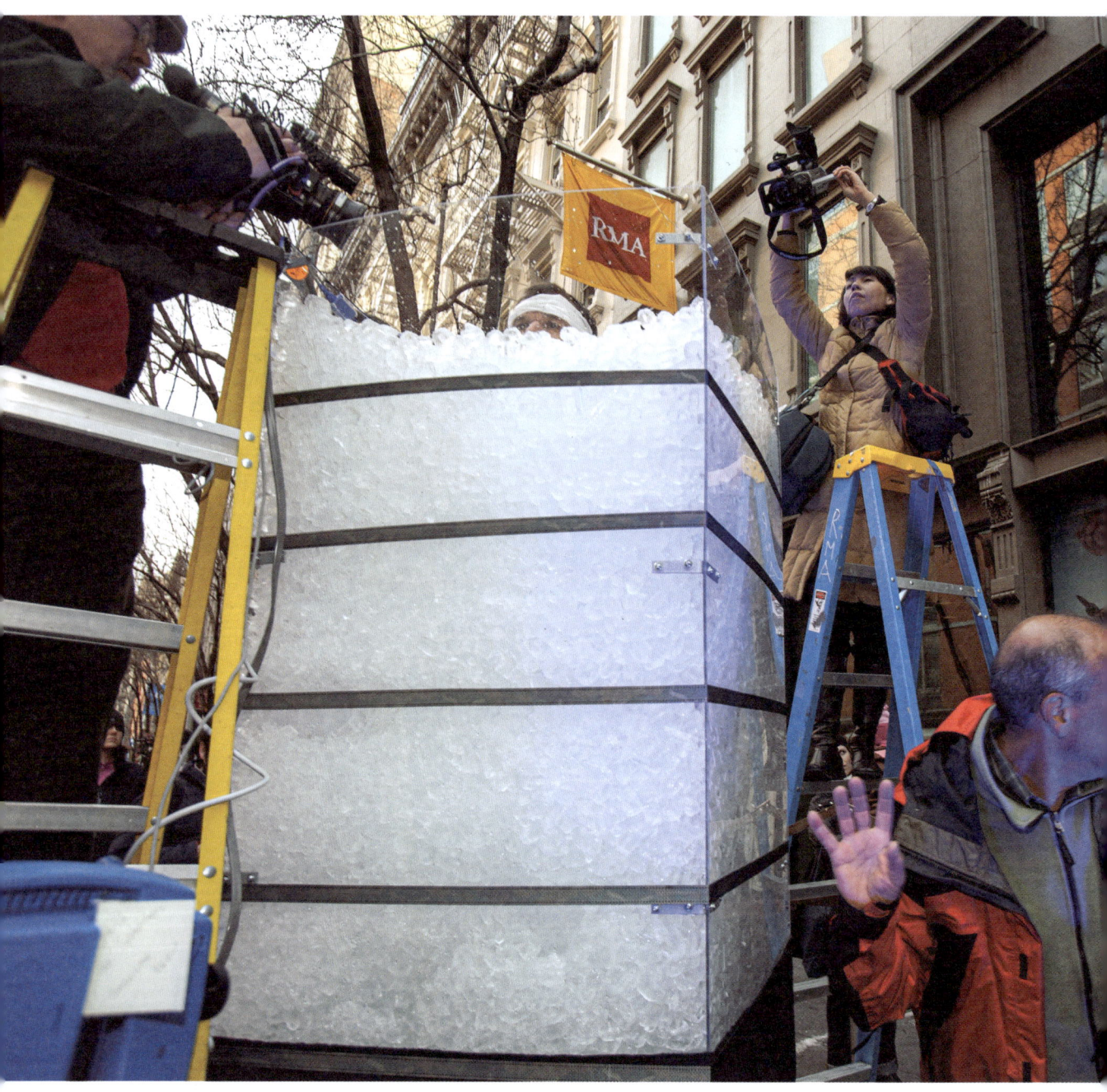

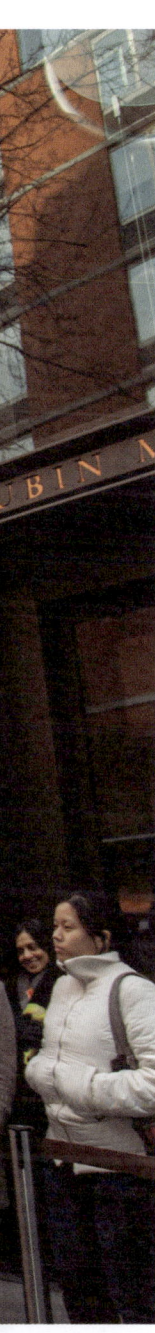

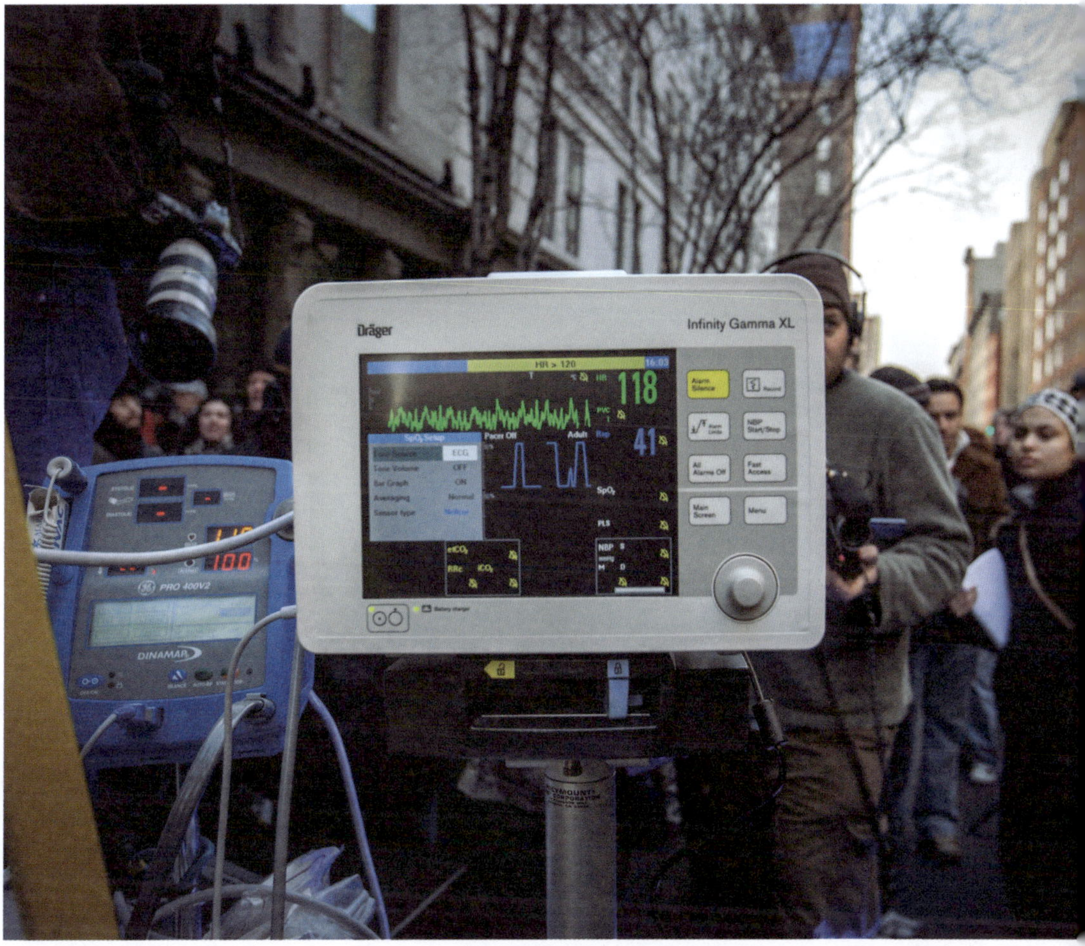

The major turning point.

Measurements were done while immersed in the ice: my heart rate, skin temperature, and a core temperature. Dr. Ken Kamler supervised. The next day I was to be tested with 307 blood markers at the Feinstein Institutes for Medical Research under the supervision of Dr. Kevin Tracey. They told me to "meditate the way I do" in the ice, but now in a seat for an hour. A week later results showed I was clearly influencing the vagus nerve, which was considered to be autonomous. Dr. Ken Kamler told me, "If you are able to reproduce these results, then that would mean huge consequences for humanity." At that moment, I became a missionary. It became conscious. I saw it in a flash.

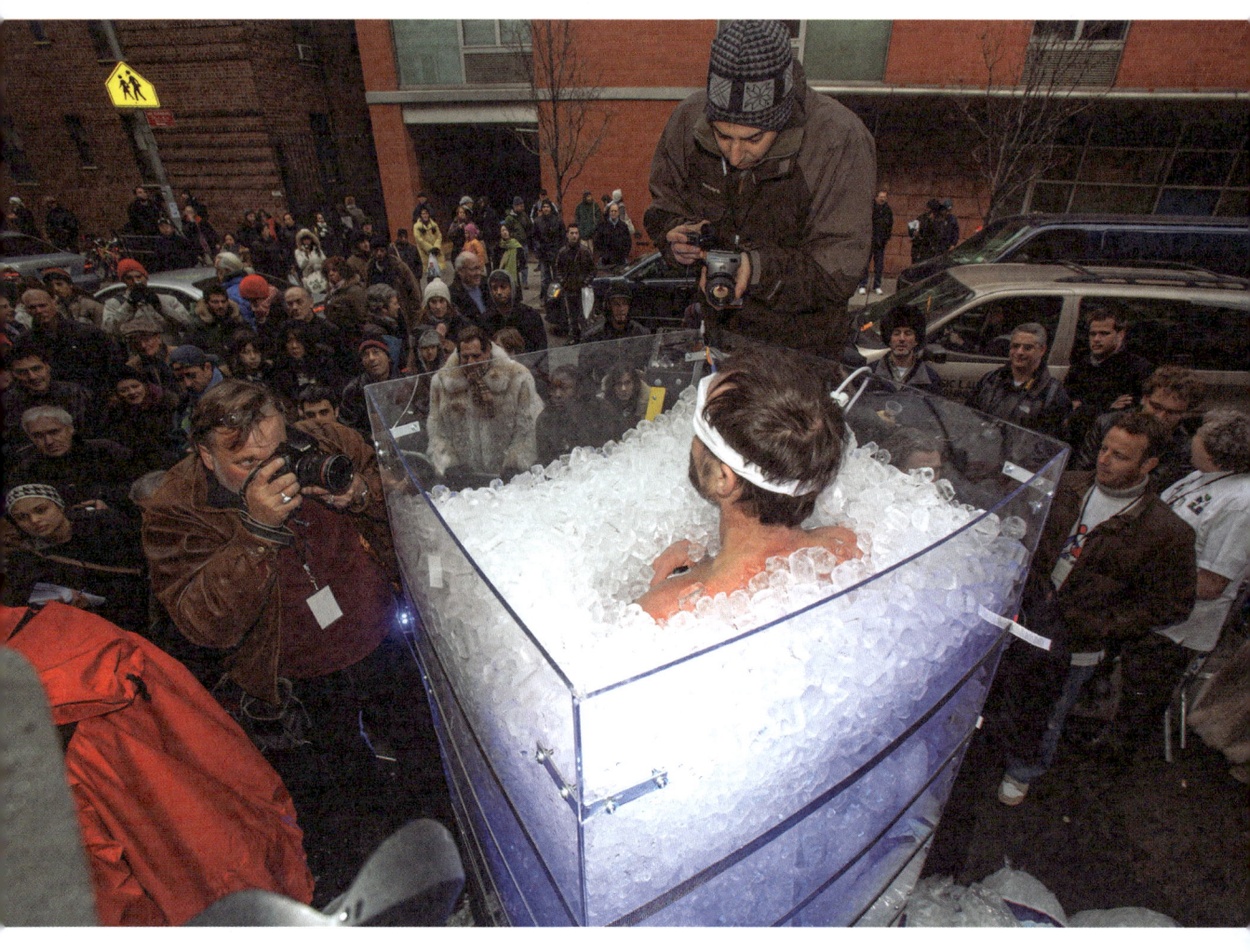

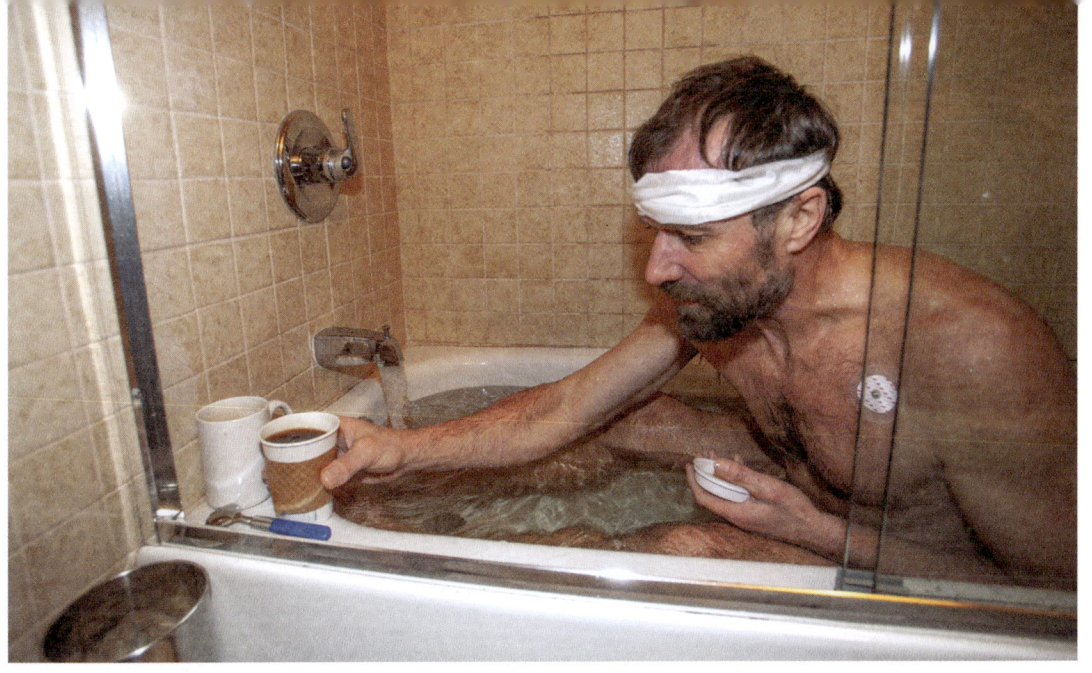

Always a coffee. This was directly after my icy record, and into a bathtub I went. What a sensation! Heat after intense cold. Did it!

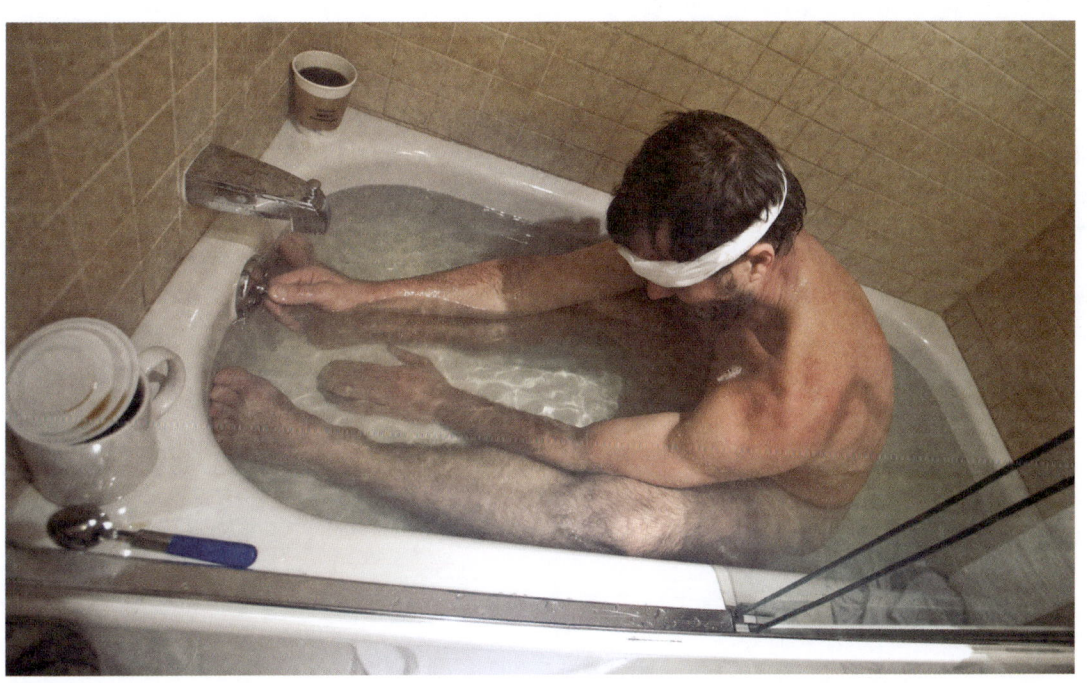

It takes a while to de-tense the body after deep contraction of the cardiovascular system exposed to cold.

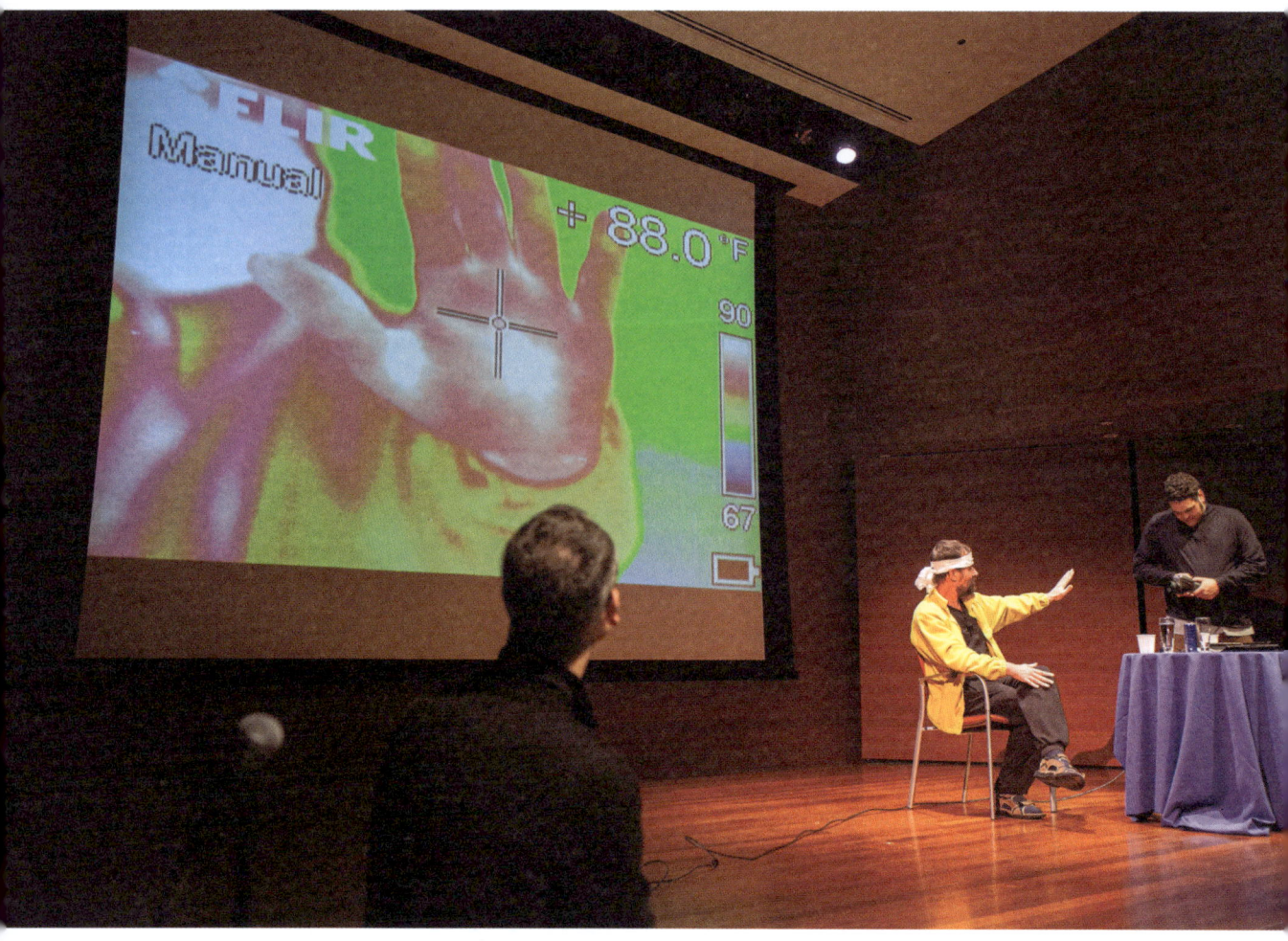

An infrared camera showed I was able to raise the temperature in my hand within 12 degrees in one minute just by using my mind. Another finding that surprised me because it was an unexpected experiment with Dr. Kevin Tracey. New areas of the brain are showing they can be controlled only if we go "out of the box." The scientific world was abuzz trying to map this new territory.

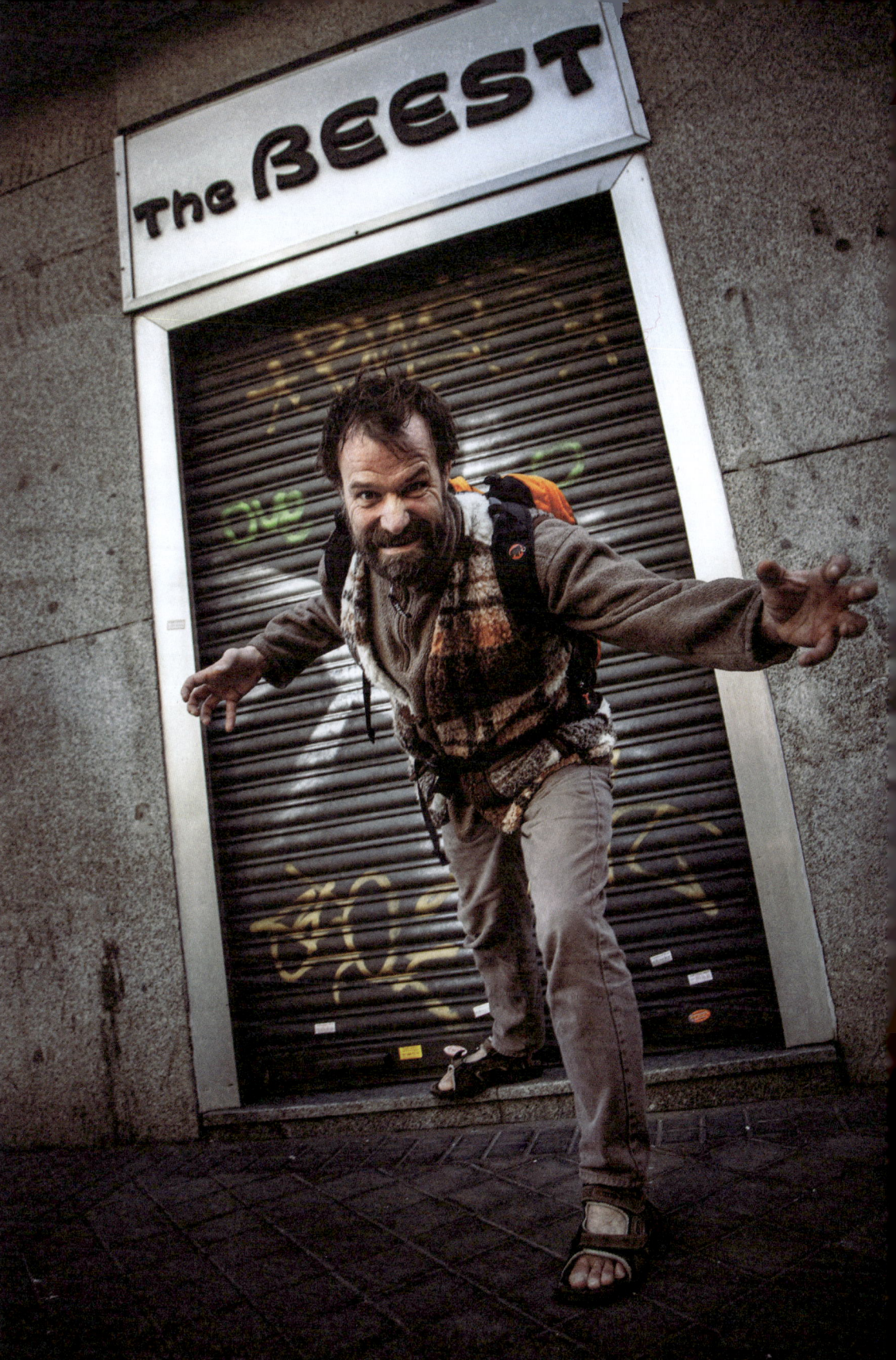

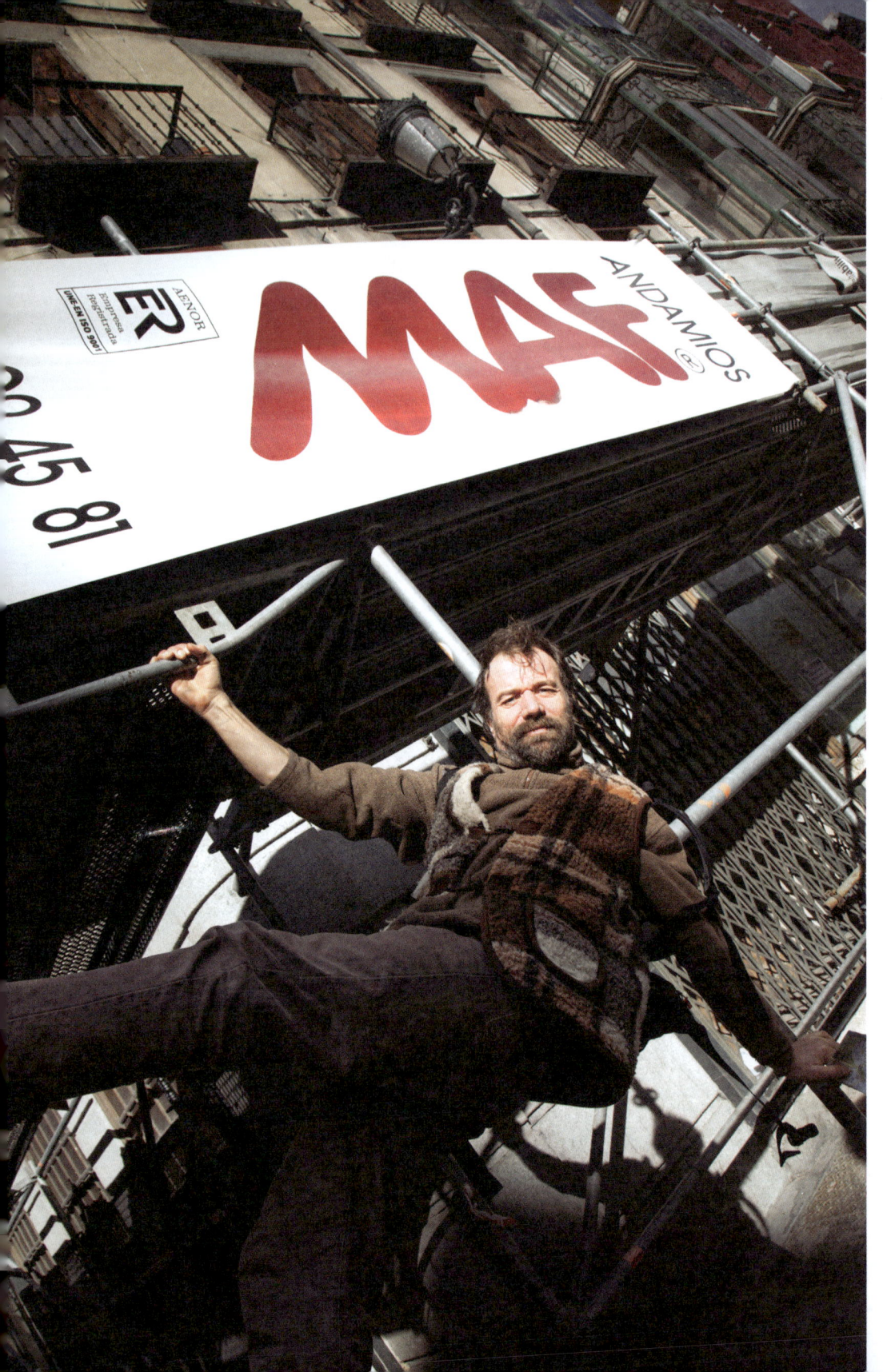

Having fun with ridiculous poses in New York in 2008.

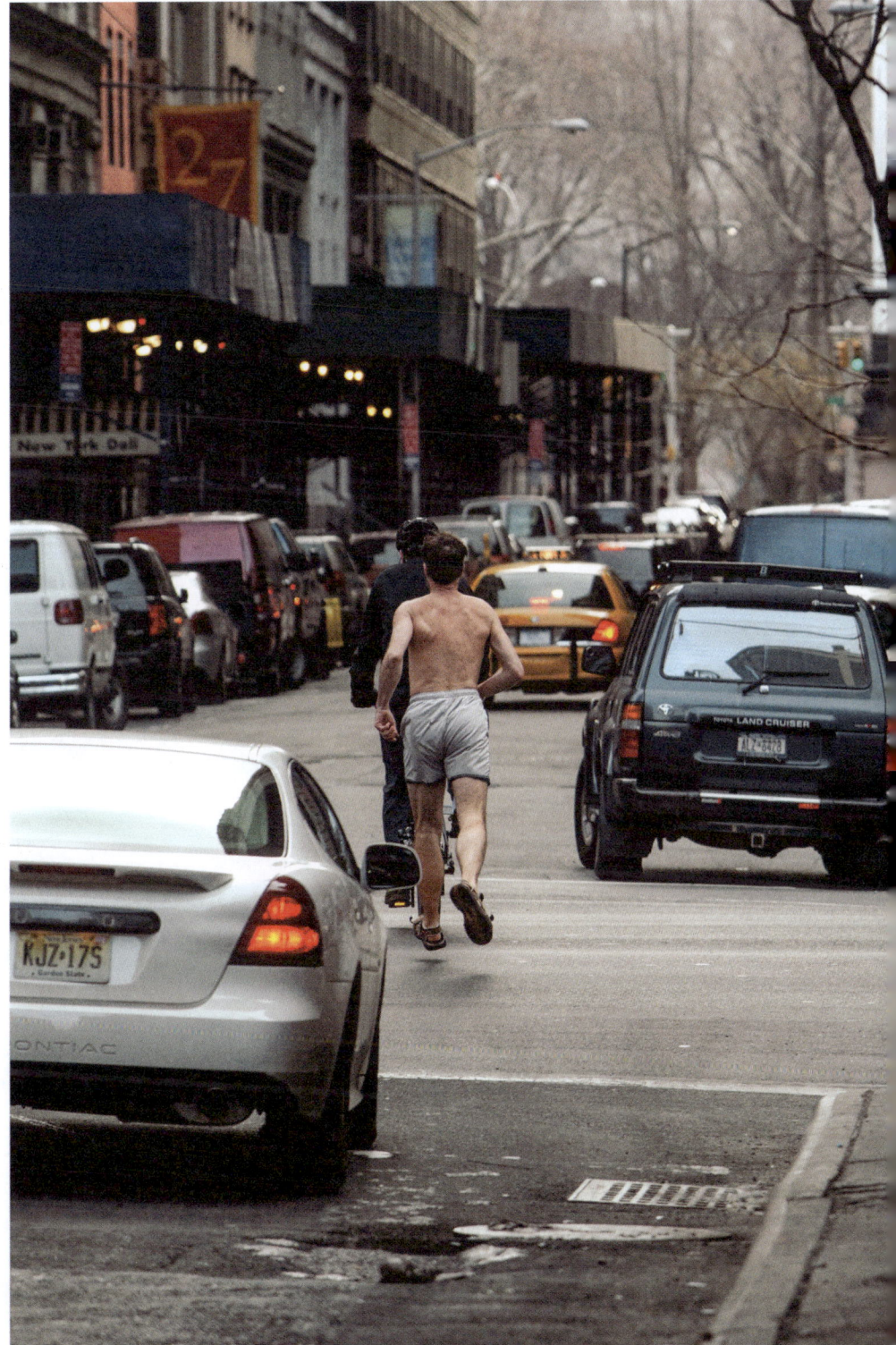

Running through chilly New York. Just do something! Sometimes something crazy isn't crazy at all when looking for new dimensions of the mind. My documentary filmmaker back then got this idea. I am always in to do something "different."

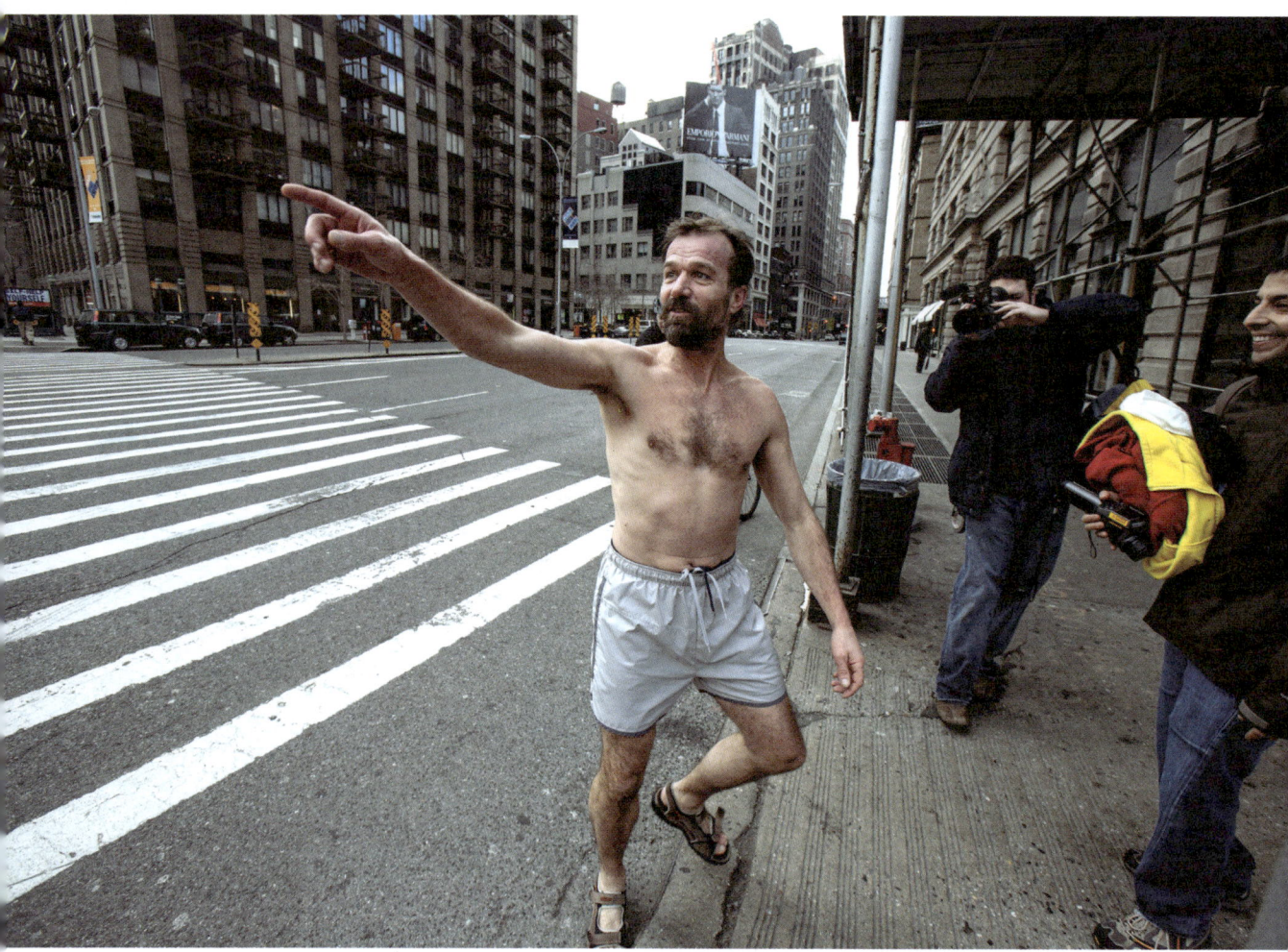

I can share my passion with anybody I meet. I'm always ready to
engage in conversation, opening up in a moment with people. I
have always been this way, famous or not, ridiculed or not, always
meeting the moment with openness and enthusiasm.

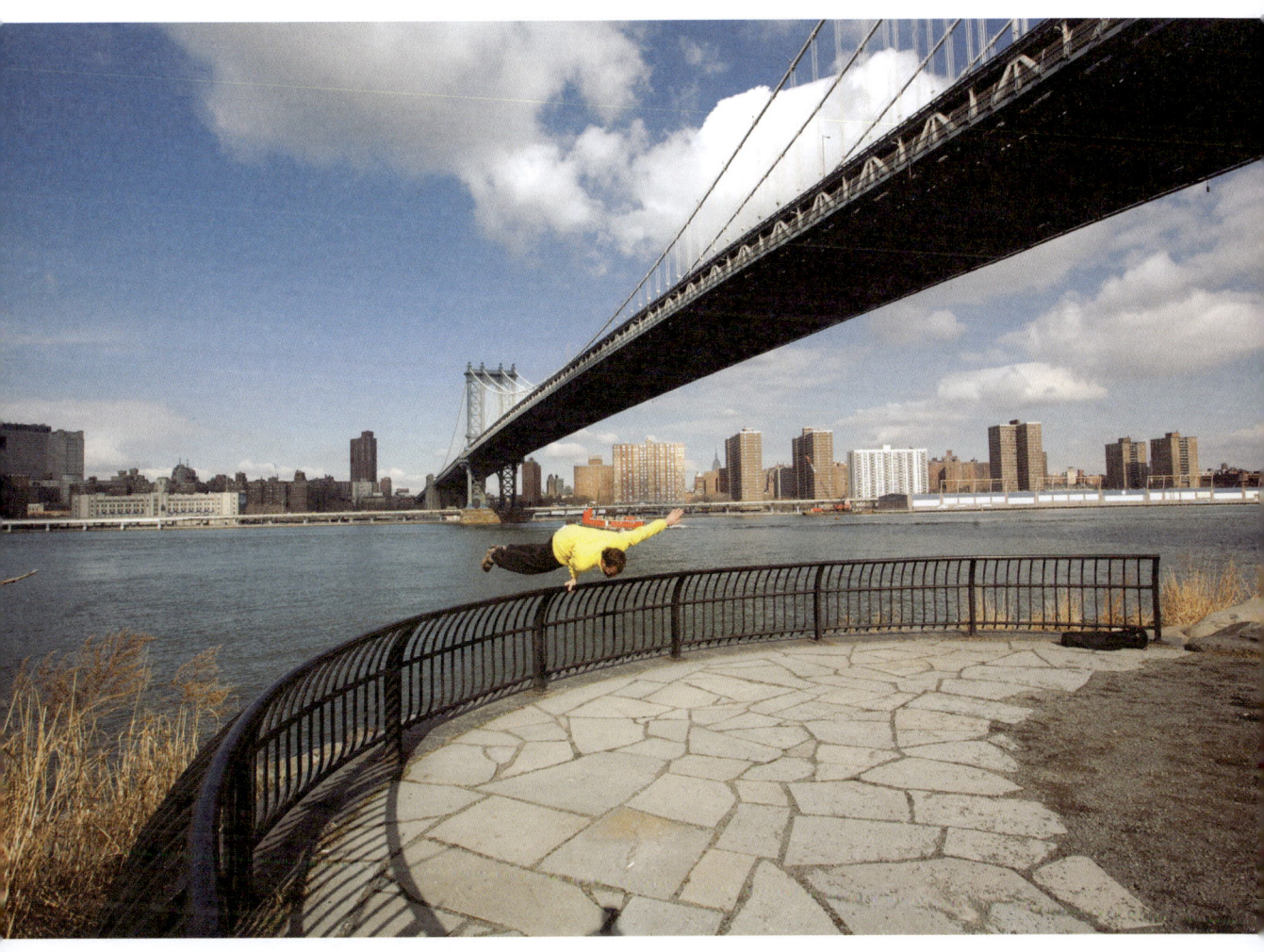

My favorite exercise. Of course, I had to display it
with the Brooklyn Bridge and Hudson River in view.

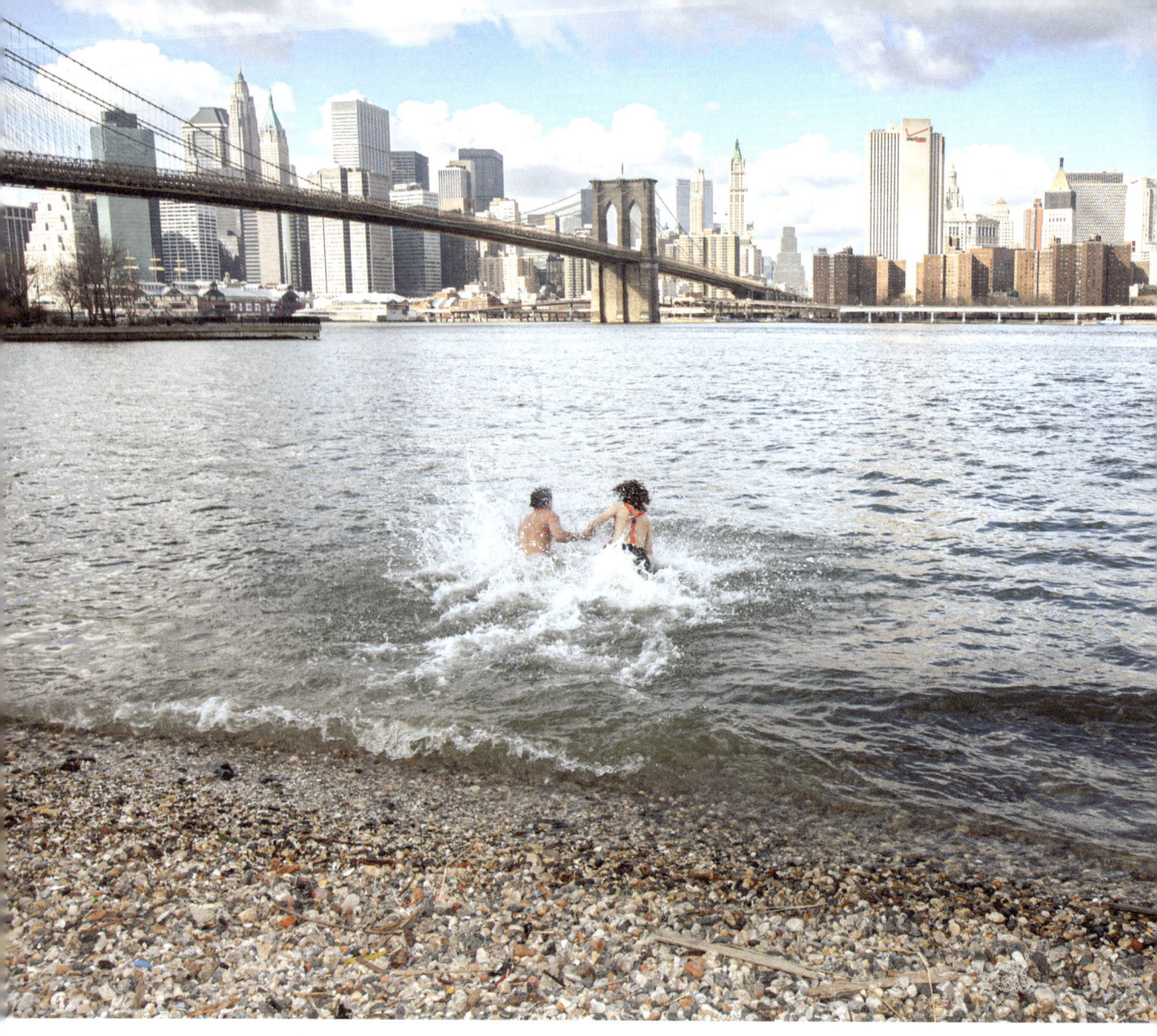

Heading into the Hudson River with a Dutch reporter. Again
and again working on more exposure. Man on a mission.

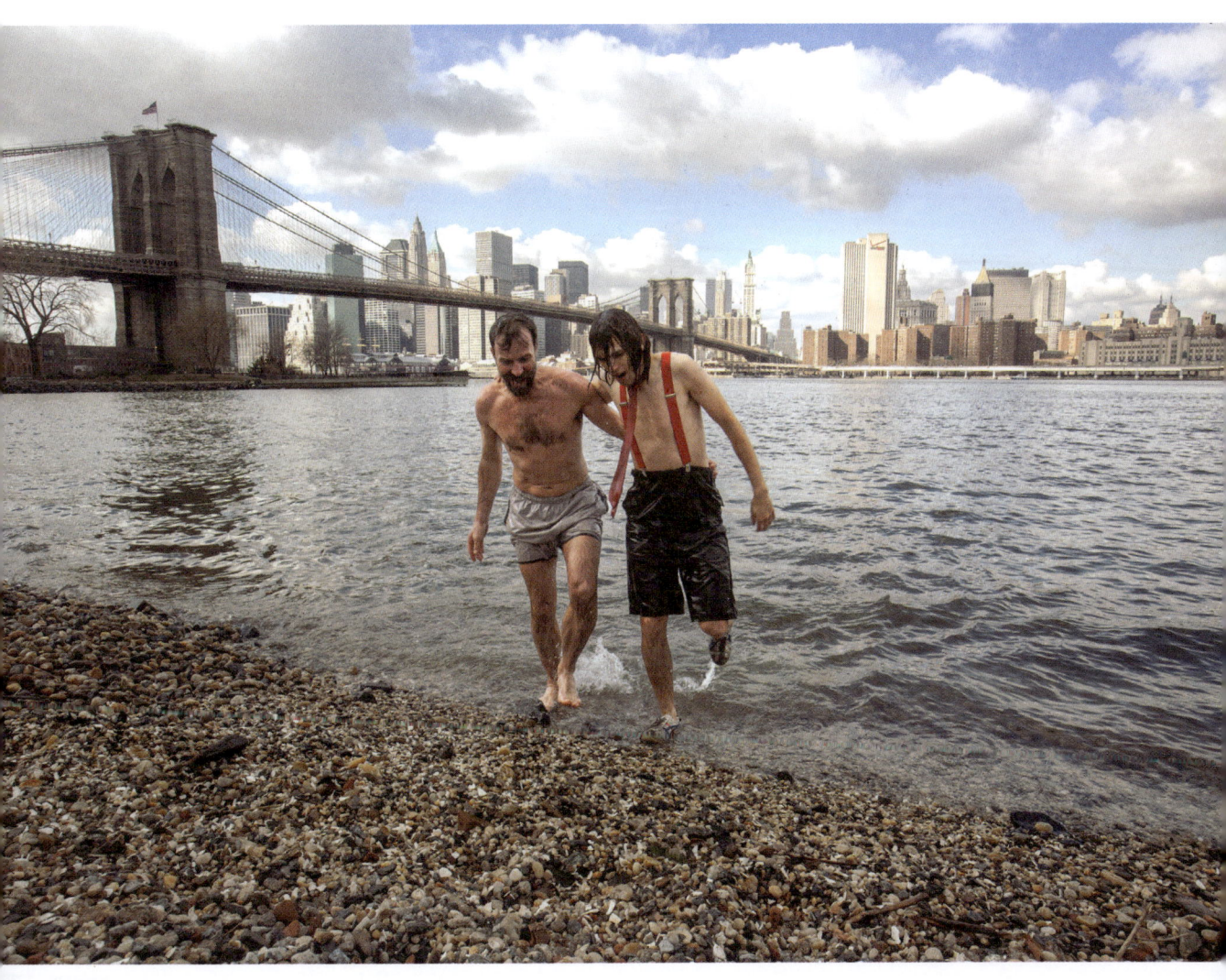

You have to go until you break the walls (existent paradigm),
or you break your balls (yielding to the existent paradigm).

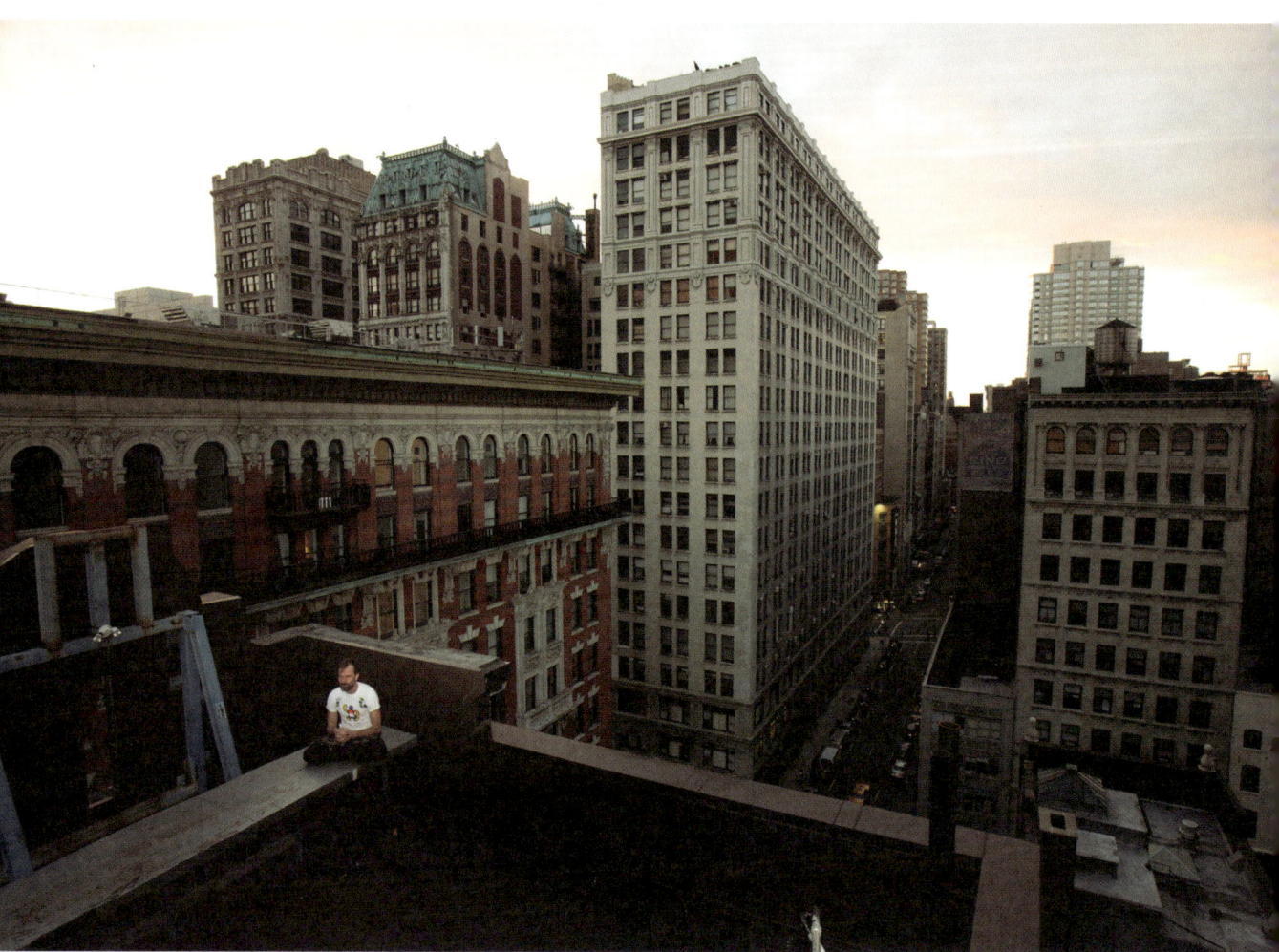

I live in Amsterdam, and suddenly I realize I am in New Amsterdam, New York.

Immense buildings. Their architecture now copied everywhere.

New York is starting to be Old York!

DOORWAY TO OUR SOUL

Yet when found the doorway we know our
Destination
Gotta pick up the bill for old paradigm
Procrastination
Something that was ours, taken by hierarchic
Powers
A debris nonetheless, but bless
Out of there
In here
Through the bridge called in Latin pons
We are able to take what is ours, our mind, and
Make the plunge
Where we go in the list of this all
Just head on to meet the clarity of your Soul
It's coming while we are going, happy days my
Friend
It all will be shown
As the dawn of a new day
Take the wings of your minds
Left, right, straight, fly away
Become lighter as you loose the debris
Of staying too long in someone else's perverted
Fantasy
Home is where the heart is
Connected through the Soul, through the mind
That is
Bliss
See you there.

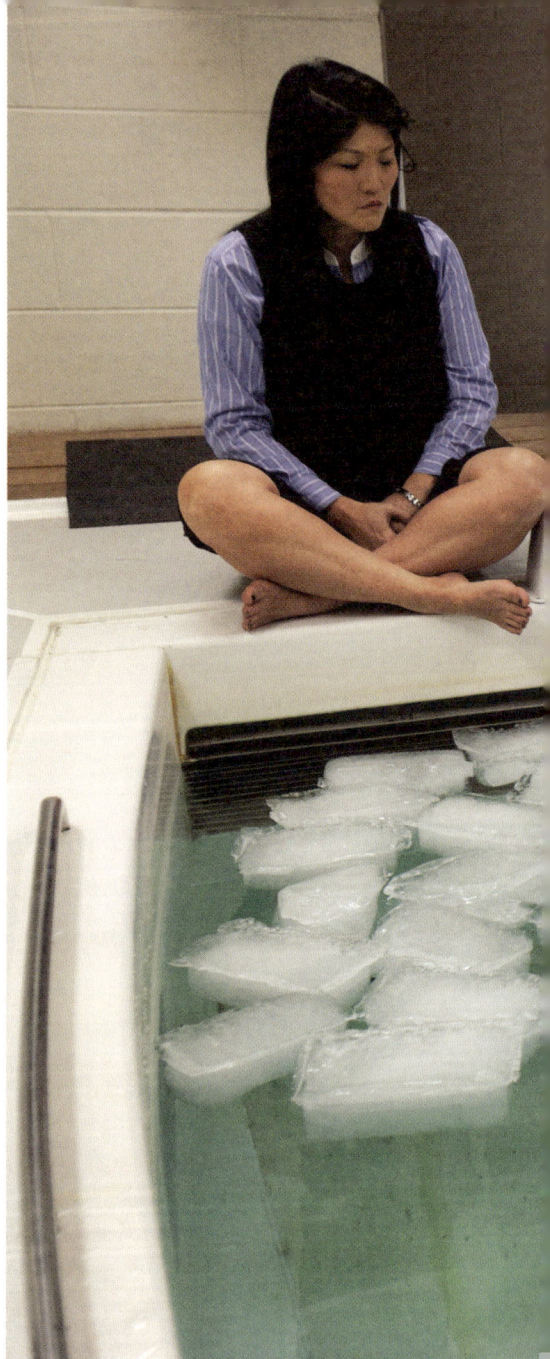

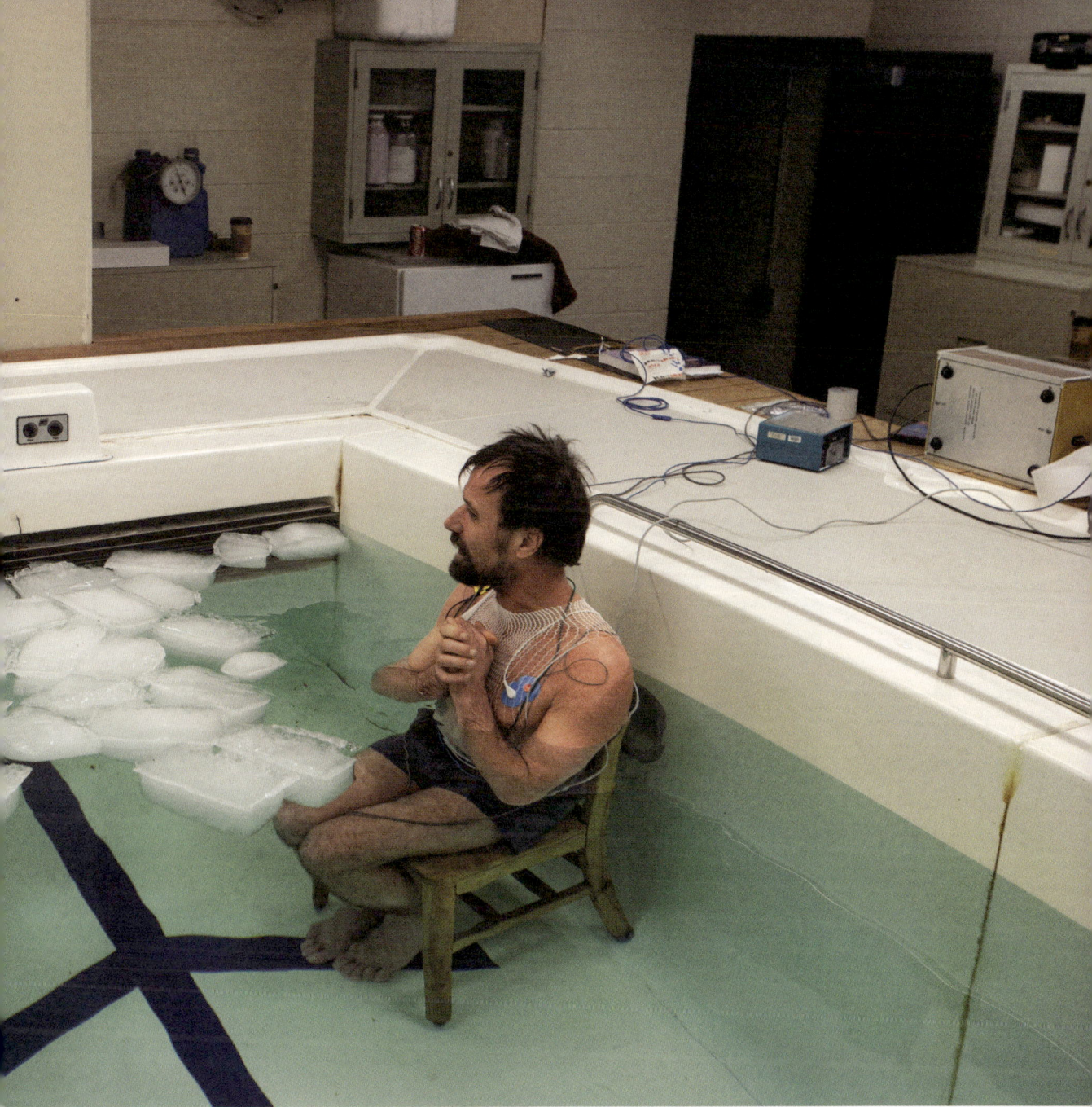

Duluth/Minnesota school of medicine.

After New York I headed to the University of Minnesota Medical School in Duluth, Minnesota. I was making a documentary. They were testing my core body temperature. I was overseen by two top thermal physiologists. I had an abnormal reaction: my body temperature remained stable. Indeed, we can do more than we think.

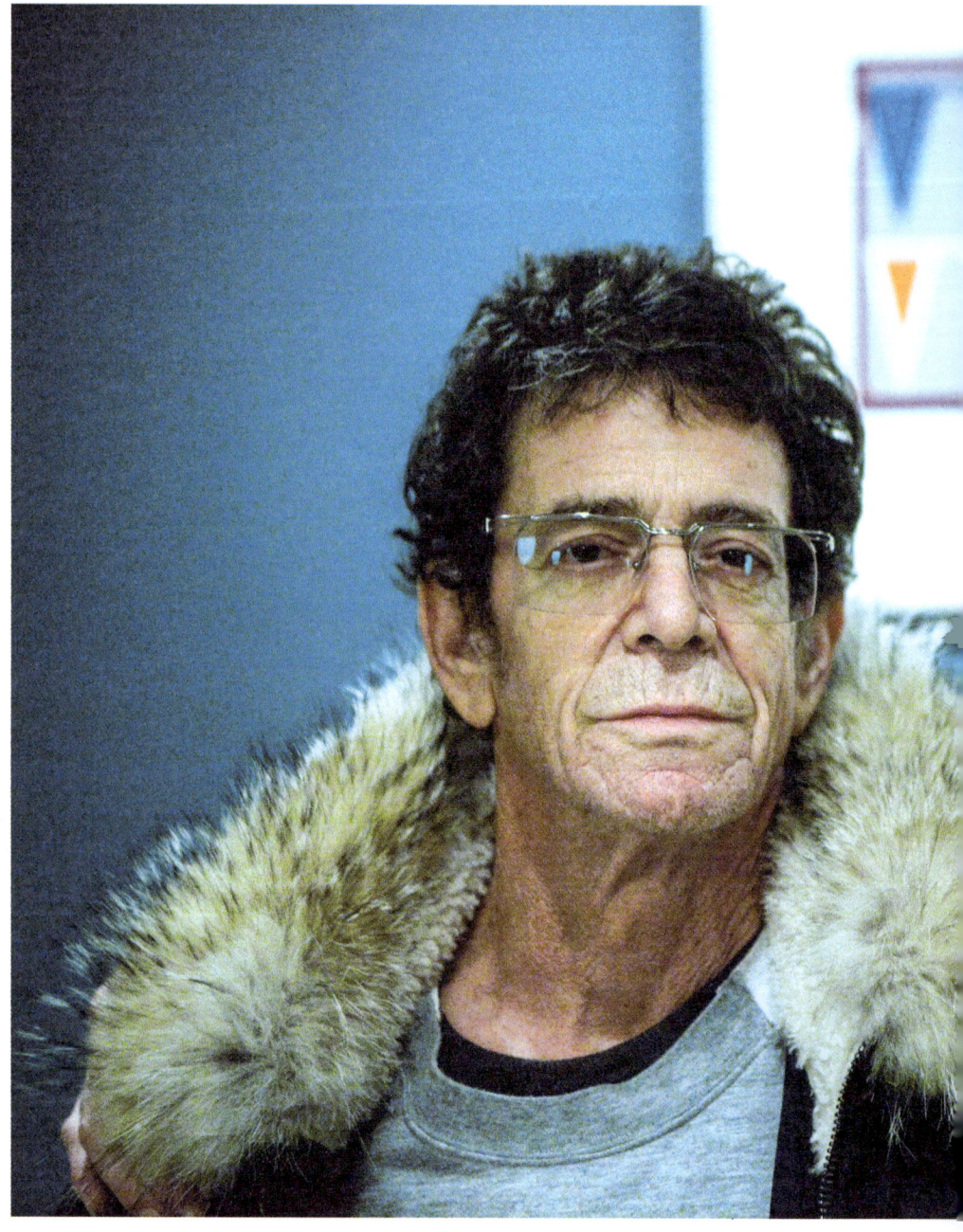

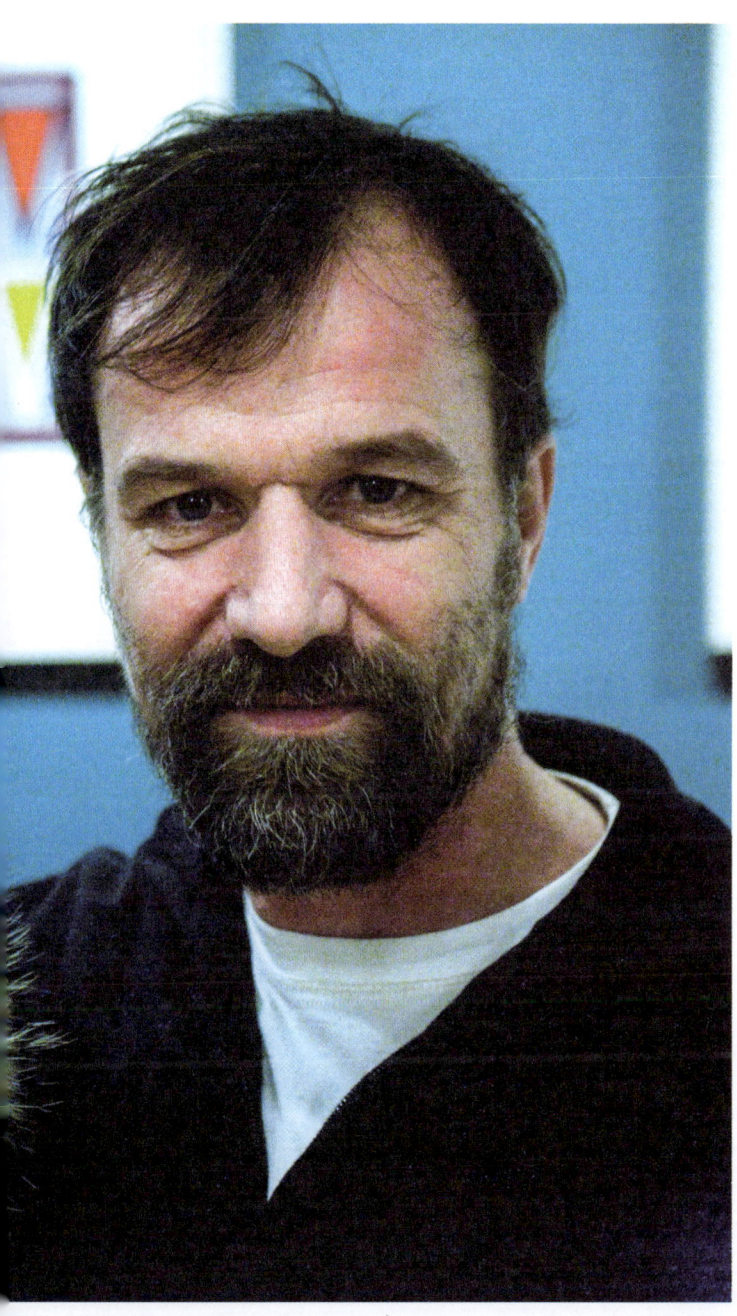

Lou Reed's wife contacted me through
the Rubin Museum of Art. I had a
three-hour conversation with him. What
a great musician and creator. I wasn't
aware of his cancer then, but the cold
and breathing can do amazing work on
cancer. It resets the body deeply. It can
boost the white cells that fight cancer.
It is great as an add-on therapy. But a
lot of research still needs to be done.

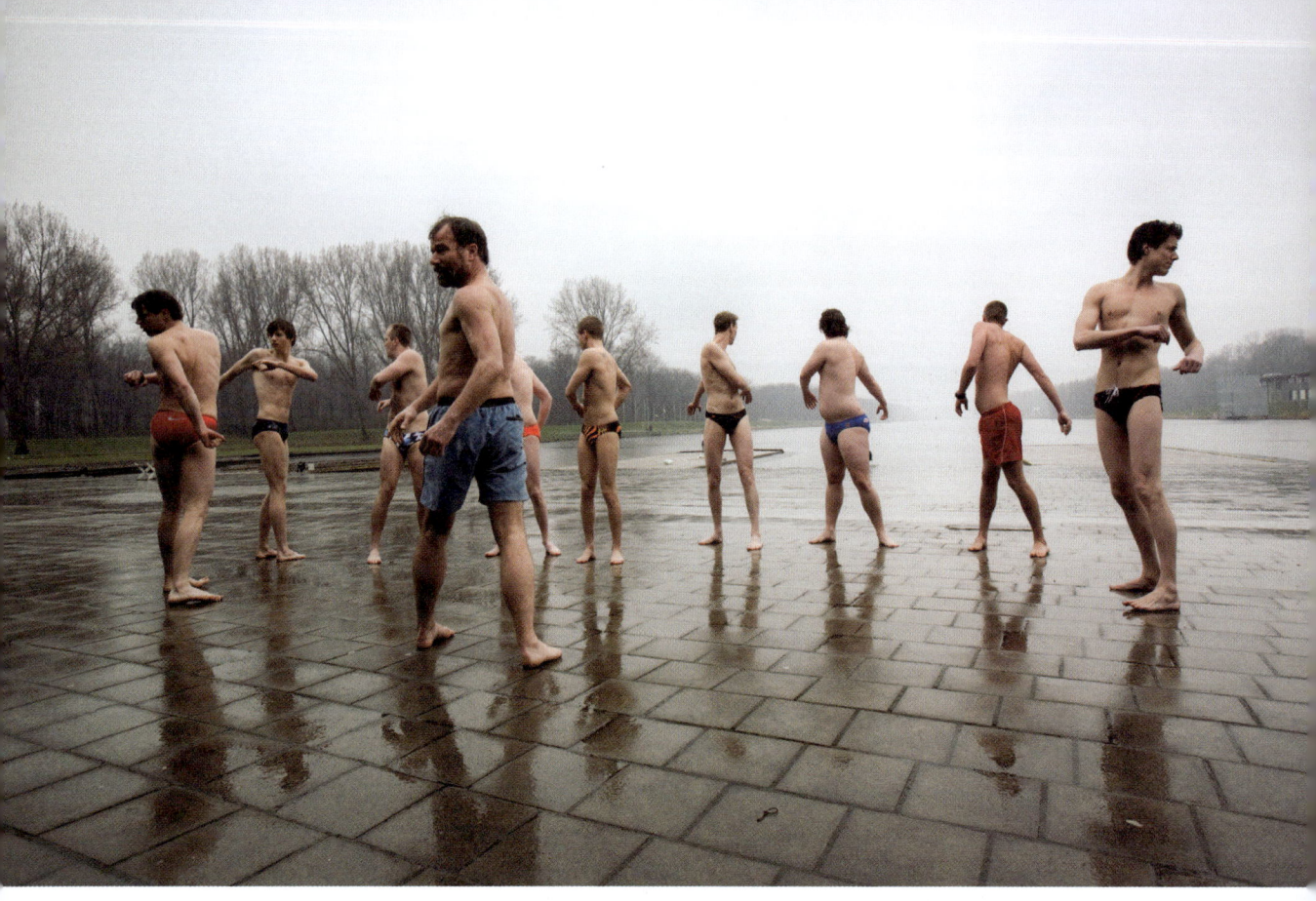

My manager back then was Walter Tiemessen, a great guy. He was a former national water polo player with an enormous hard shot, nicknamed "the Bomber." He had a water polo team and asked me to train them.

Mens sana in corpore sano;

A healthy mind in a healthy body.

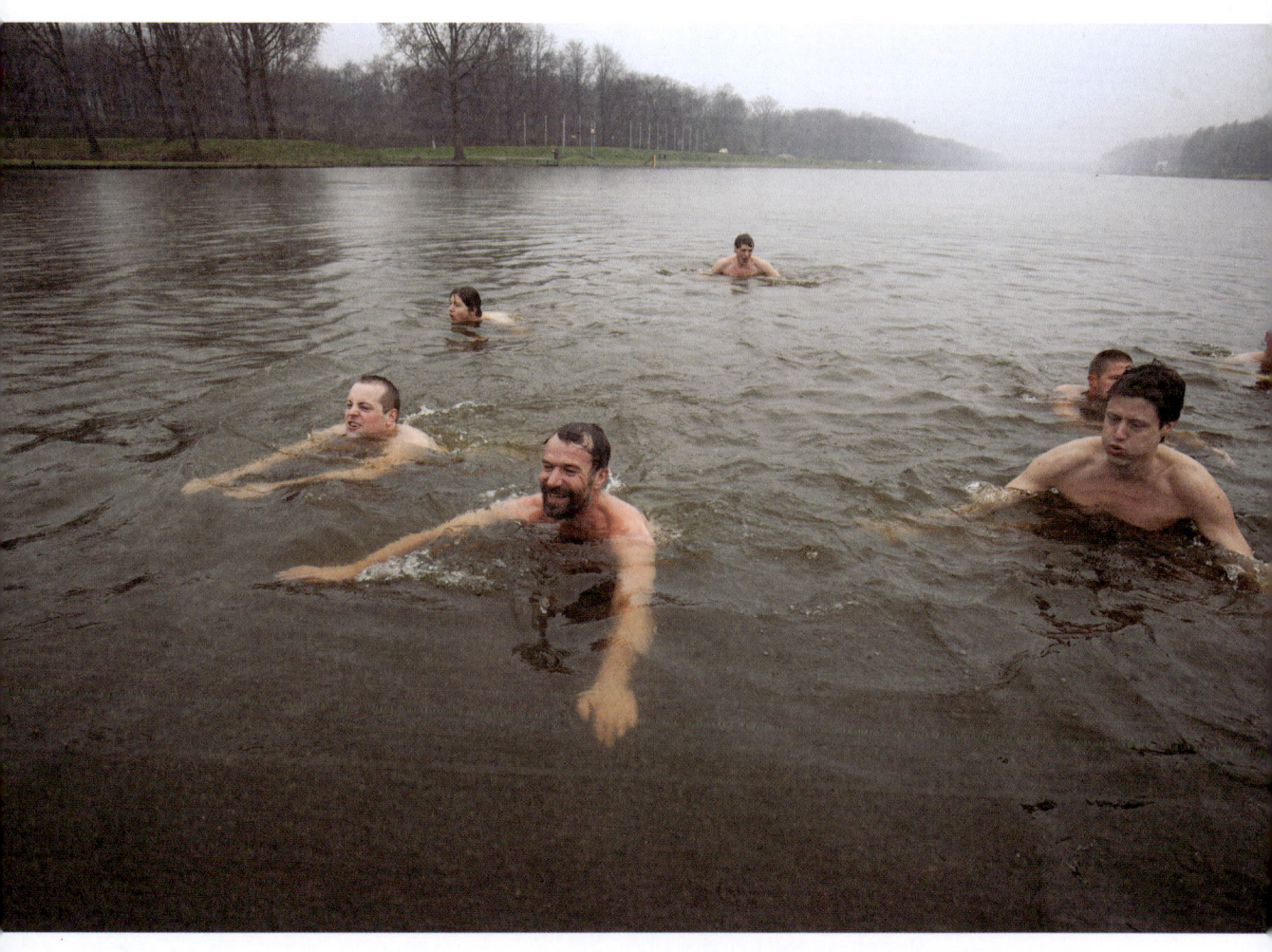

Cold-water training brings you right back to who you are and
what you are. Thermogenesis is the best cardiovascular fitness
workout. Do it for yourself; you will never ever regret it.

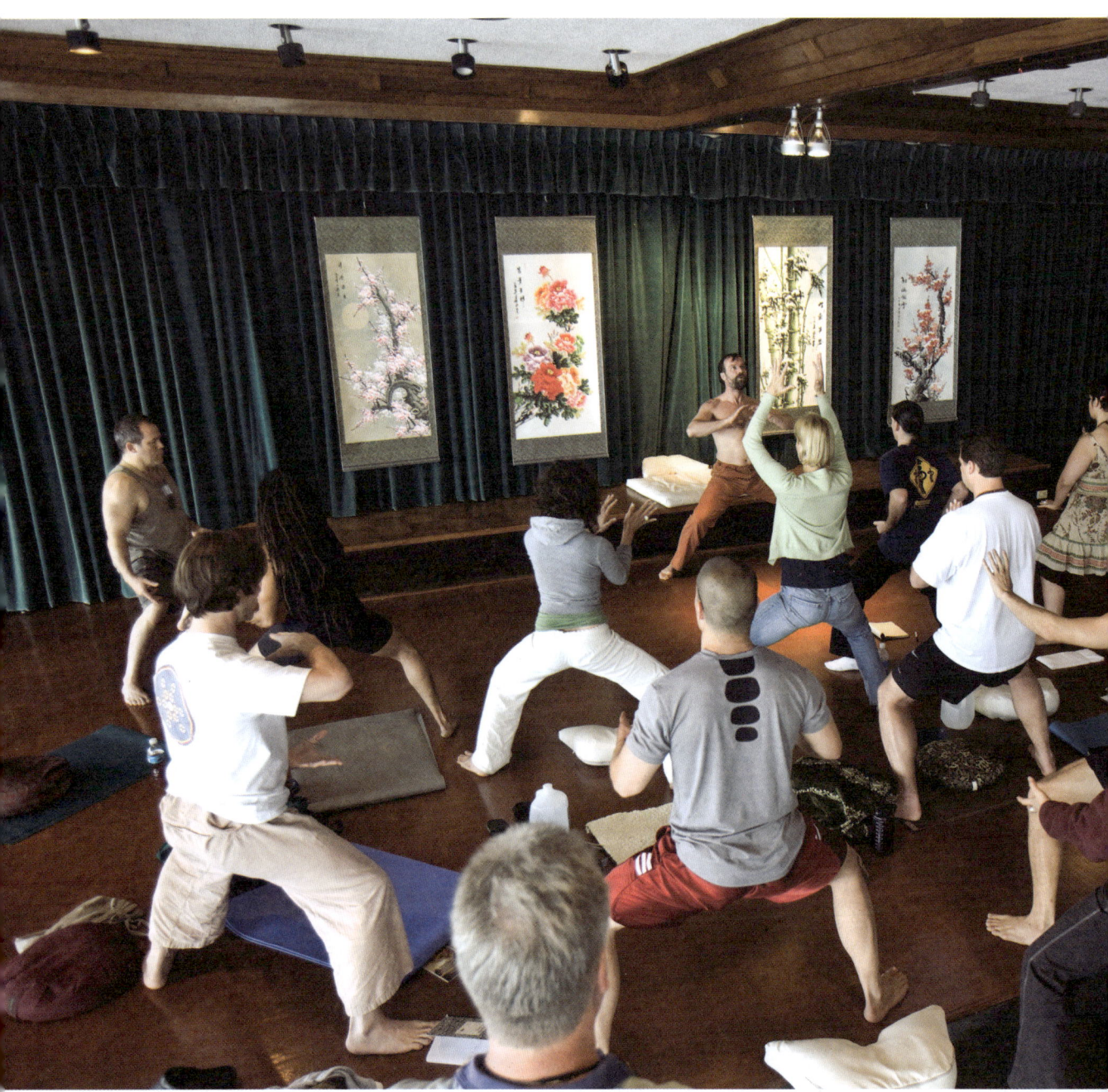

In Miami, teaching the horse stance. I had become known to the world more and more as the Iceman, and I had a certain methodology. People were interested, curious, intrigued by it all. Back then the Wim Hof Method was not known, but my methodology already existed.

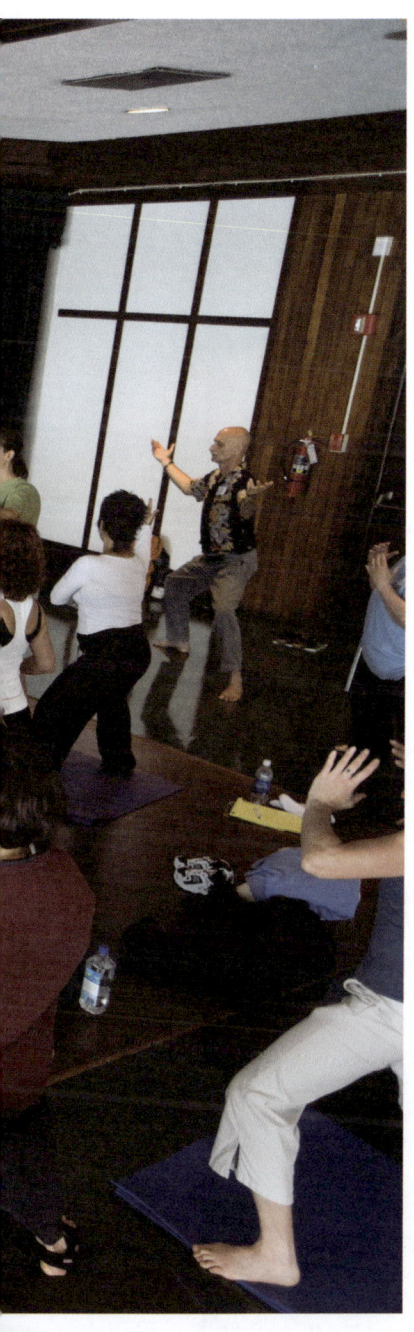

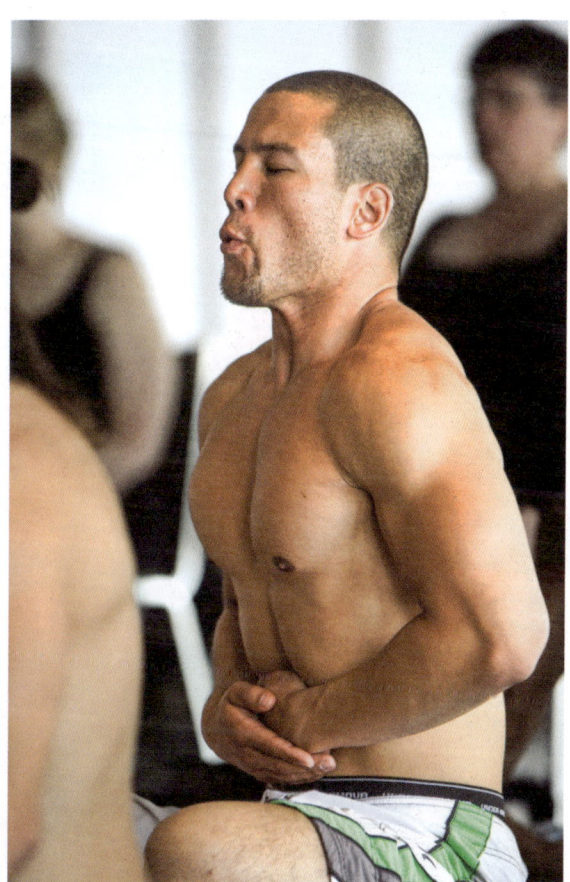

Consciously using your diaphragm
while breathing deeply stimulates the
body. Simultaneously, you massage
the intestines. Our gut! Our God!

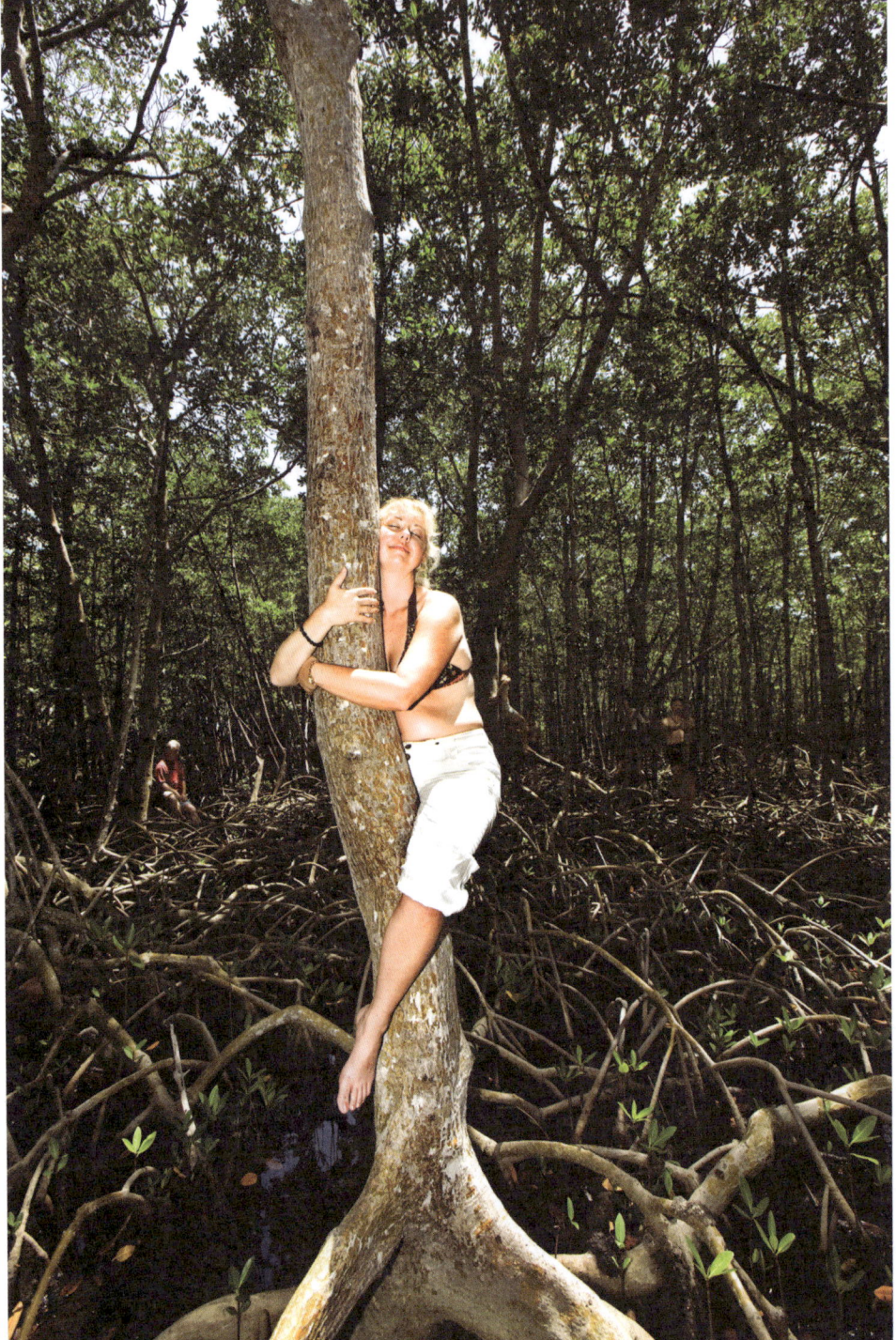

The mangroves near Miami.

Tree hugging. The trees exhale oxygen and inhale CO2. We exhale
CO2 and inhale oxygen. We are one and should embrace it.

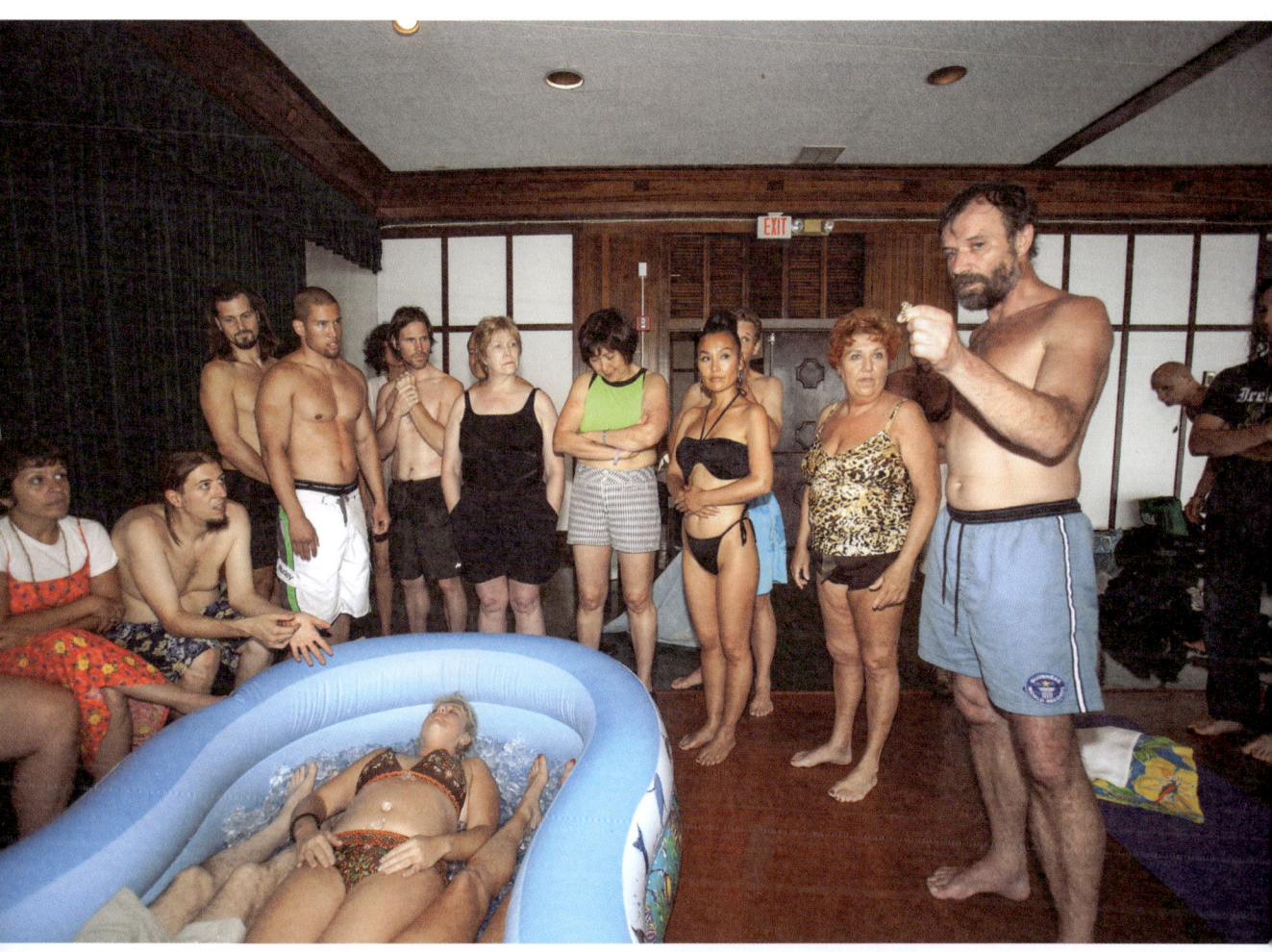

Icy water unites people, as it is a common force that brings the collective spirit to the surface. In our society, we have all these extension tools to make our lives comfortable, but they take away the need to help each other with nature's hostile elements.

Good memories of the retreat in Miami County. Lots of love and willingness to learn about natural ways.

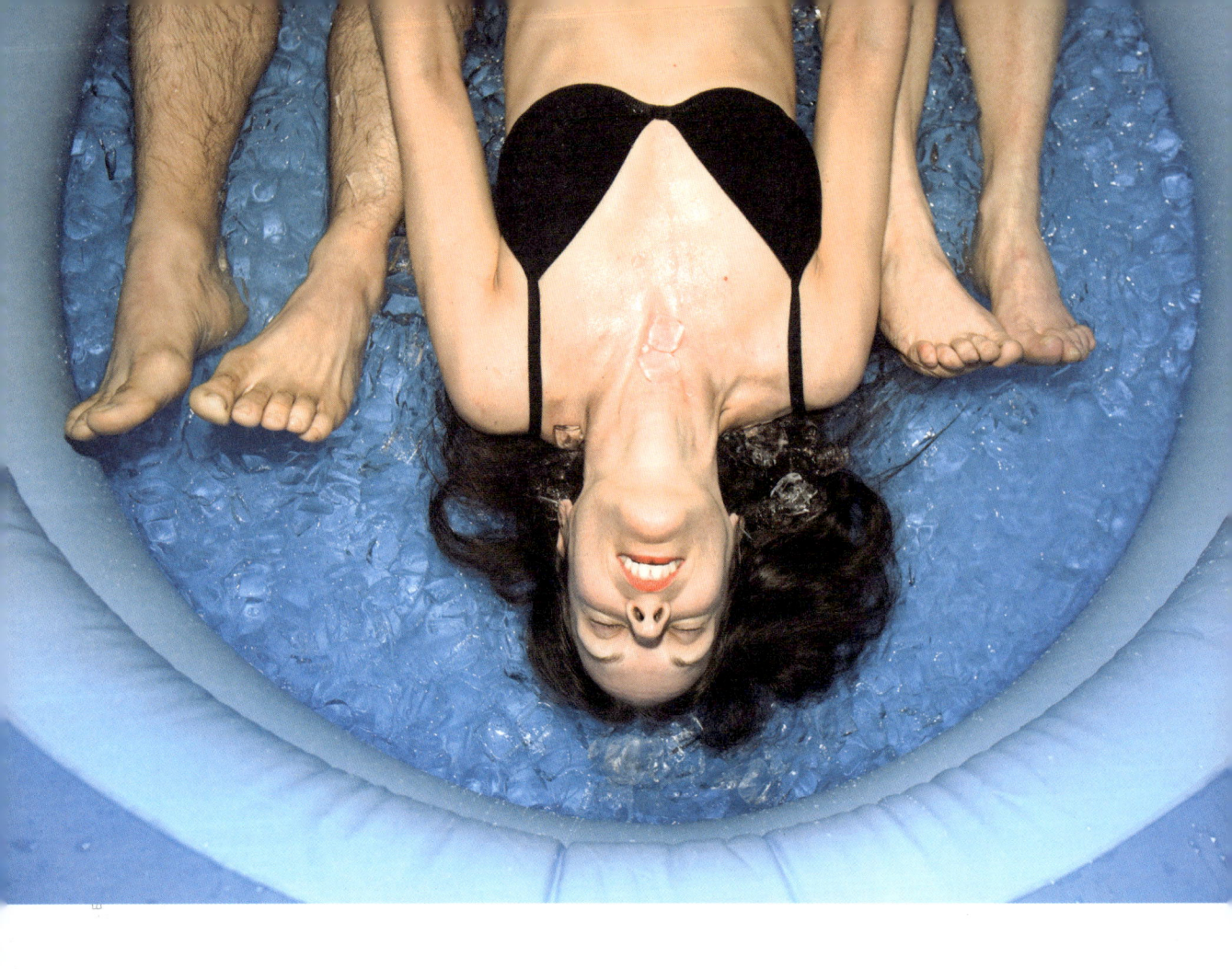

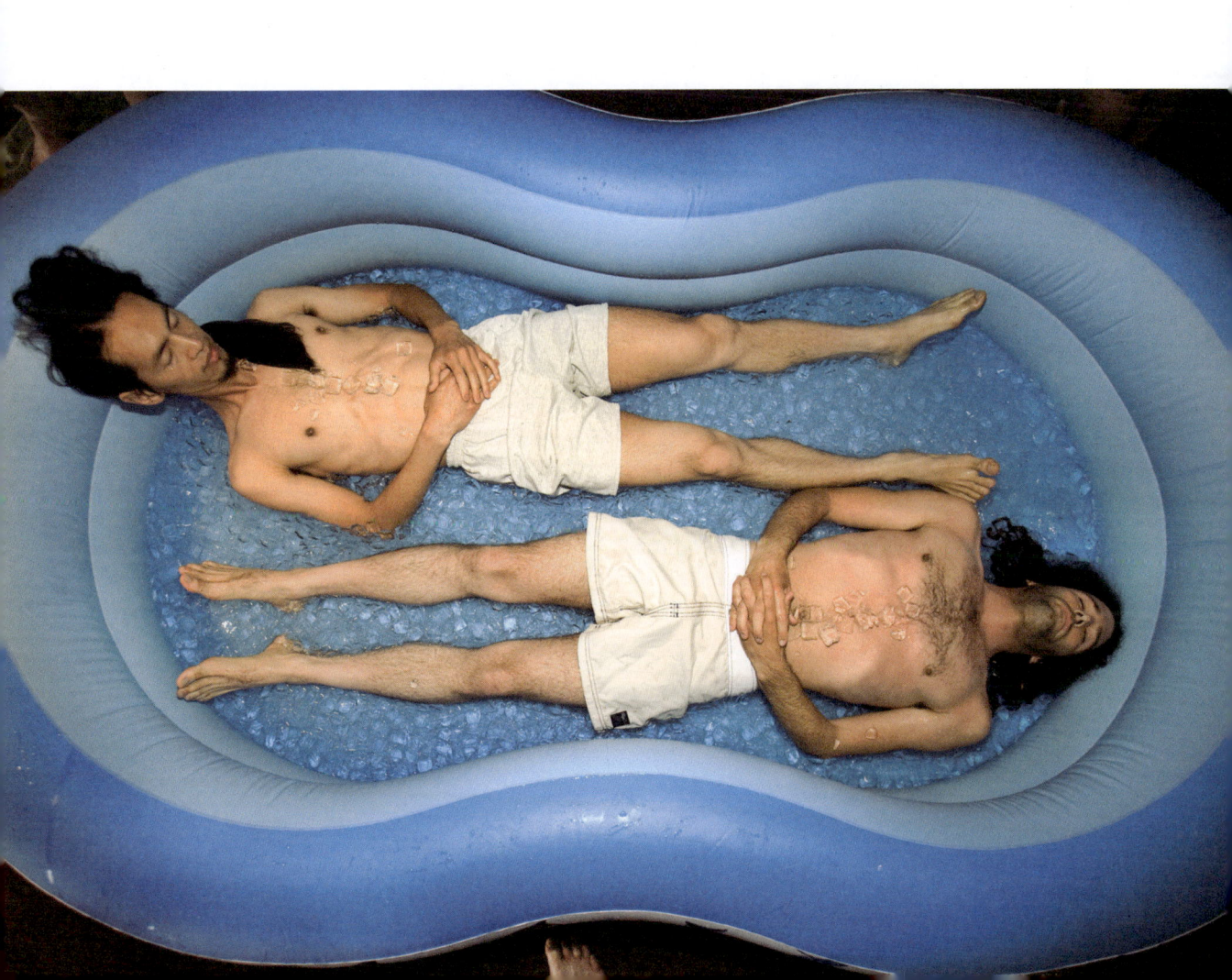

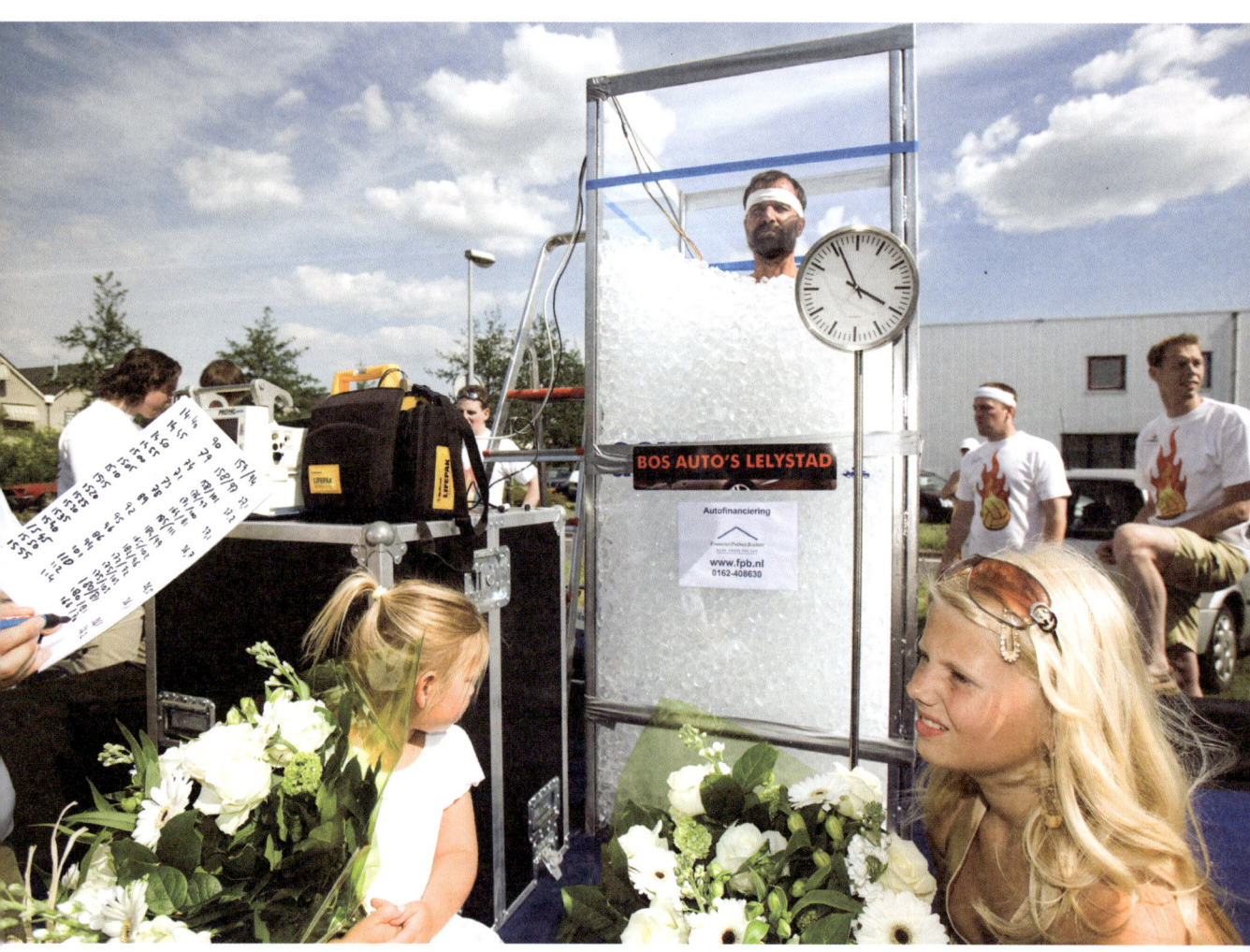

The life of an Iceman. The record is about to be broken in
the Netherlands. Another successful one serving as another
stepping stone in my mission of happy, strong, and healthy.

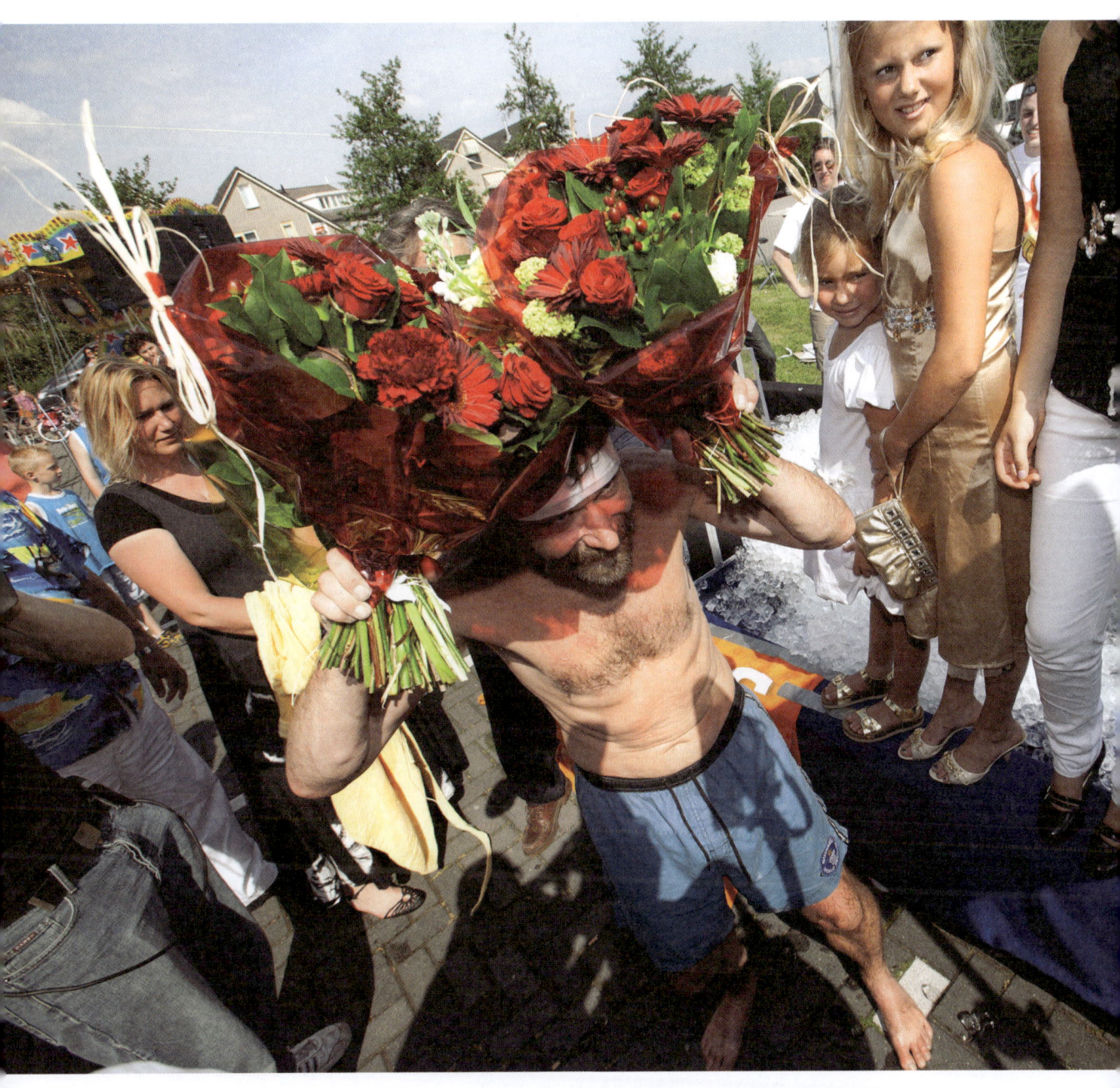

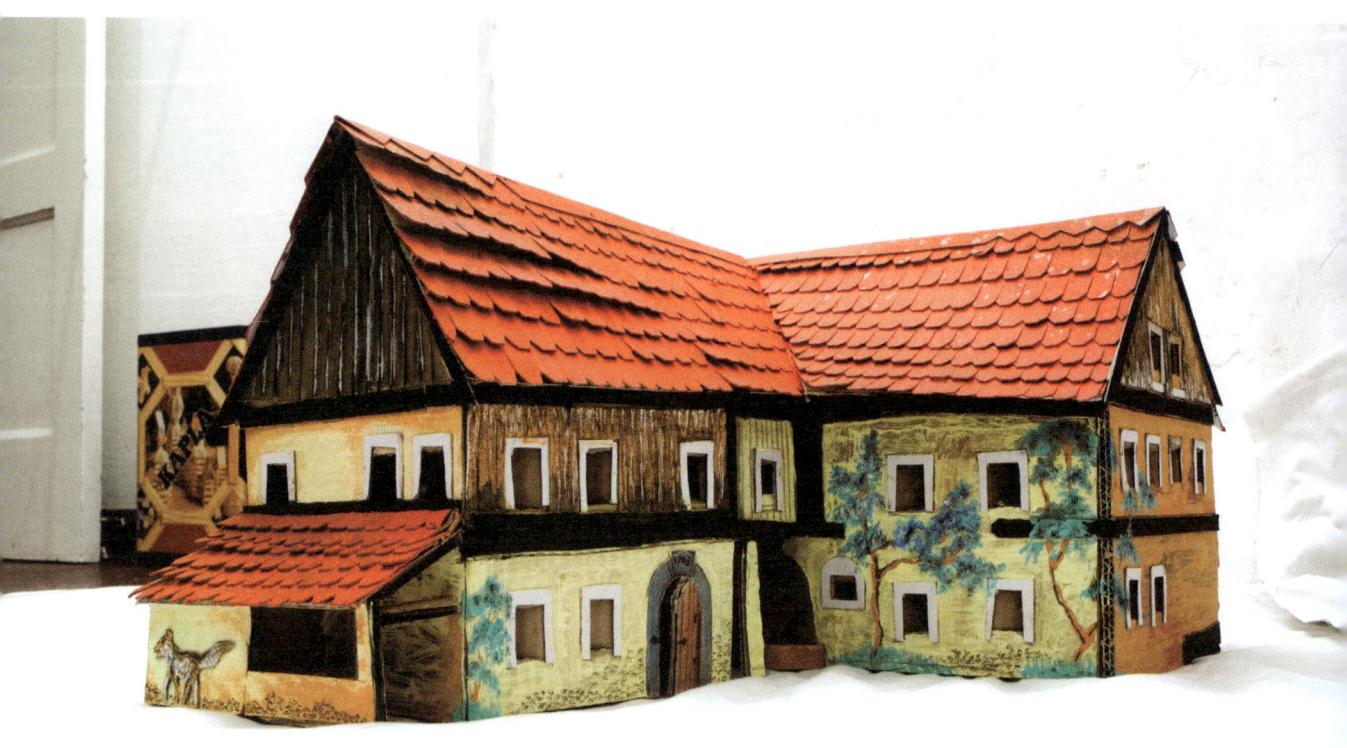

Exploring creativity and pushing your limits isn't just about
pushing yourself physically. It's about exploring all things and
staying curious. I made a cardboard maquette of a house in
Poland. It's called "the Kuznia," a Polish word that means "smithy"
in English. Cardboard is great! You just need creativity.

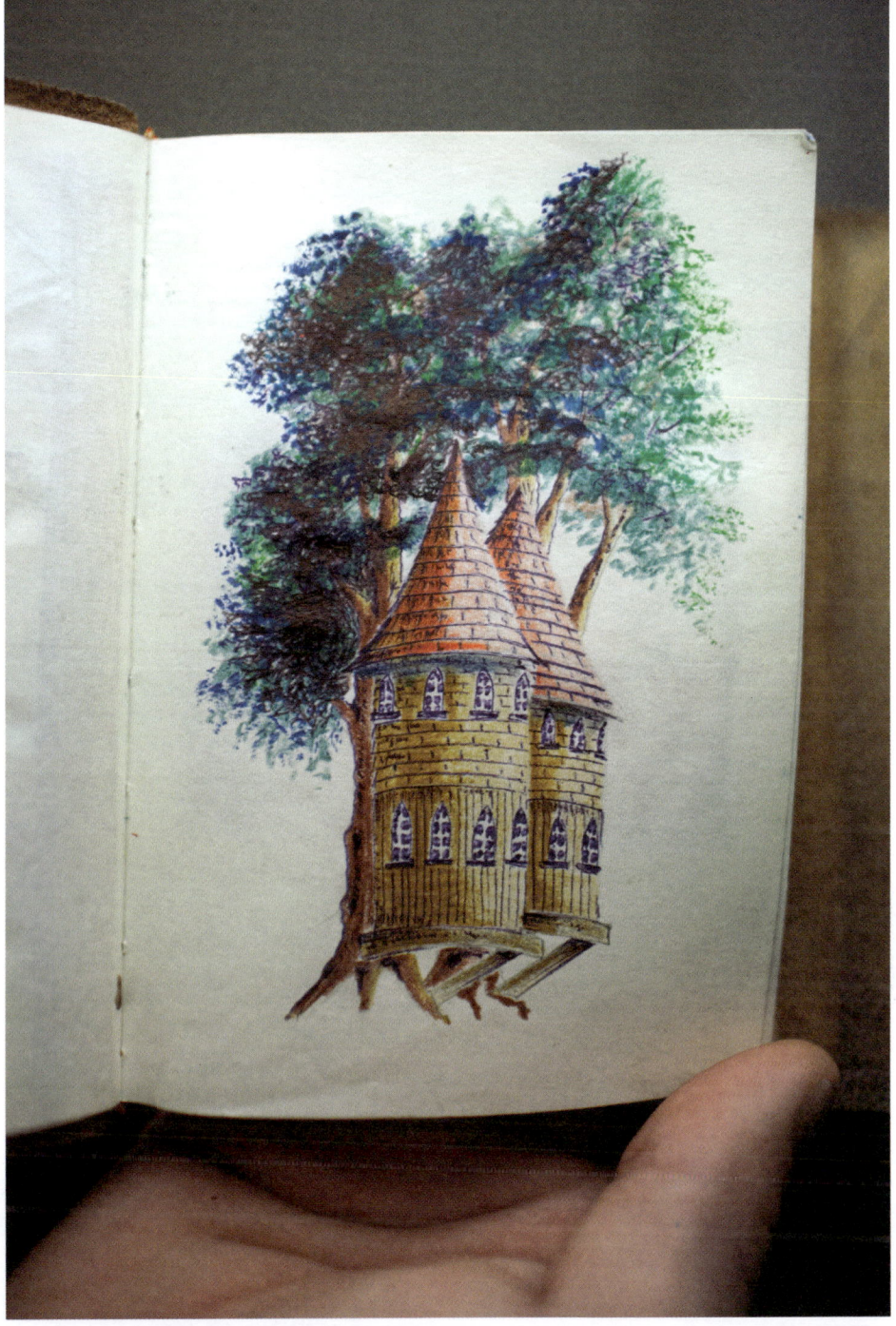

Ideas are one step closer to reality. Here I wanted to make treehouses from recycled wood, but I ended up making bunk beds in the shape of a castle instead. Ideas have their own power. If you start with something, then it becomes tangible. The next step is to make it bigger, but you don't necessarily have to do that because you have already manifested your idea.

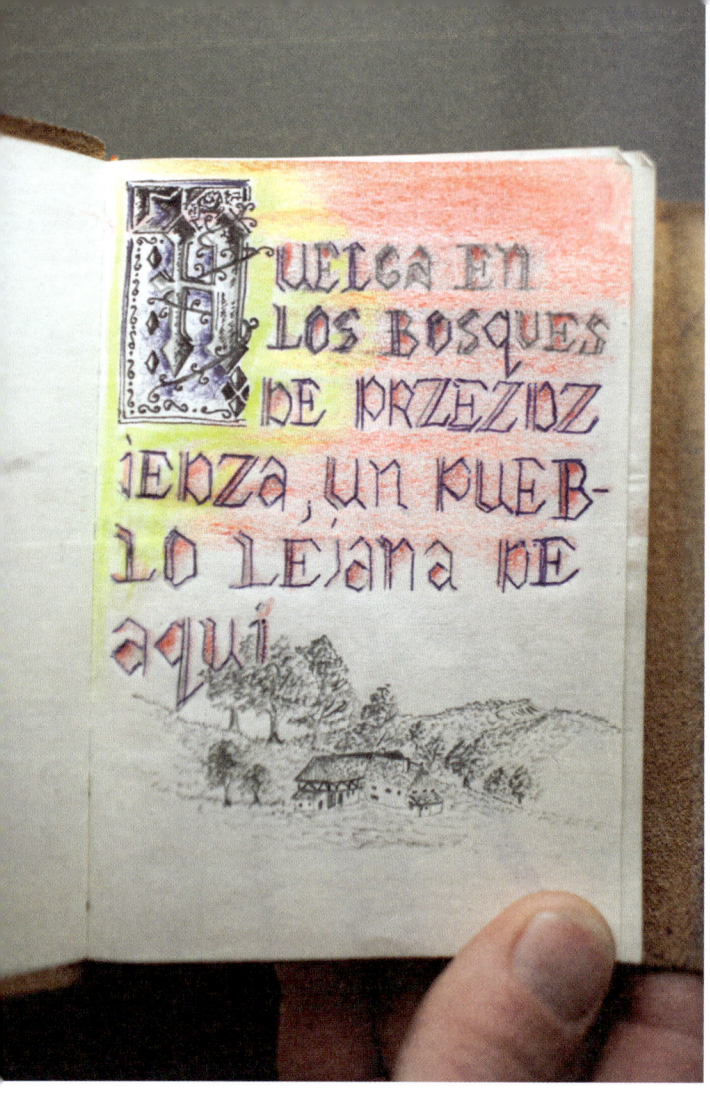

My notebook, making and seeing
tales starting in my imagination.

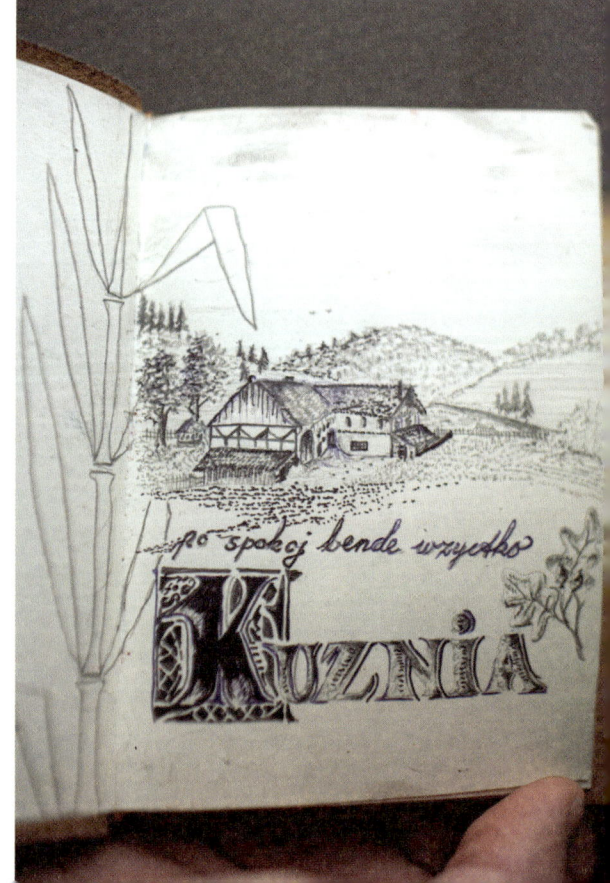

FREEDOM

Living without responsibility for others
Dancing, drinking, traveling, no fathers or
Mothers
Then rise in love. Or fall
Suddenly you are incentive with pregnancy
Natures course, no longer fantasy
Ho, ho, ho it's really serious
Gone freedom, responsibility period
The belly grows, so are the worries
Then when delivery
A miracle happens
Ties are tied directly
To a deeper understanding invincibility
So strong a new discovery
Within yourself, spiritual infinity
Love unconditionally
As it says, without lies, tied to a boundless
Energy
My baby, innocent being unaware
Changed me with the speed of light
To be there
Where I always looked for outside, worldwide
While it is here, when I look at him, a new beginning
Where I don't need to go nowhere
Because all you need is that care
A loving stare
There is more than meets the eye
Freedom caused by my baby
That's why.

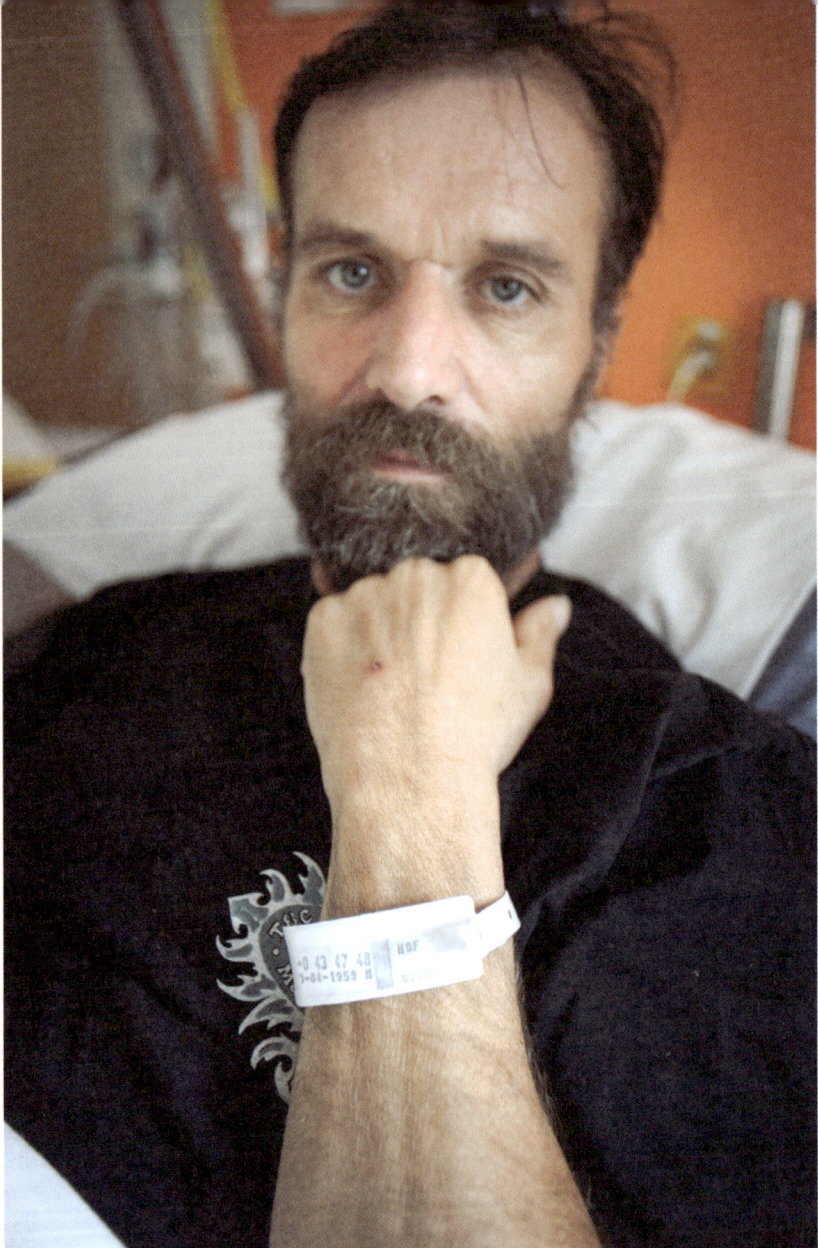

This is after two and a half weeks of no food. My intestines ruptured while doing an extreme enema in Vondelpark in Amsterdam. They had to open me up, clean me out, and sew me back up. I had totally miscalculated the power of the fountain. It almost killed me. My microbiome was completely washed away after the operation. I remember feeling very inflamed, and I had my partner bring frozen water bottles to roll over my back. I needed the cold. I could not really do my breathing because of the operation, so I did conscious breathing instead, which also helped. The doctors told me I would not be able to go back to my former life of trying for records. But four months later, I was back in the ice doing a world record and went on to do eight more.

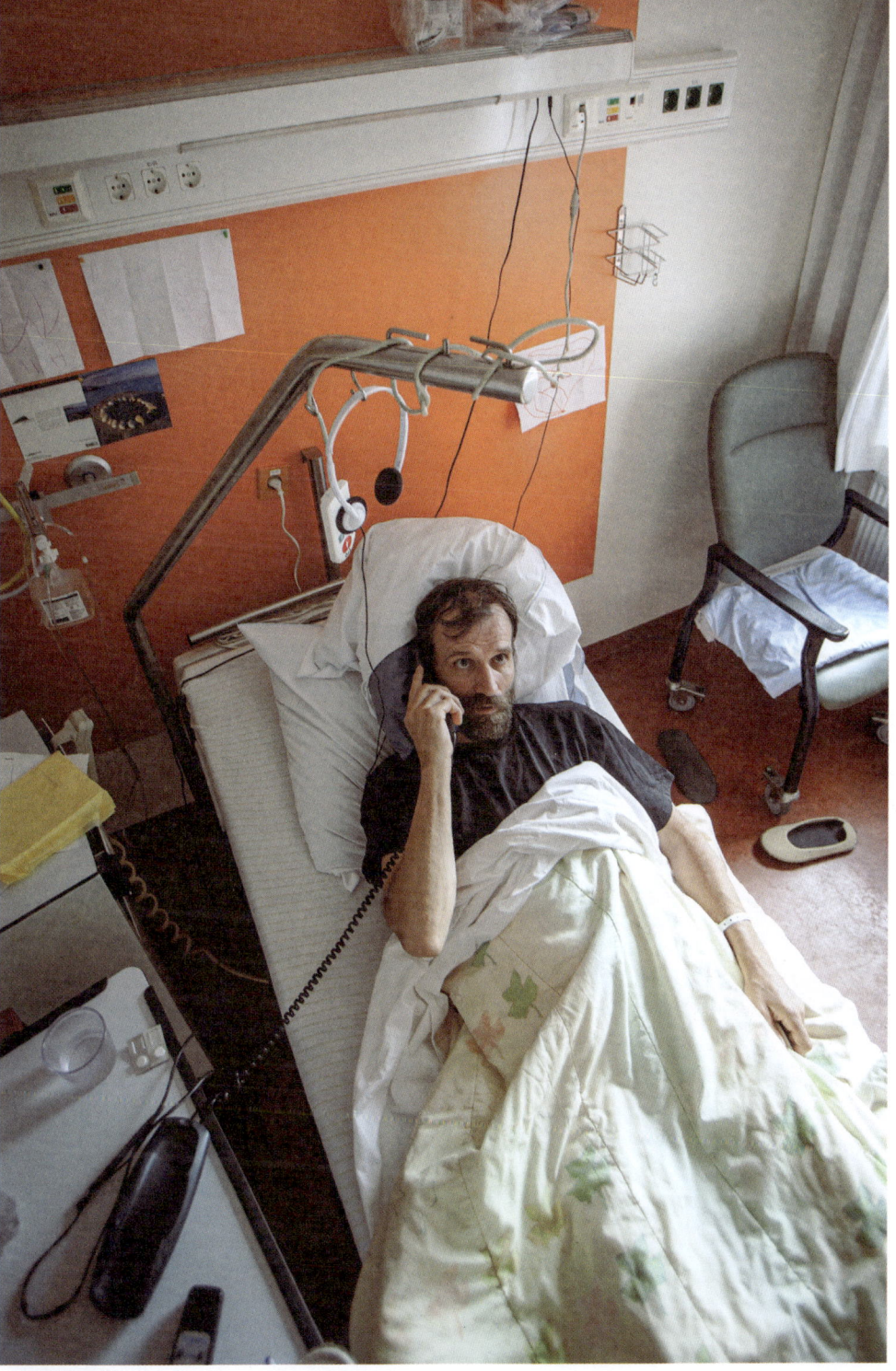

My abdomen was still fully open, yet
life goes on and calls upon me.

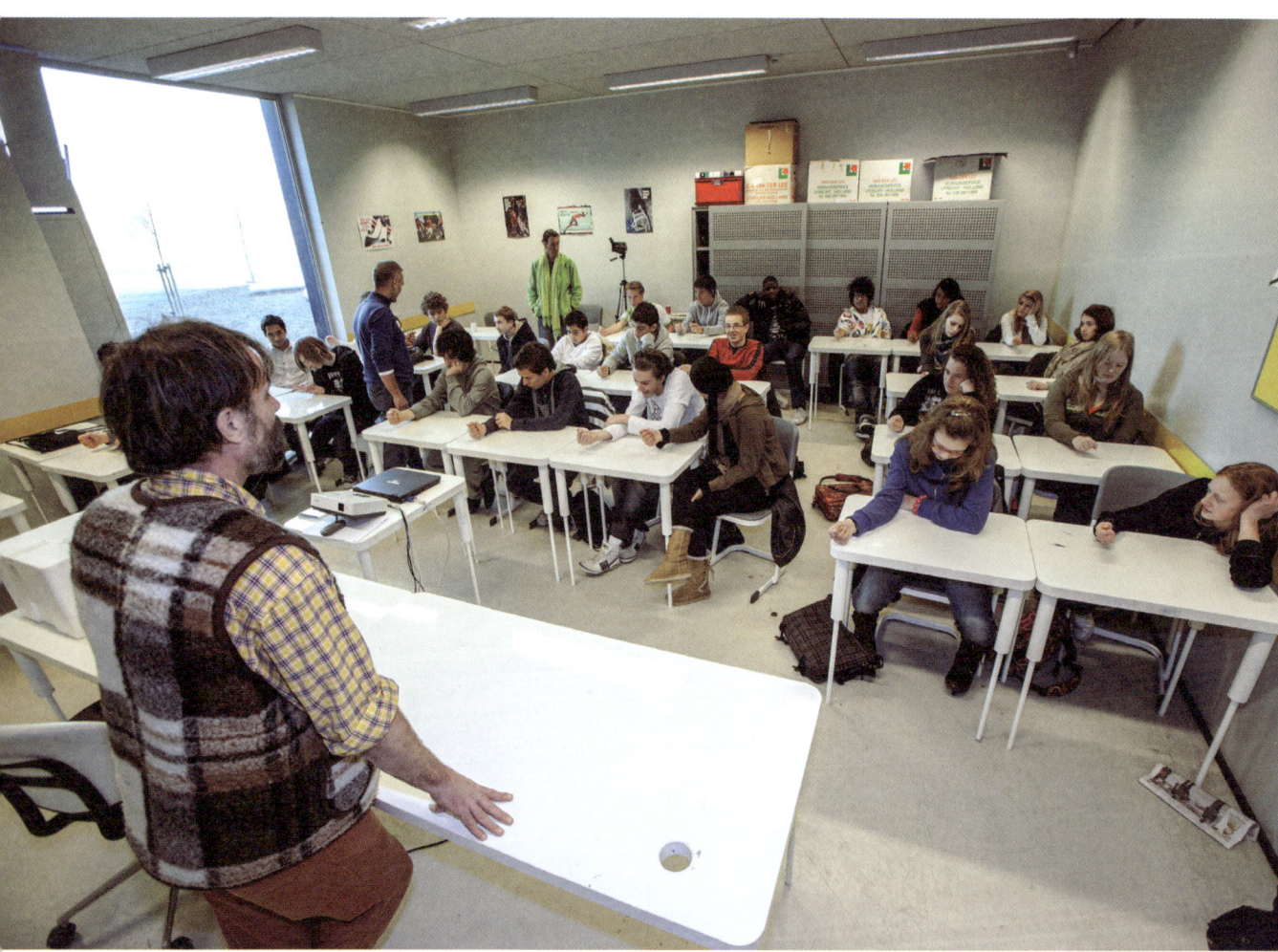

I believed in my mission and went back to spreading it. This time with high school students. In the beginning, it was quite difficult to get through to the pupils. I loved every minute of it anyway.

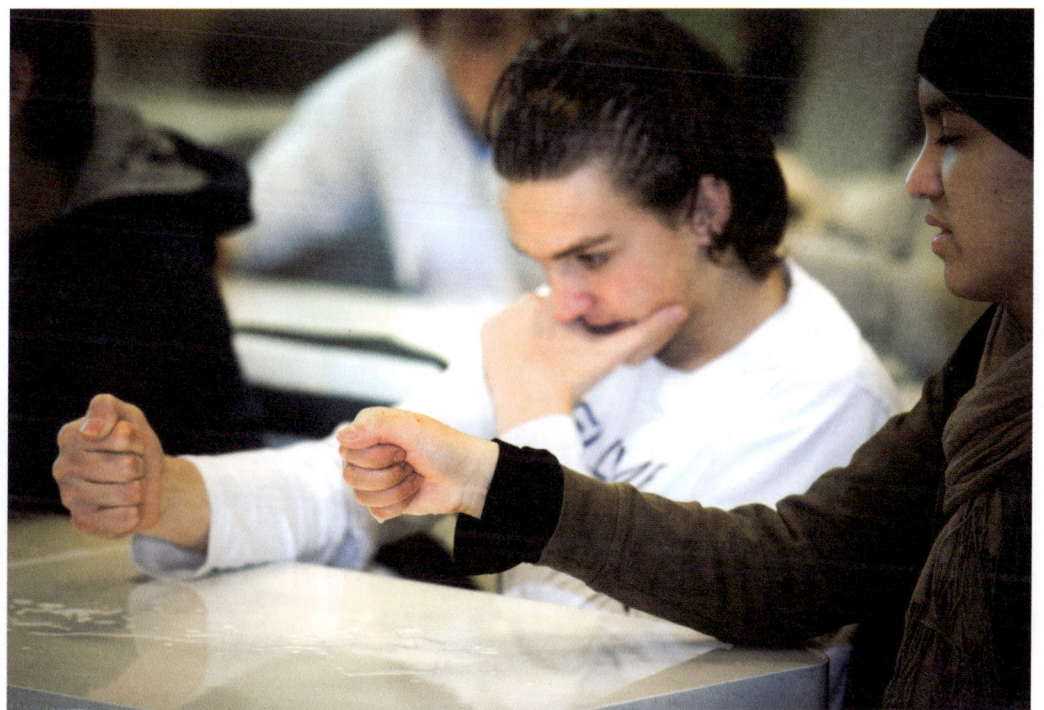

How to melt an ice cube with the power of your mind. A way to connect with the deep brain, the hypothalamus/thermoregulator.

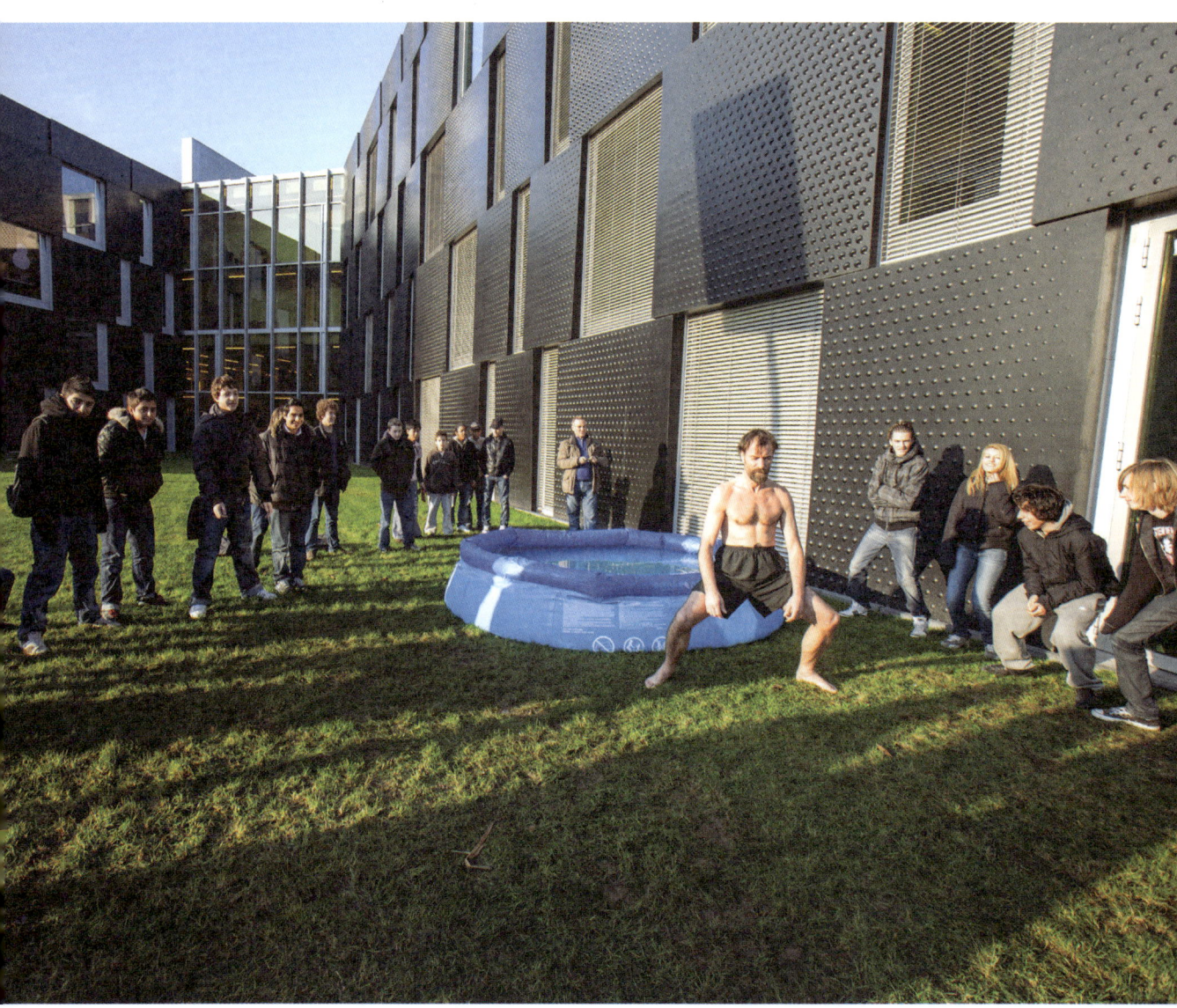

The horse stance looks funny, especially when people look at it without trying it. This was 2011. In 2022, I did it with fifty thousand people at a festival, and the following year, I did it with eighty thousand people at Defqon.

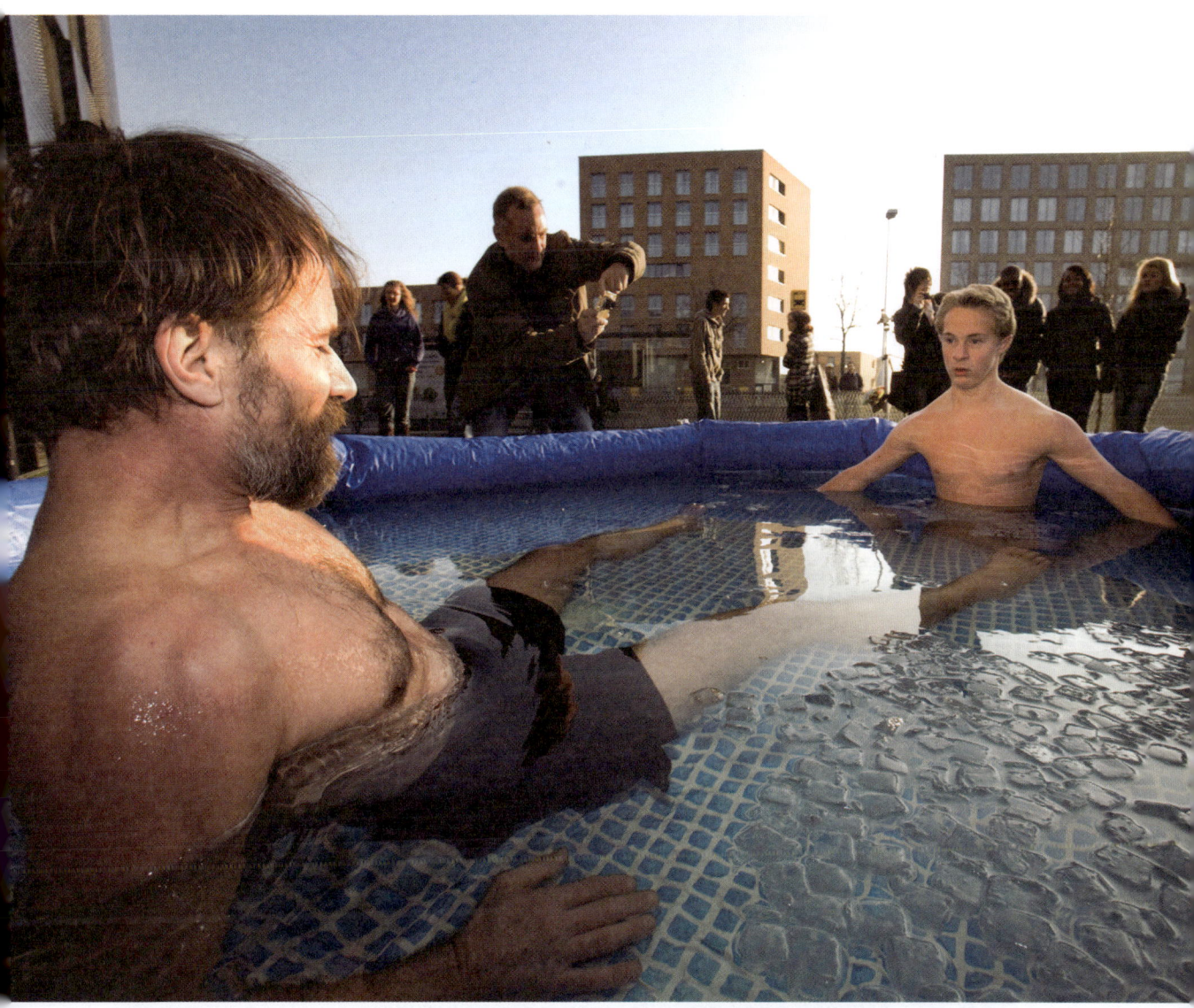

Only one followed me into the pool then, in 2011.

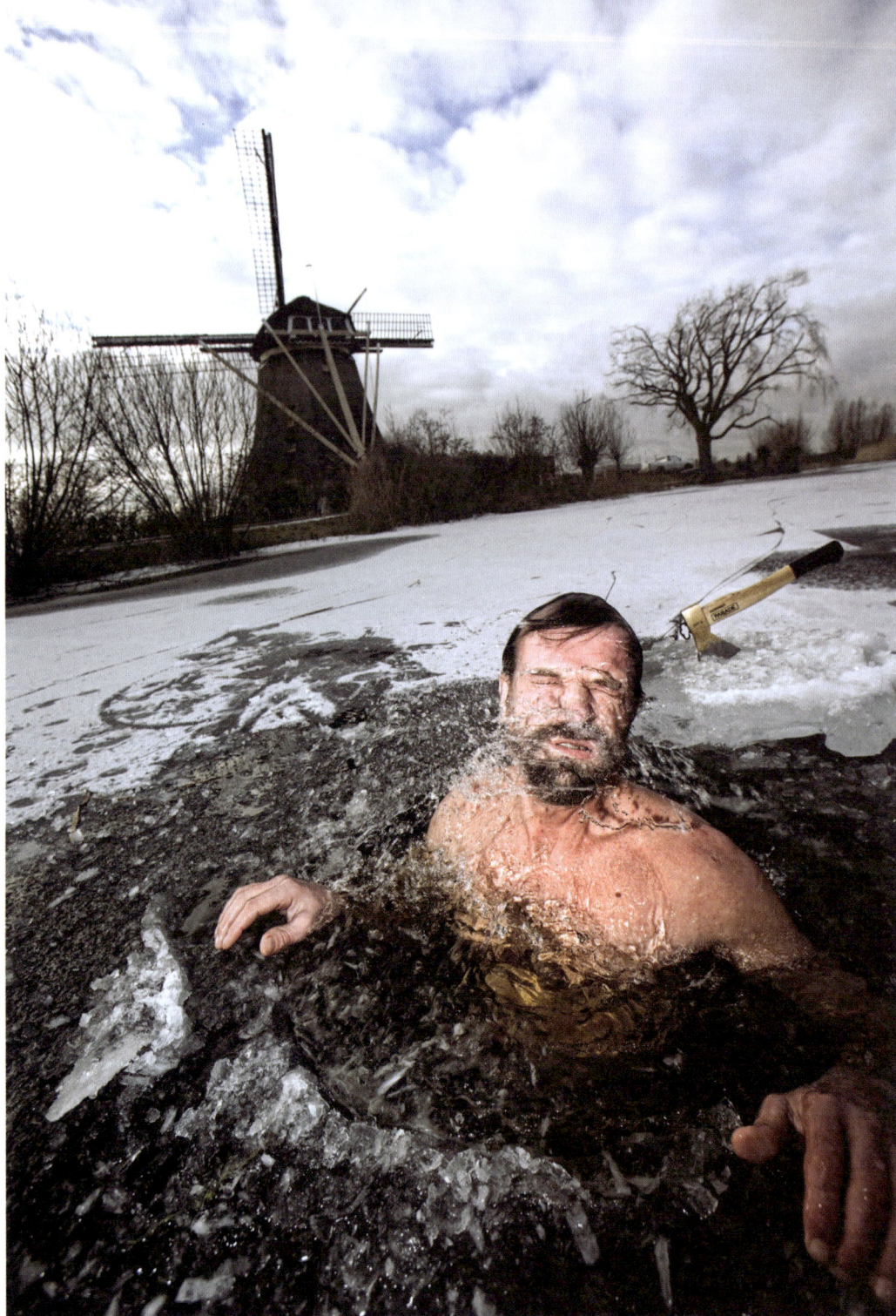

The Netherlands, windmills, and only one Iceman. Not anymore!

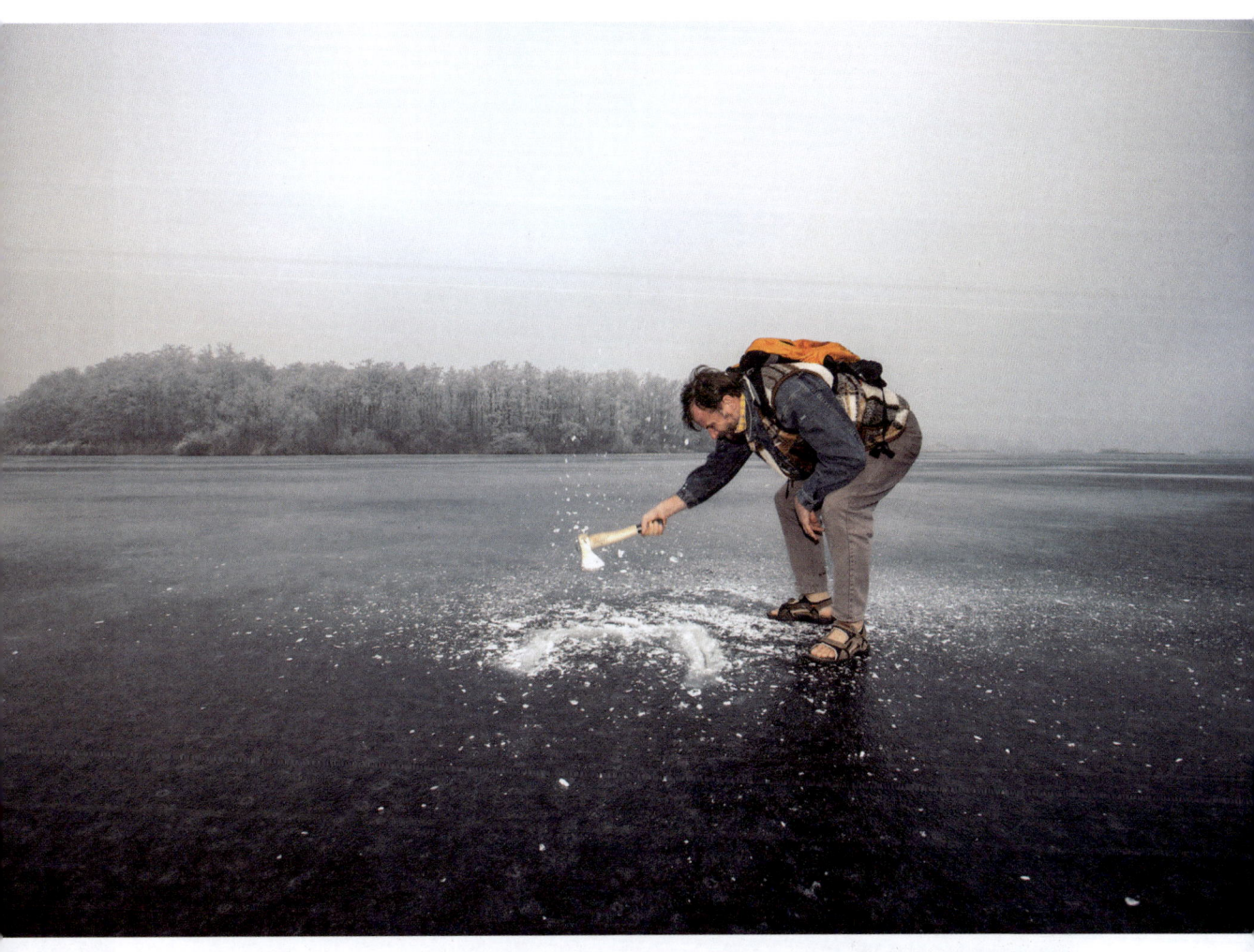

Back in the lakes. I still stuck with my training, as I always had. My winter routine never left me, in good times or bad times. Discipline. This is what I did for years in the winters, with nobody around, all alone in the water, training. In winter, life retreats back to the core. As with cold water, there is a solace you can experience, a silence there. It's beautiful and deeply cleansing.

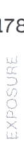

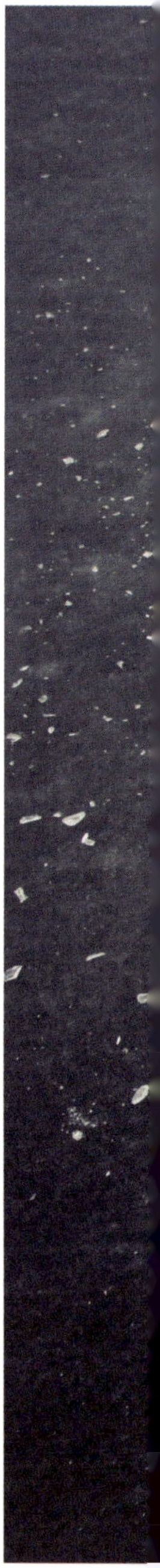

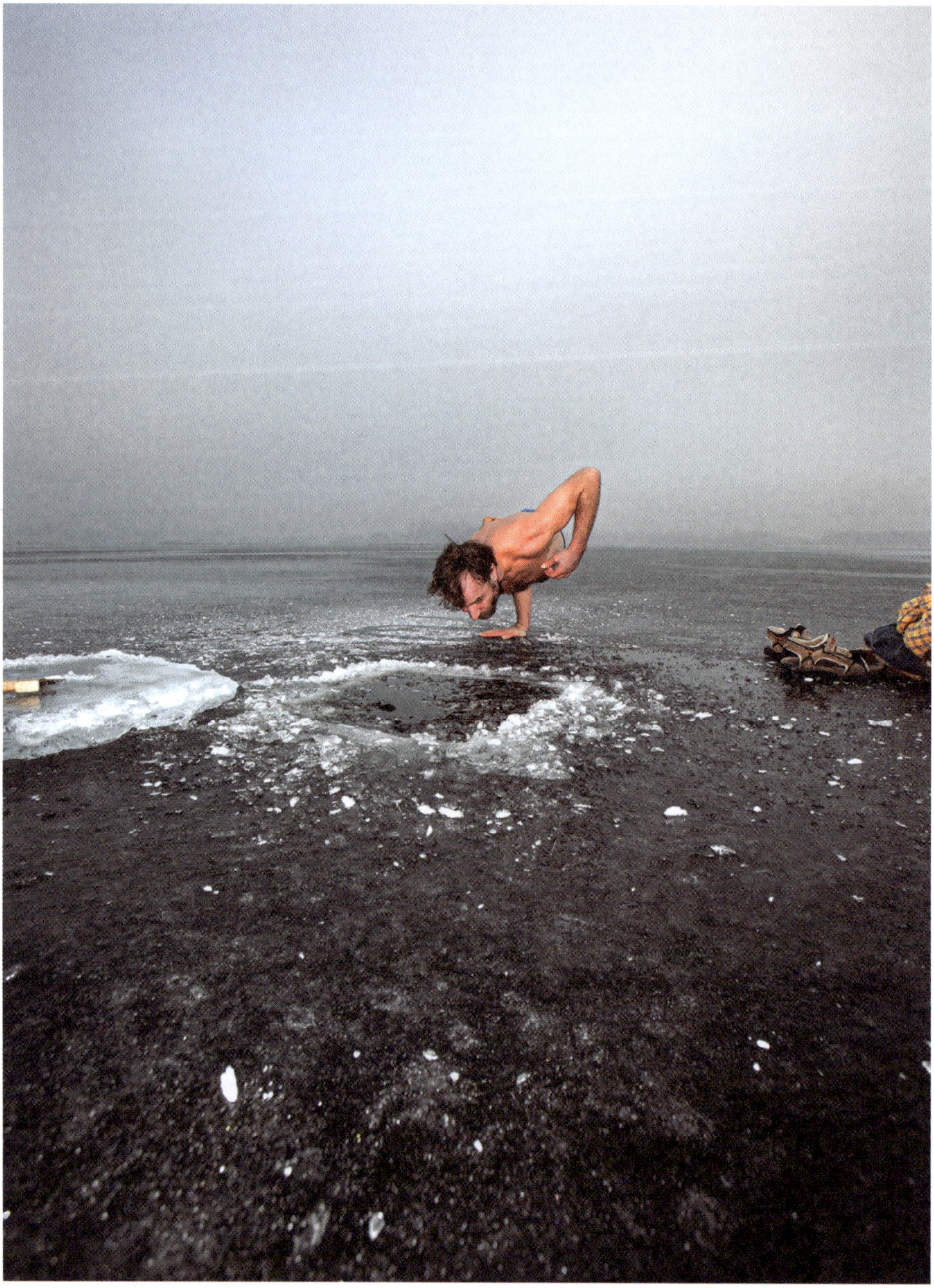

If you have been doing a posture for years, then you know exactly how you feel when you do it. It is all about control and flow. Here I am on the ice, freezing temperatures, but it's the same posture I did on rocks. In-depth control over a posture makes you flexible in mind and body. Eka Hasta Sarira Uttanasana, One-Limb Body-Lifting Posture.

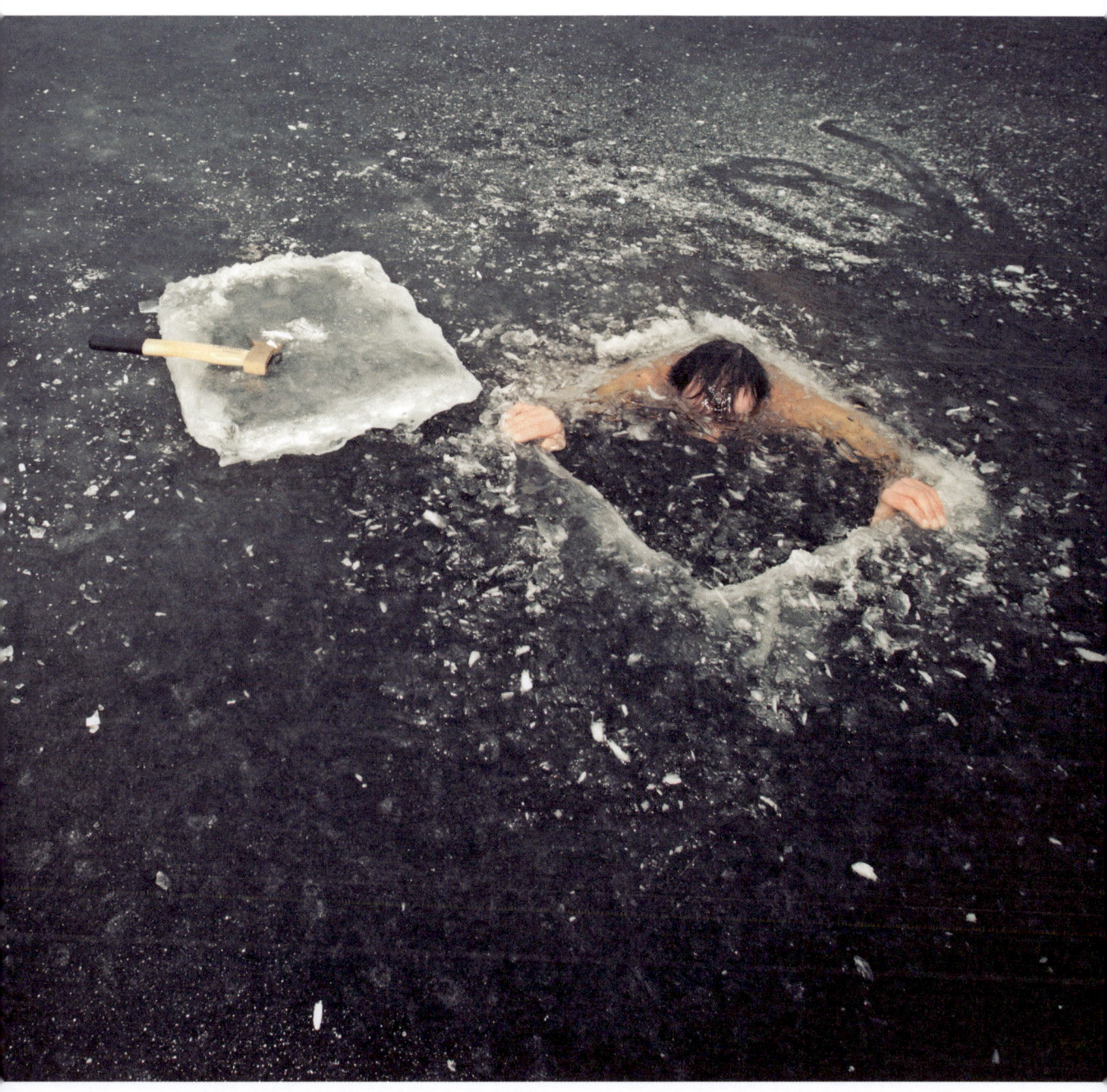

Ice water immersions make you stop ruminating—no doubt.

NATURE KNOWS, HOW IT GOES

Flows,

We have fears, beyond belief

So invest into belief

Then fear, will disappear

Forever, together

The Soul is the whole

Separation is no longer

Reconnect stranger and stranger

Manifest like a rock

Time will be gone

Runs like a Swiss clock

Precisely there

Priceless aware

Stole my heart like a charming thief

Belief

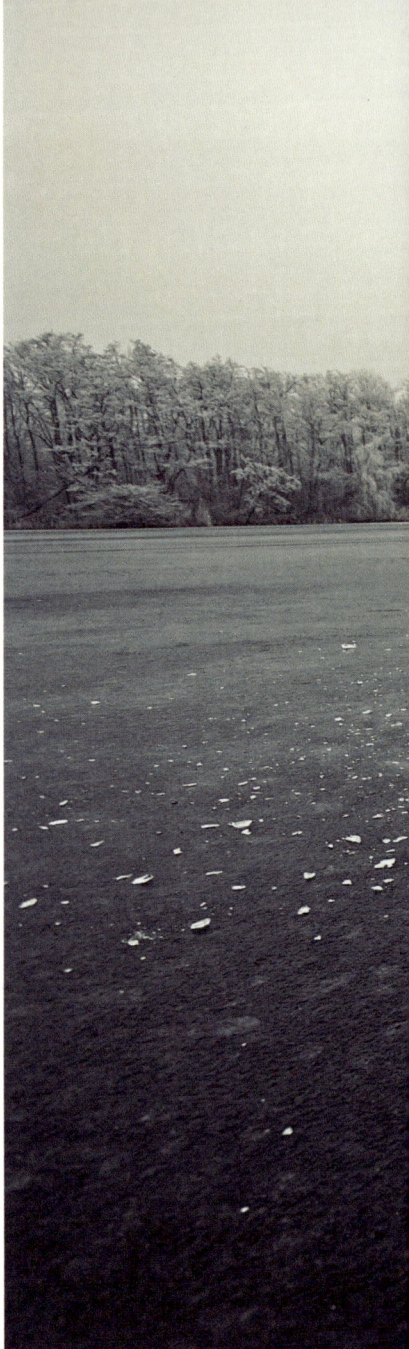

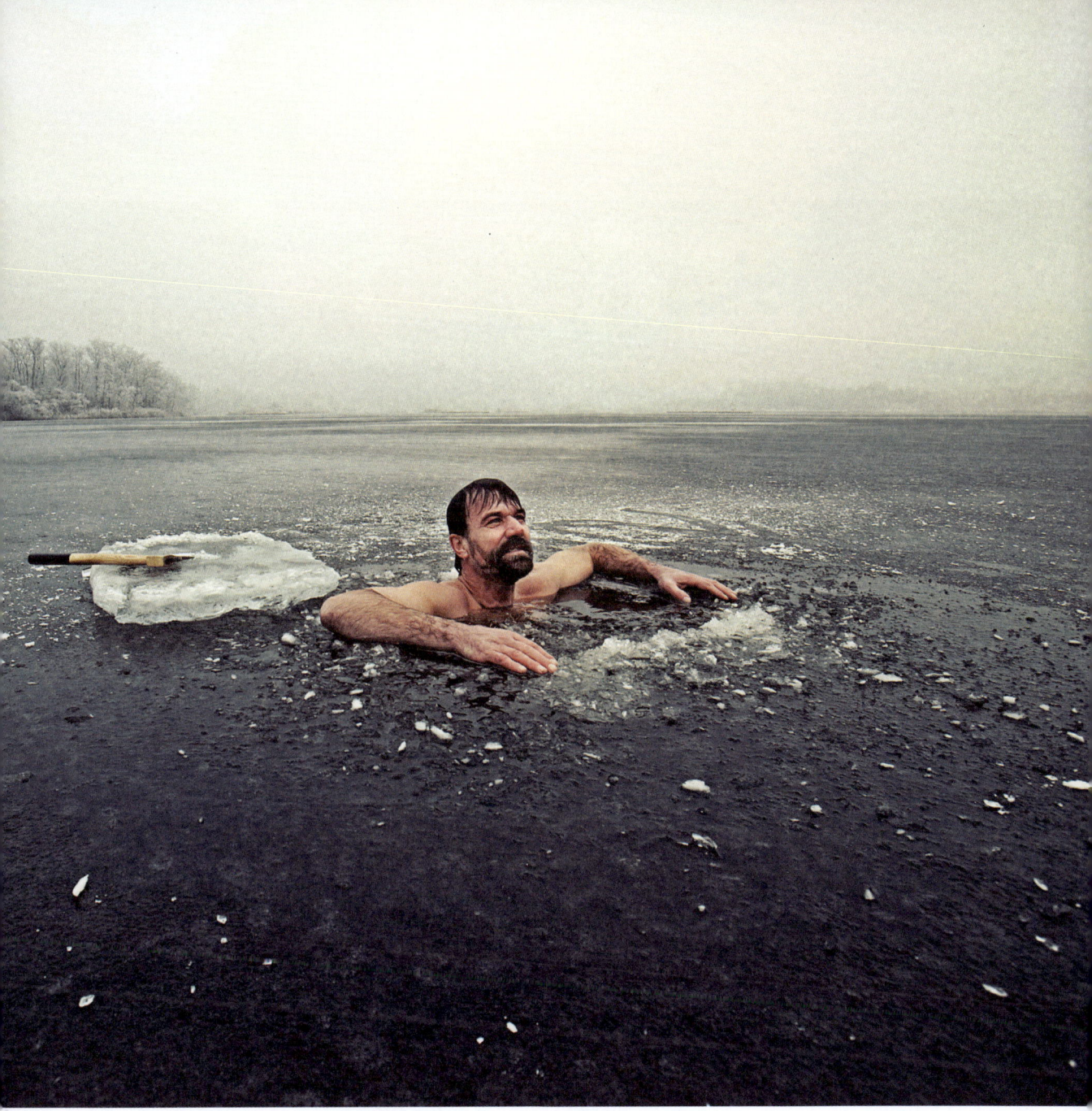

Refreshed.

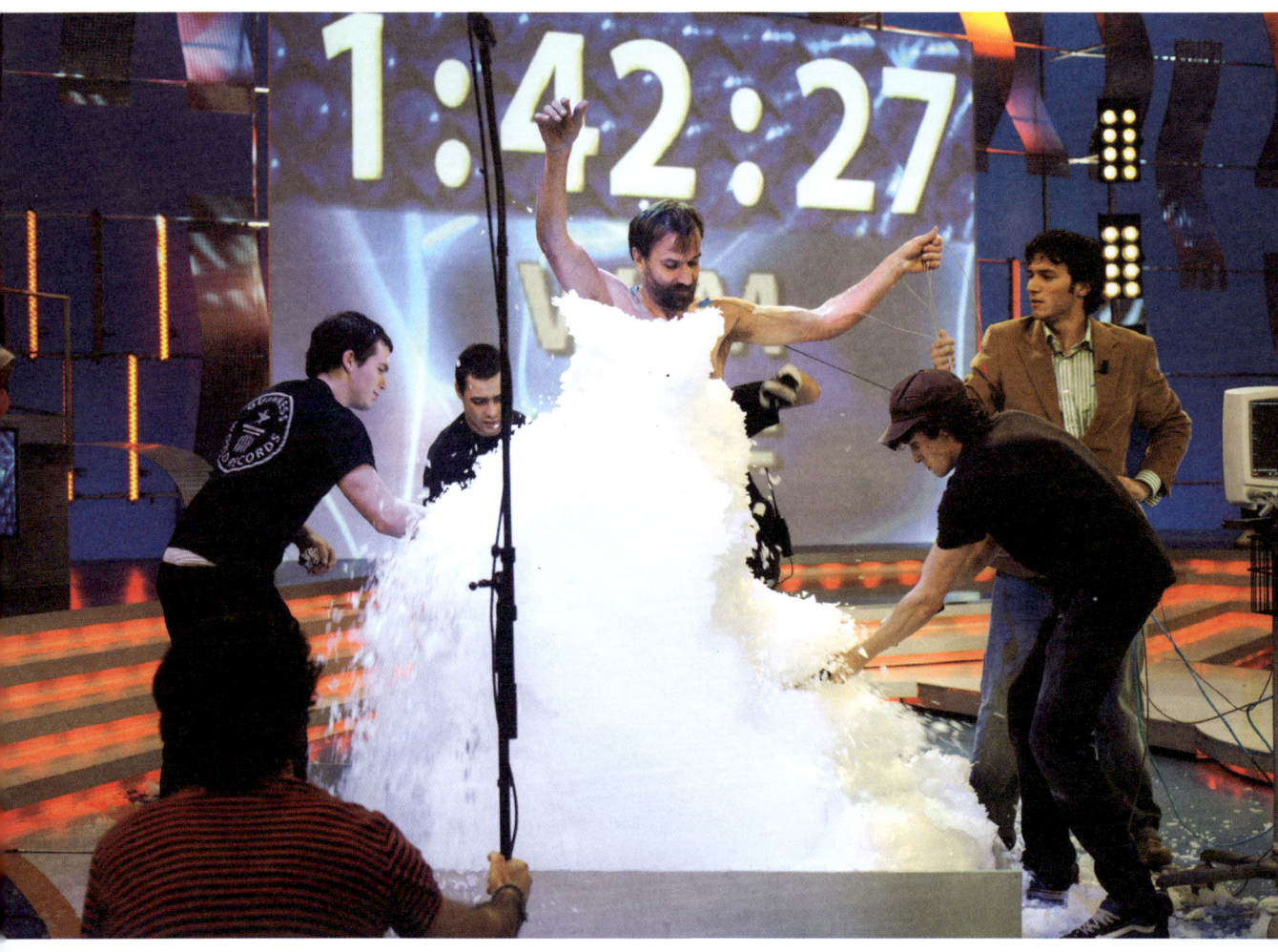

Another Guinness World Record, in Madrid.
Feeling deeply accomplished.

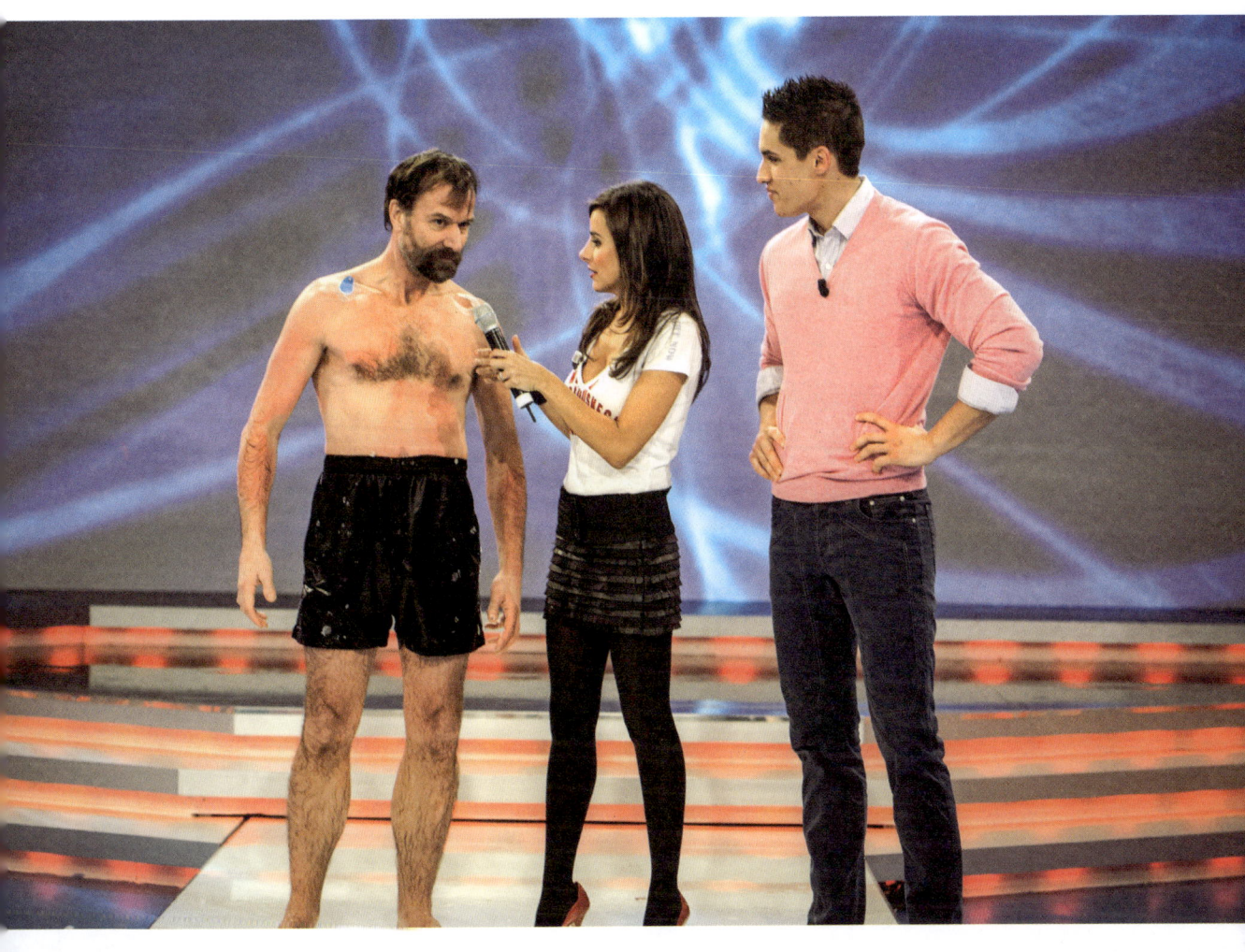

In many shows I got to appear in shorts. Crazy stuff!

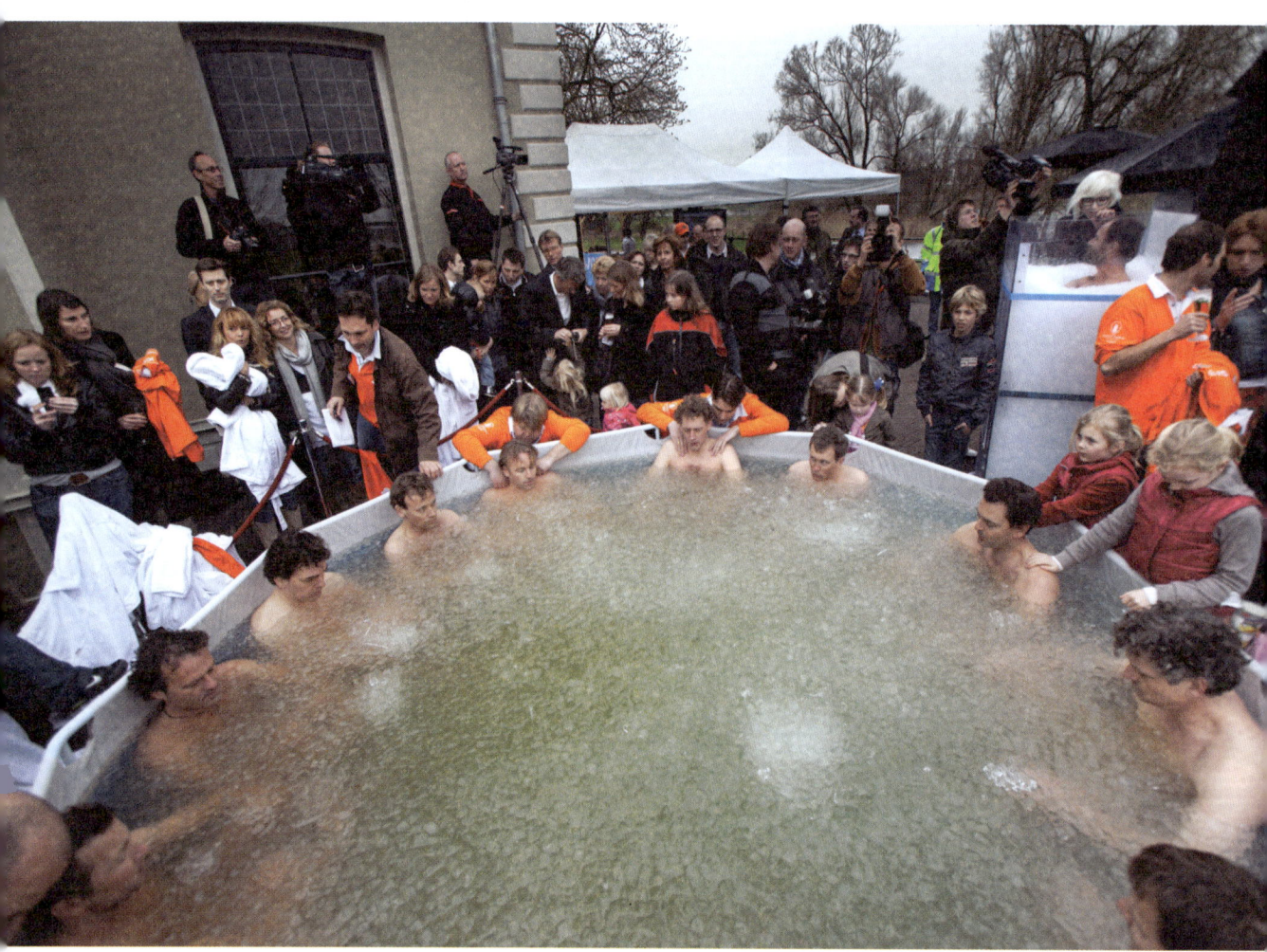

Me in an icebox. But more impressive are the people there doing five minutes in the tub. Cold immersion has spread and has by far outreached the world-record circus act I was in. To dare inspires people to recognize the courage in themselves and to see and feel the need to join.

Like an army of unconditional being, no words, feeling strong and good.

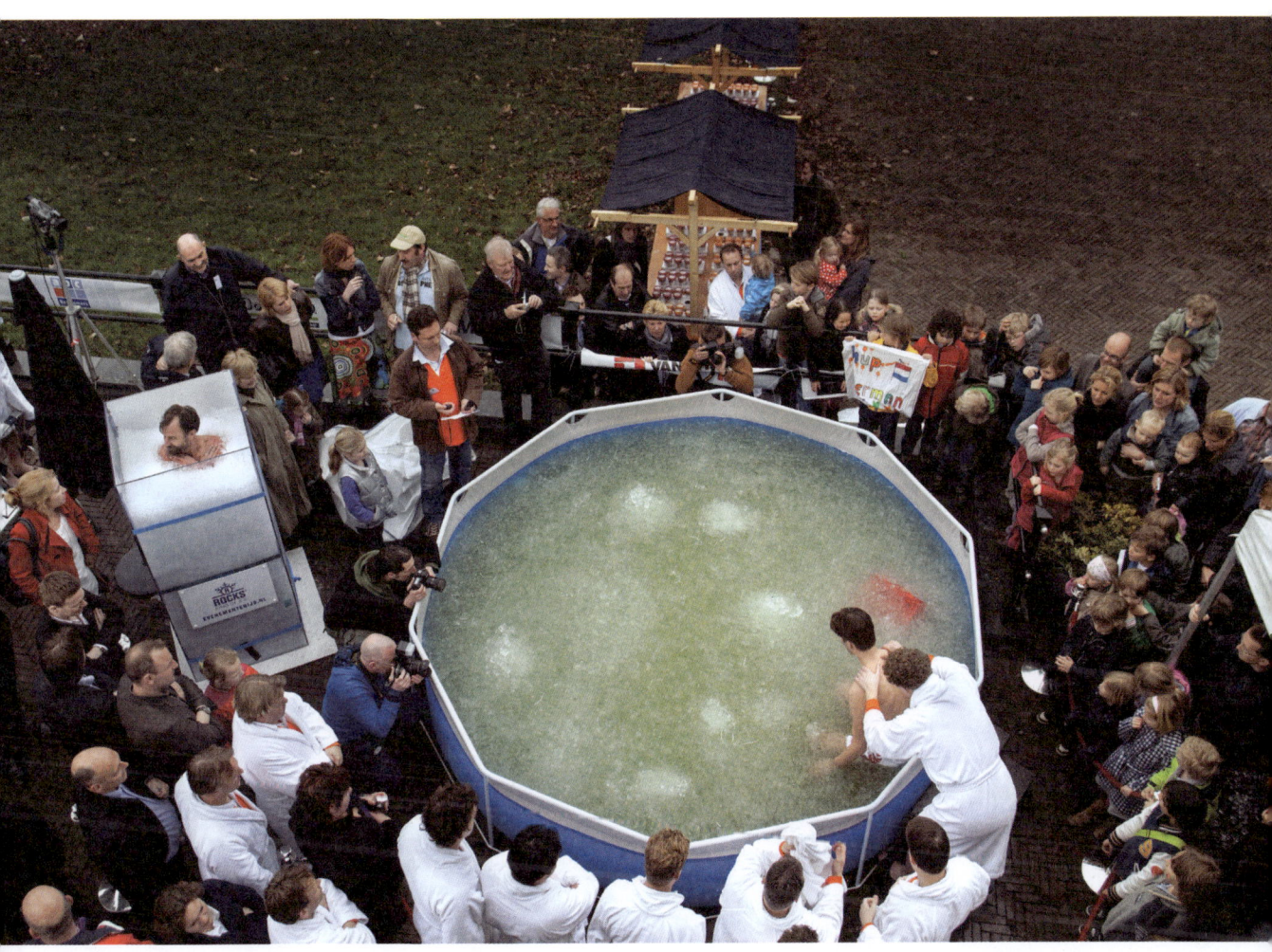

The icy water is no longer a challenge for one daredevil. Now, we all dare the devil.

Cool me down! When you go into the ice, you feel yourself and your thoughts vanish like snow in the sun.

REDWOODS

Sequoia, gigantea rhododendron

Far out, far on

Cherokee tree, being free

Giants who stood the torture of time

We cut most of them, cutting with our past

Forgot how wisdom grows, we are going too fast

The bark suffered many wildfires

Impervious, to all that

Though the intent of many liars

Killing old wisdom, too sad

That growing majestically to the sky

An unforeseen grace

Is telling us to shamefully bow and cry

That our days

Are numbered, if not come up with answers

And show why

We voraciously hunt, blunt

Keep on going with staggering ignorance

Looking around, deeply stunned

Where to go from here

When nothing is left

But outward-oriented stupidity

Bow down, humbly back to your roots

Nothing sentimental

Like bamboo it shoots

Mycelium old wisdom

Has come

To reveal our oneness

In harmony for our children

To play upon her deep embrace

Cut the ignorance, deeply and all

timelessness, our beautiful Soul

Has come to say goodbye

If we do not leave these gentle giants

Natural wisdom growing tall

Receiving messages from the sky

Deeply rooted, we don't know why

Post our rage, blinding cage

The saga has come, let's get things straight

Respect your mother.

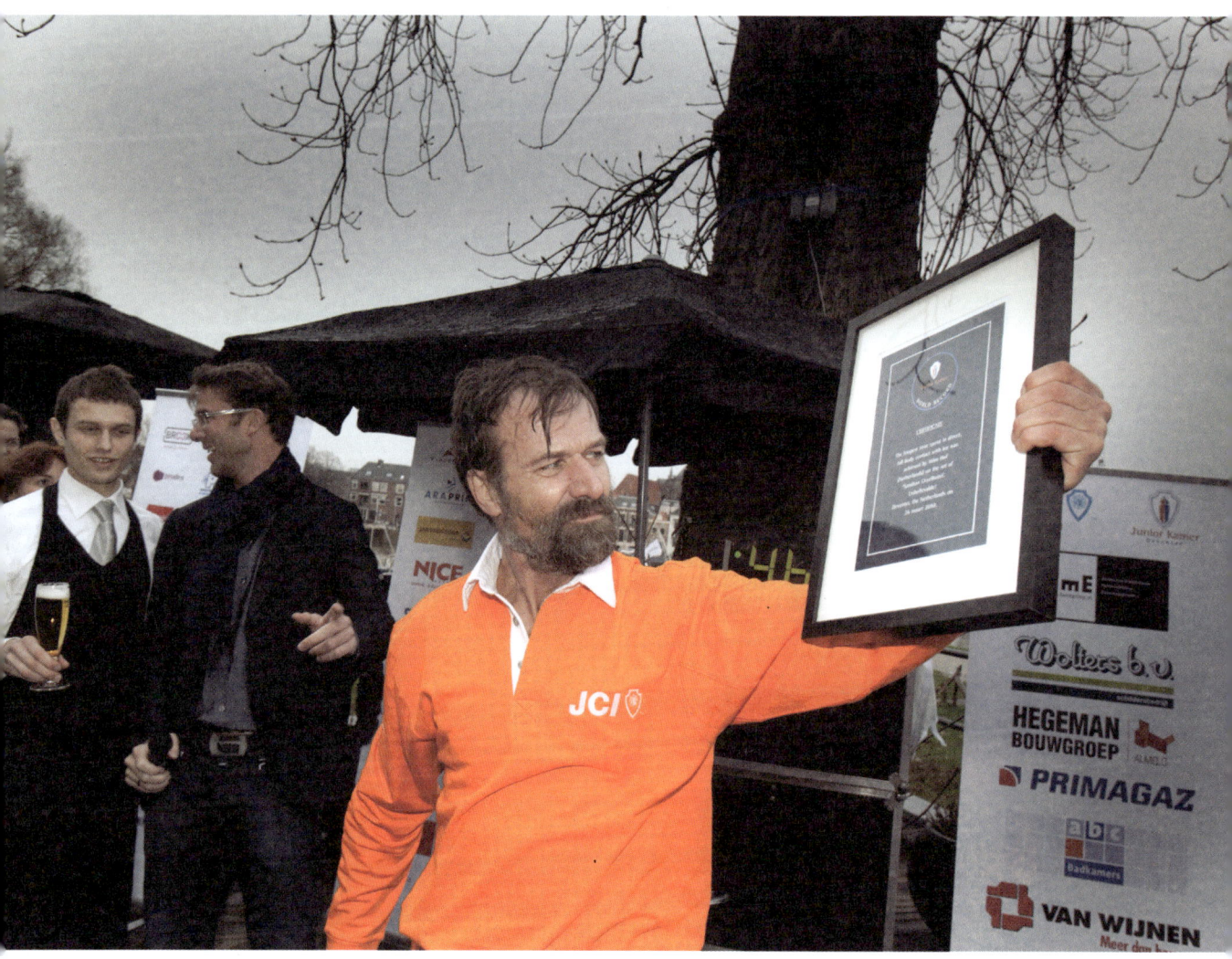

Always proud to get certificates, records, diplomas, honorary statements.

Recognition is feeling seen in true value—but we are so much more than what we can see or be.

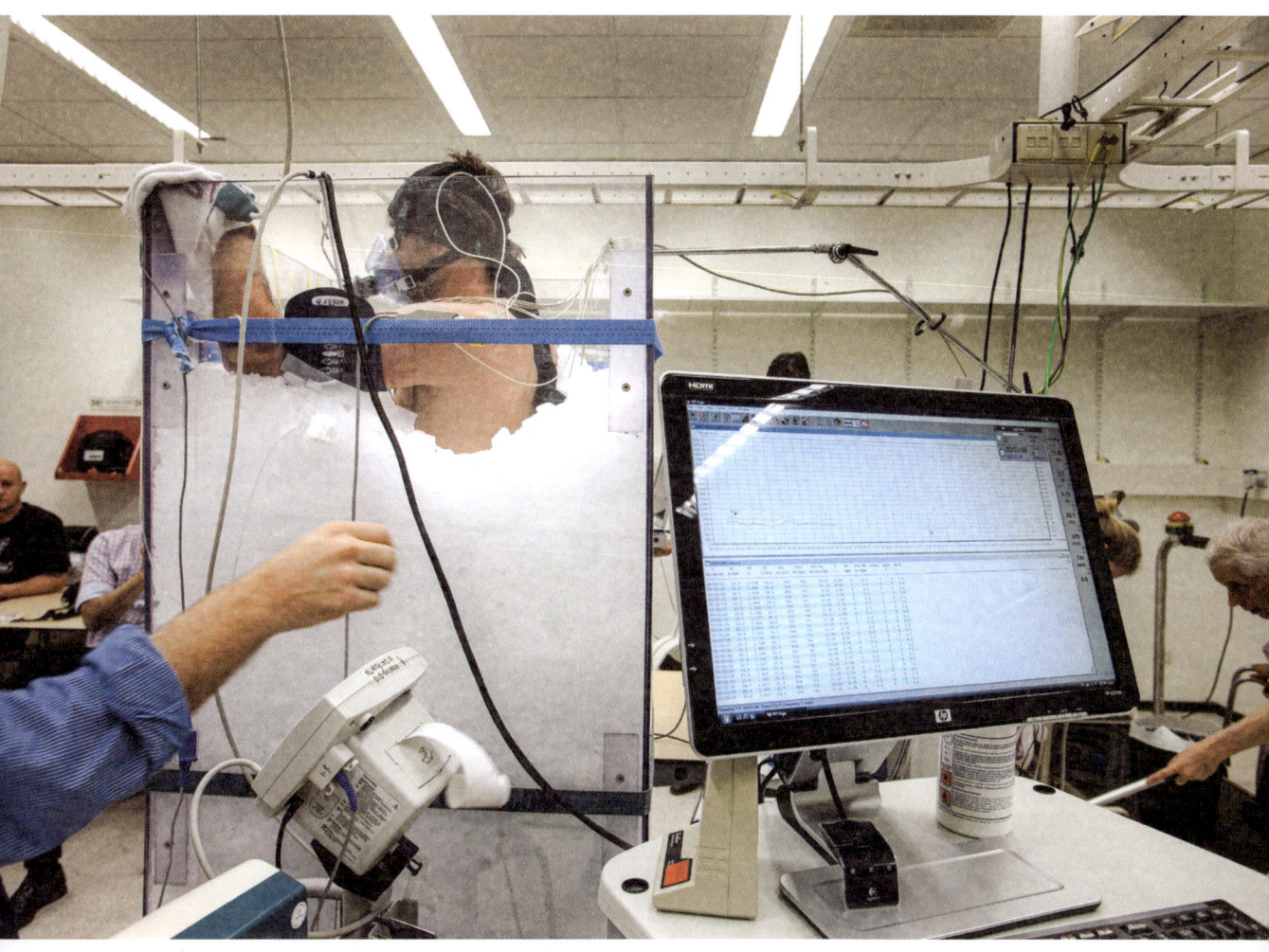

This was another pivotal moment. Radboud University, in Nijmegen, Amsterdam, 2010. Thirty-seven vials of blood were taken, and I was in the ice for eighty minutes. I was to perform under the supervision of Dr. Maria Hopman for an event the next day. They tested the blood ex vivo by exposing it to endotoxin; there was zero reaction. The cold shock proteins are so strong that nothing wrong can enter the cell. It should have set off alarm bells in the scientific community! However, this study did in fact set off a series of events that have changed the books.

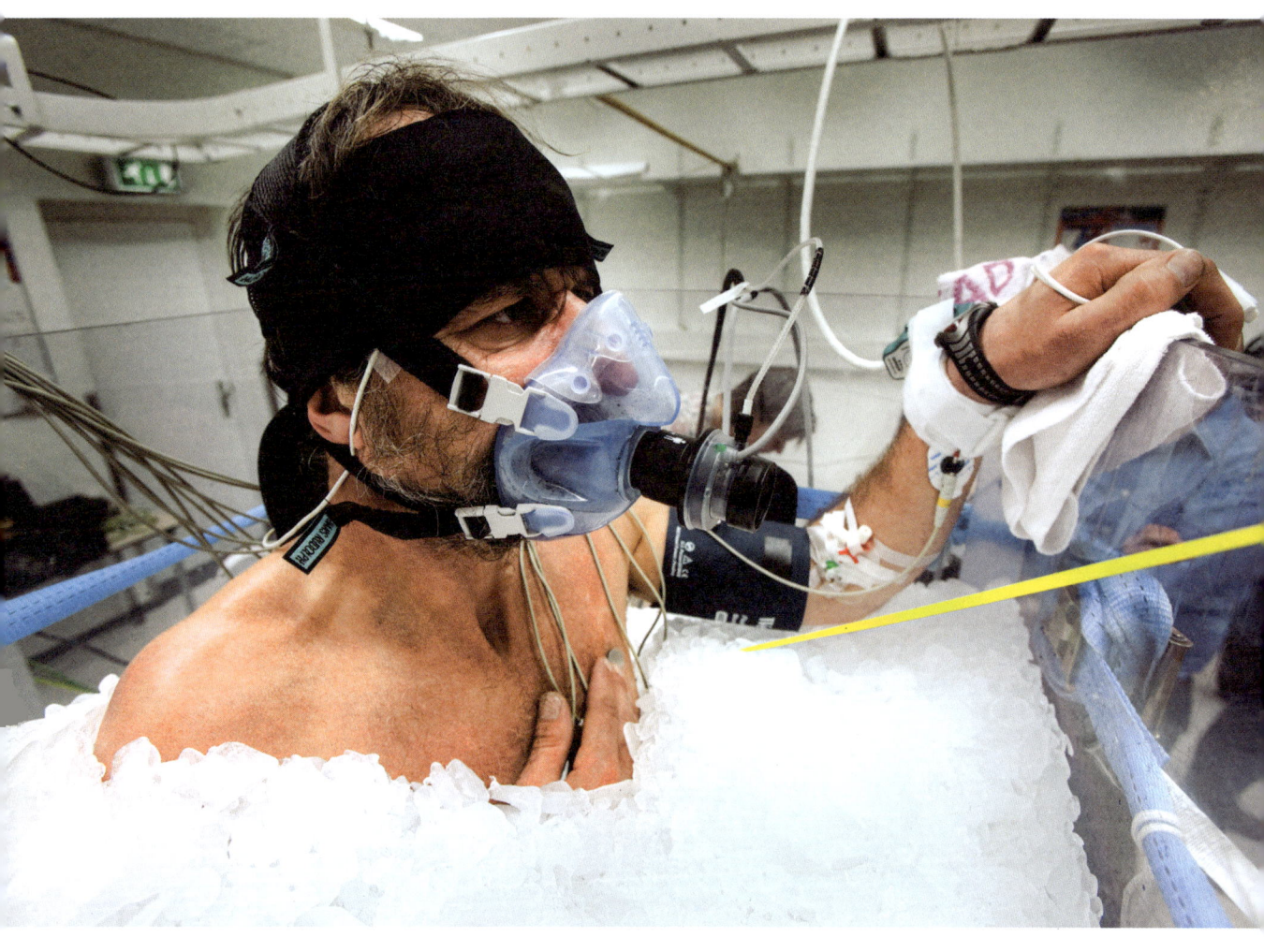

Professor Netaya asked me humbly if I would be willing to
be injected (in vivo) with endotoxin. I said absolutely yes!

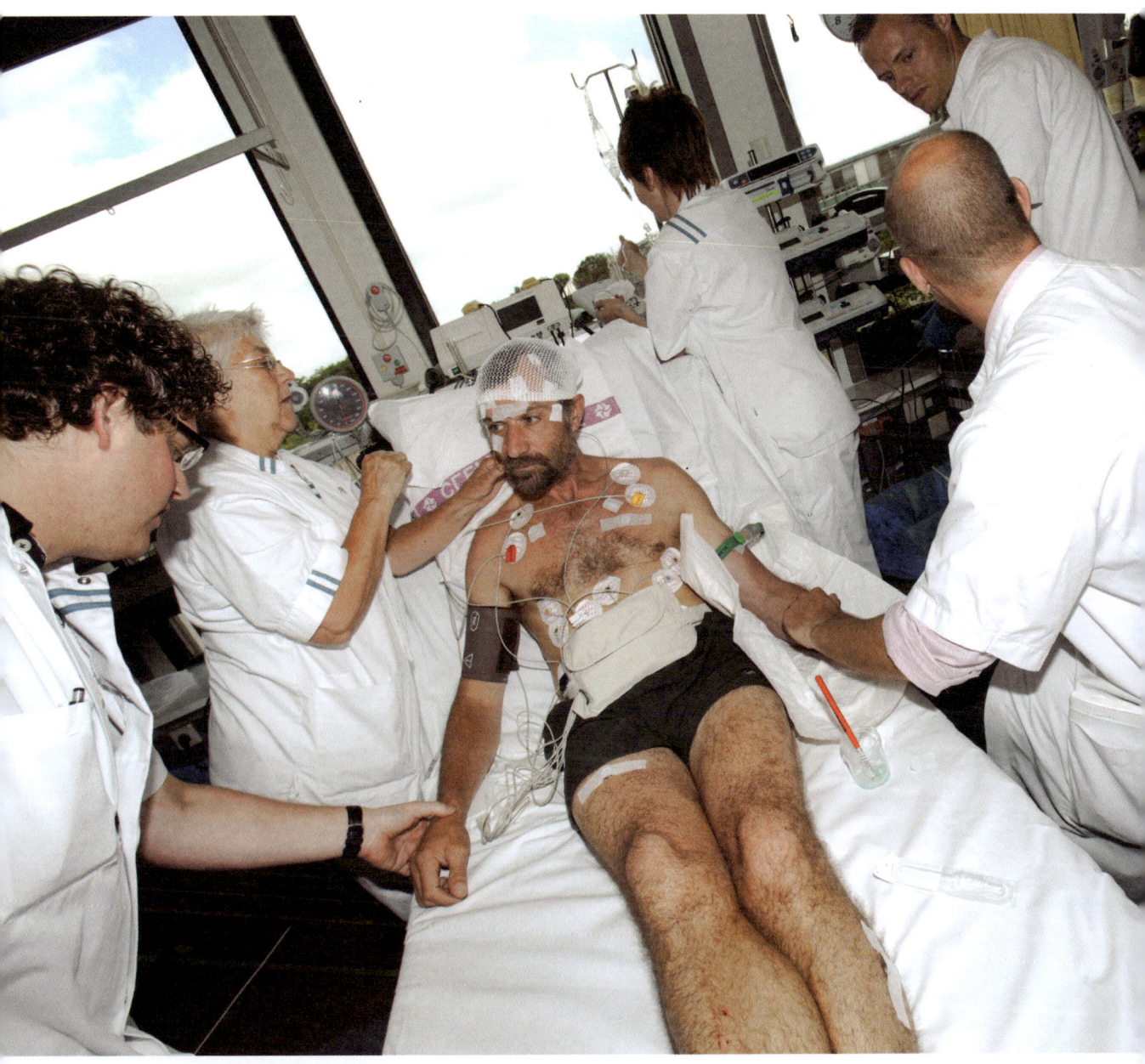

Endotoxin experiment in vivo. I'll volunteer anytime.

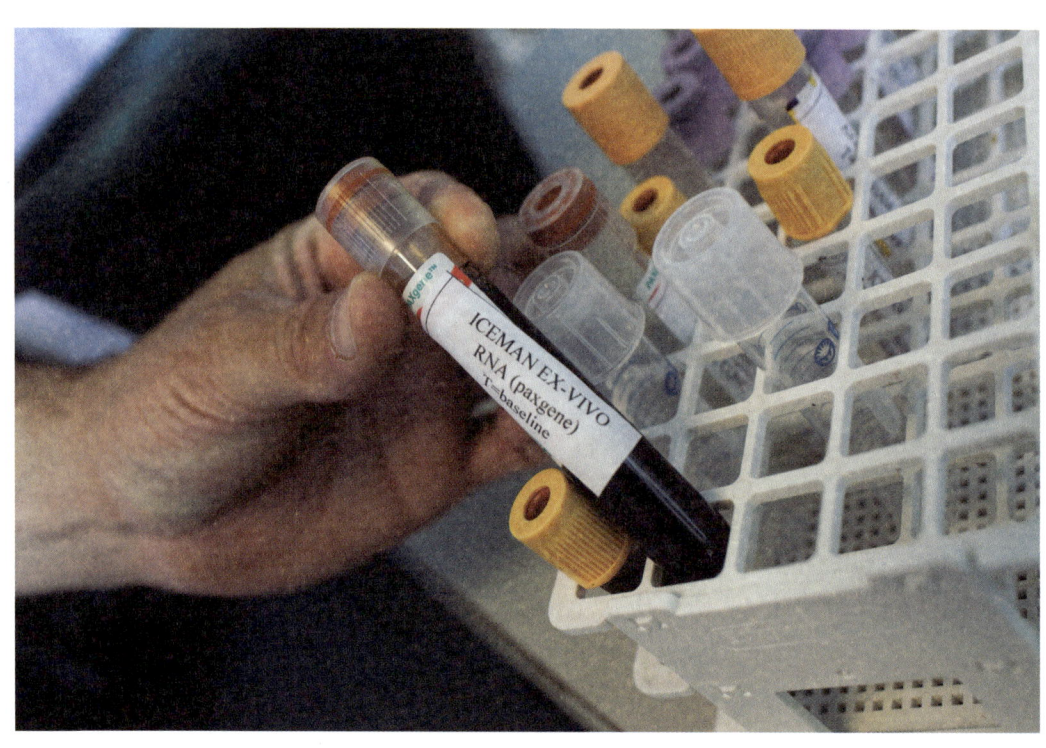

192

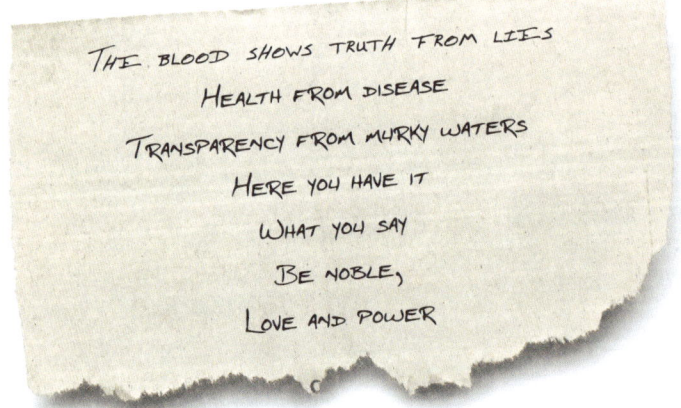

THE BLOOD SHOWS TRUTH FROM LIES

HEALTH FROM DISEASE

TRANSPARENCY FROM MURKY WATERS

HERE YOU HAVE IT

WHAT YOU SAY

BE NOBLE,

LOVE AND POWER

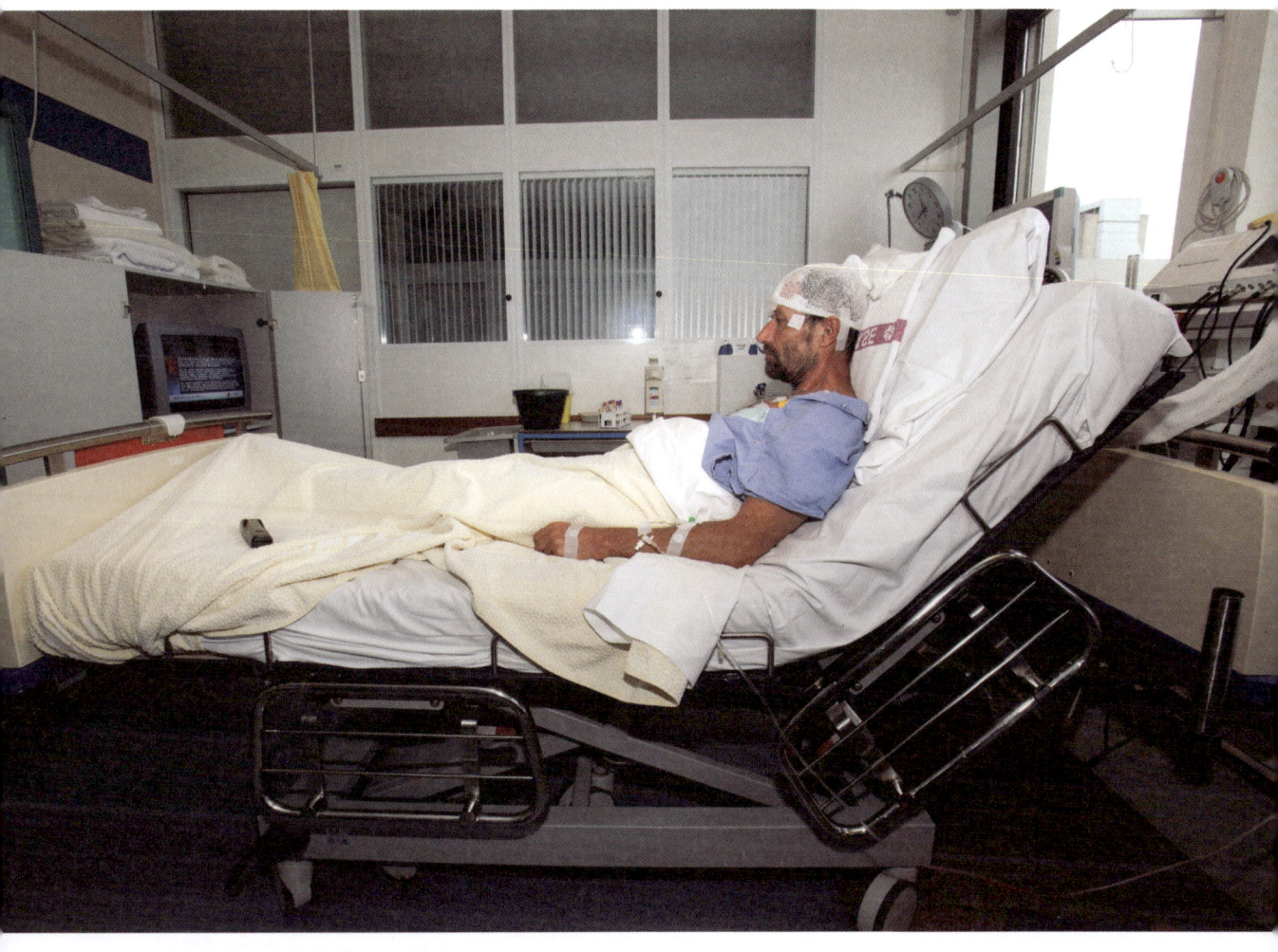

I showed voluntary control over the autonomic nervous system and innate immune system. "But you are an anomaly, an exception, a freak of nature," they said. I responded, "Anything I can do, anybody can do." That resulted in a comparative study which led to the incredible finding. Yes, anybody can influence their own systems!

Give your best,

and the best will come

Patients. Patience, so close

Heal the gaps we suffer from

where faith comes back full force.

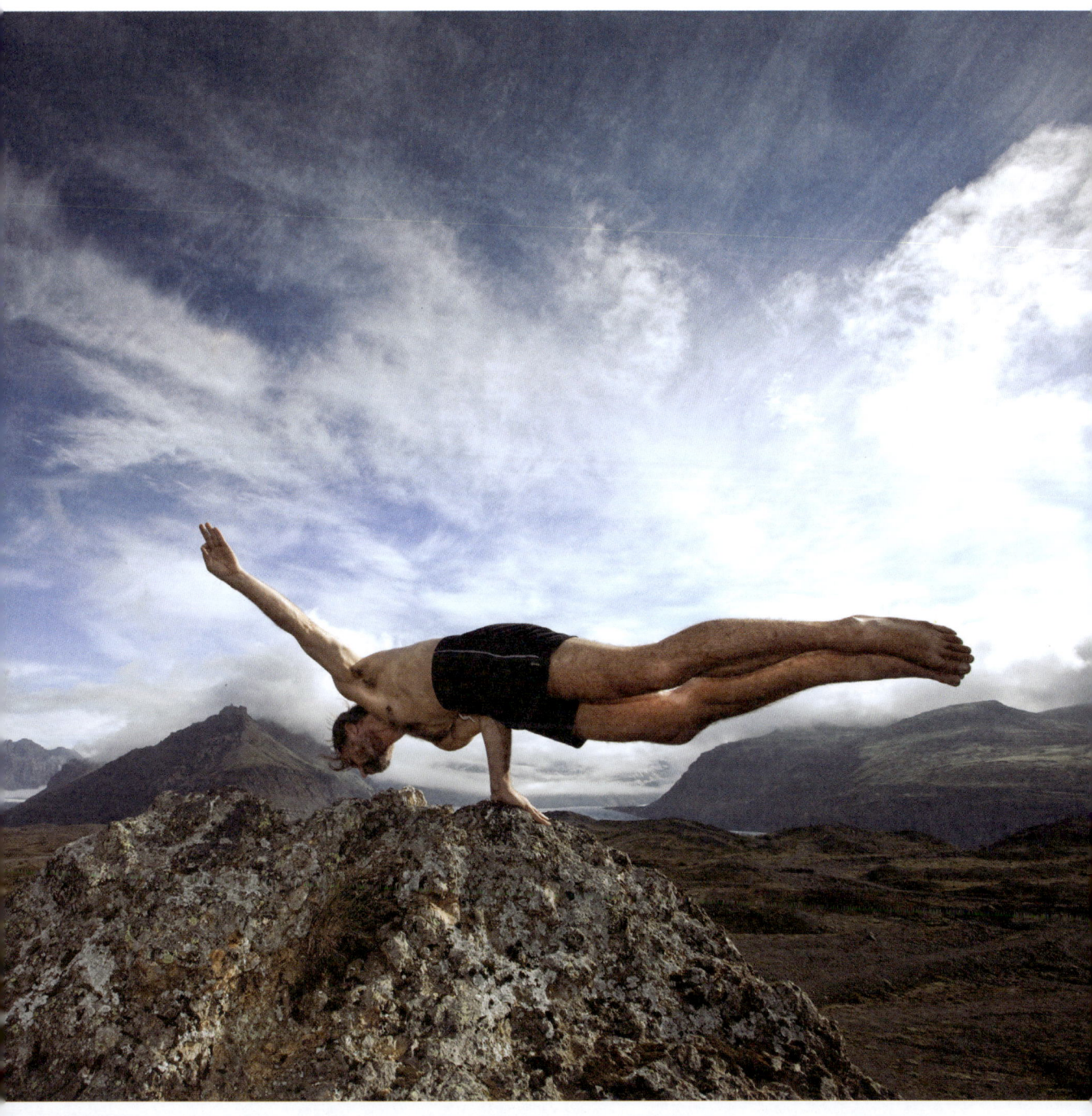

Iceland, summertime. Almost twenty-four
hours of light. Strange phenomenon.

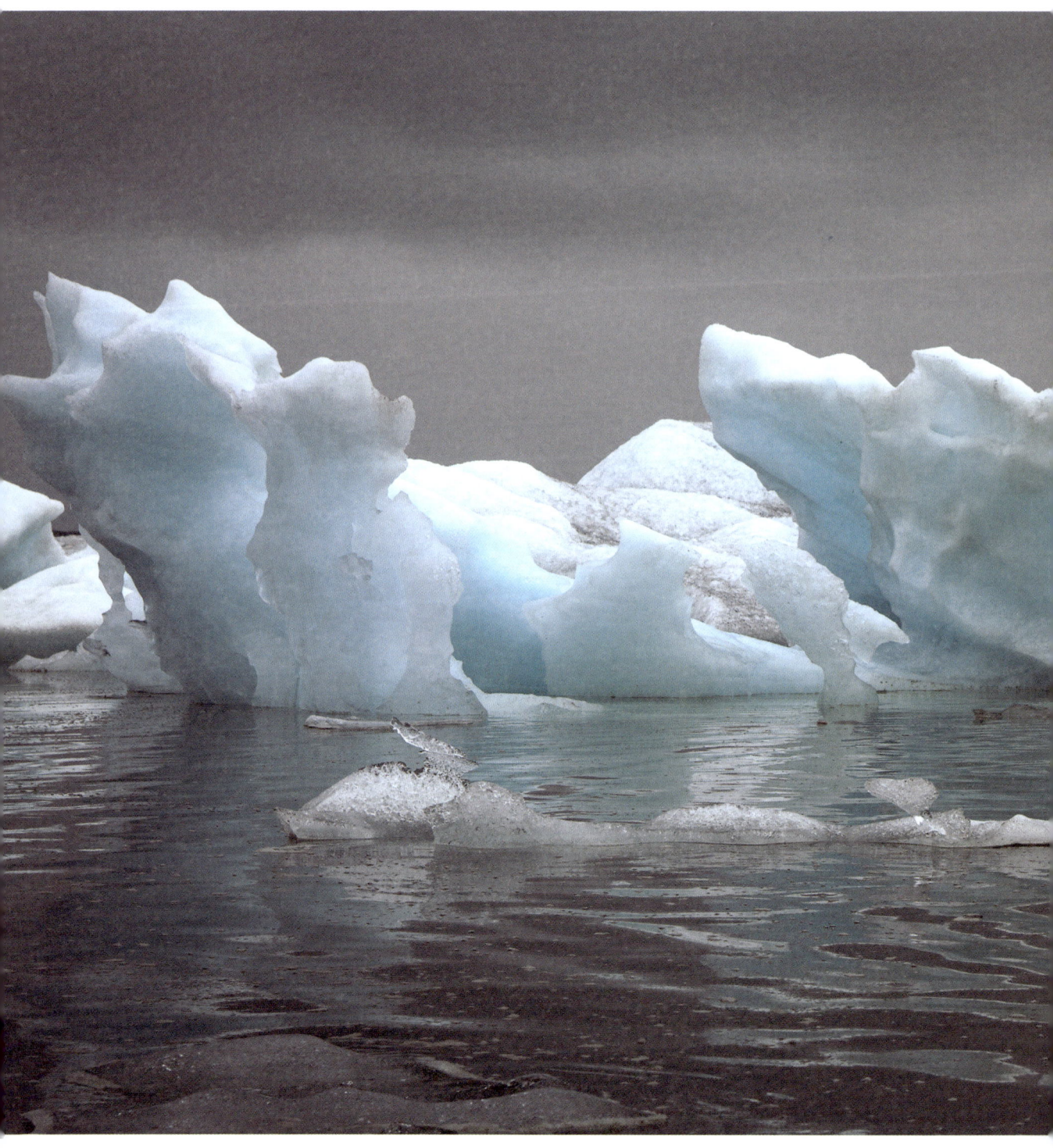

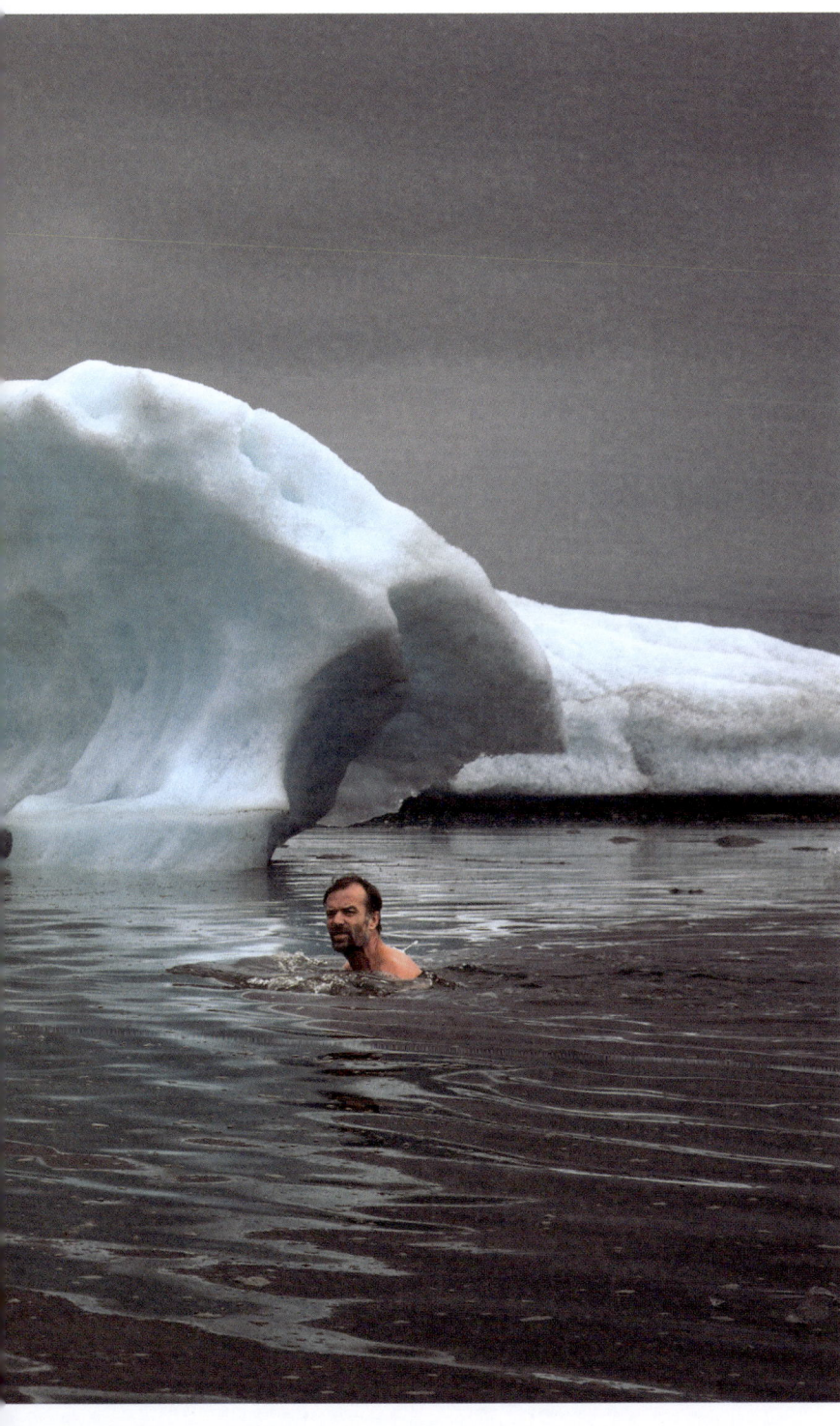

The beauty of icy
sculptures made by
the hands of nature.

It changes twenty-four
hours a day. An ongoing
display of cold beauty.

I want to be part
of that anytime.

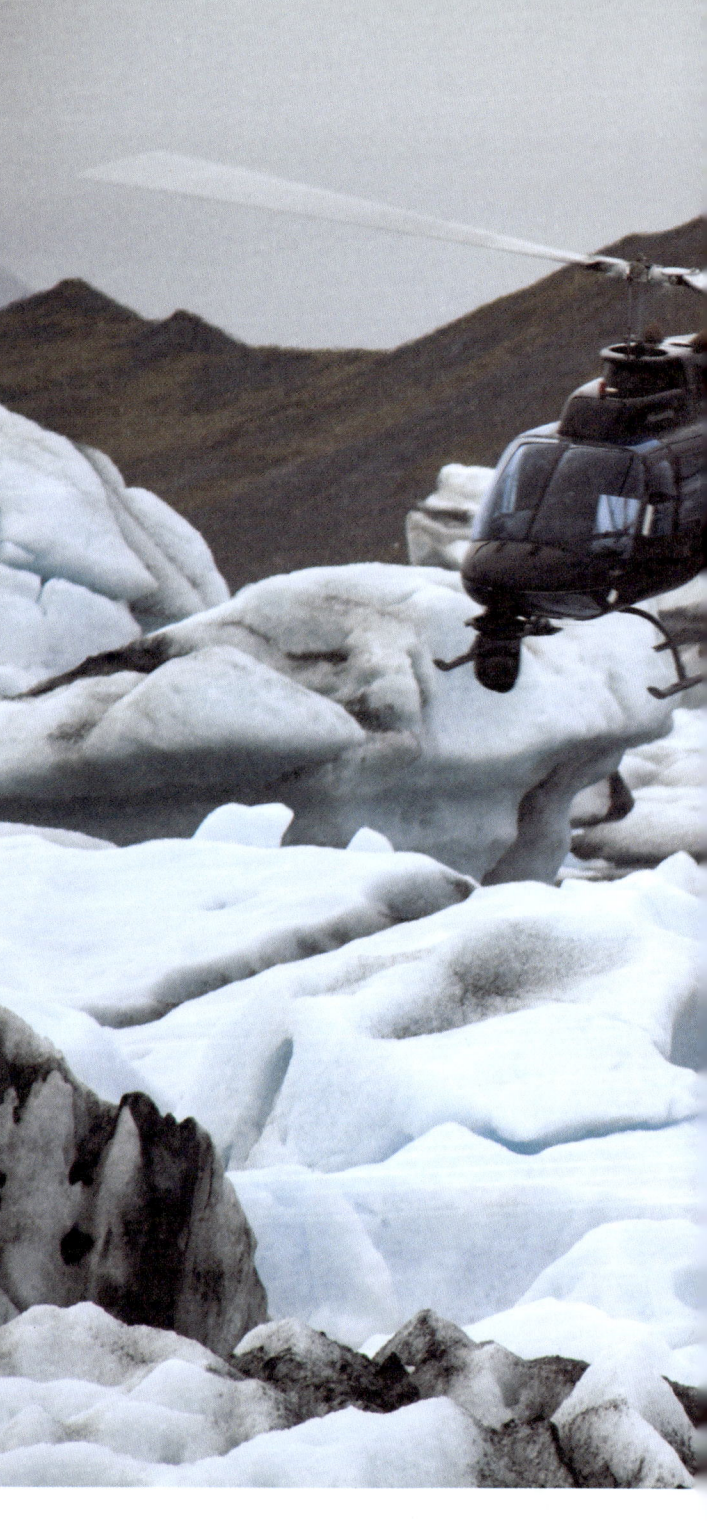

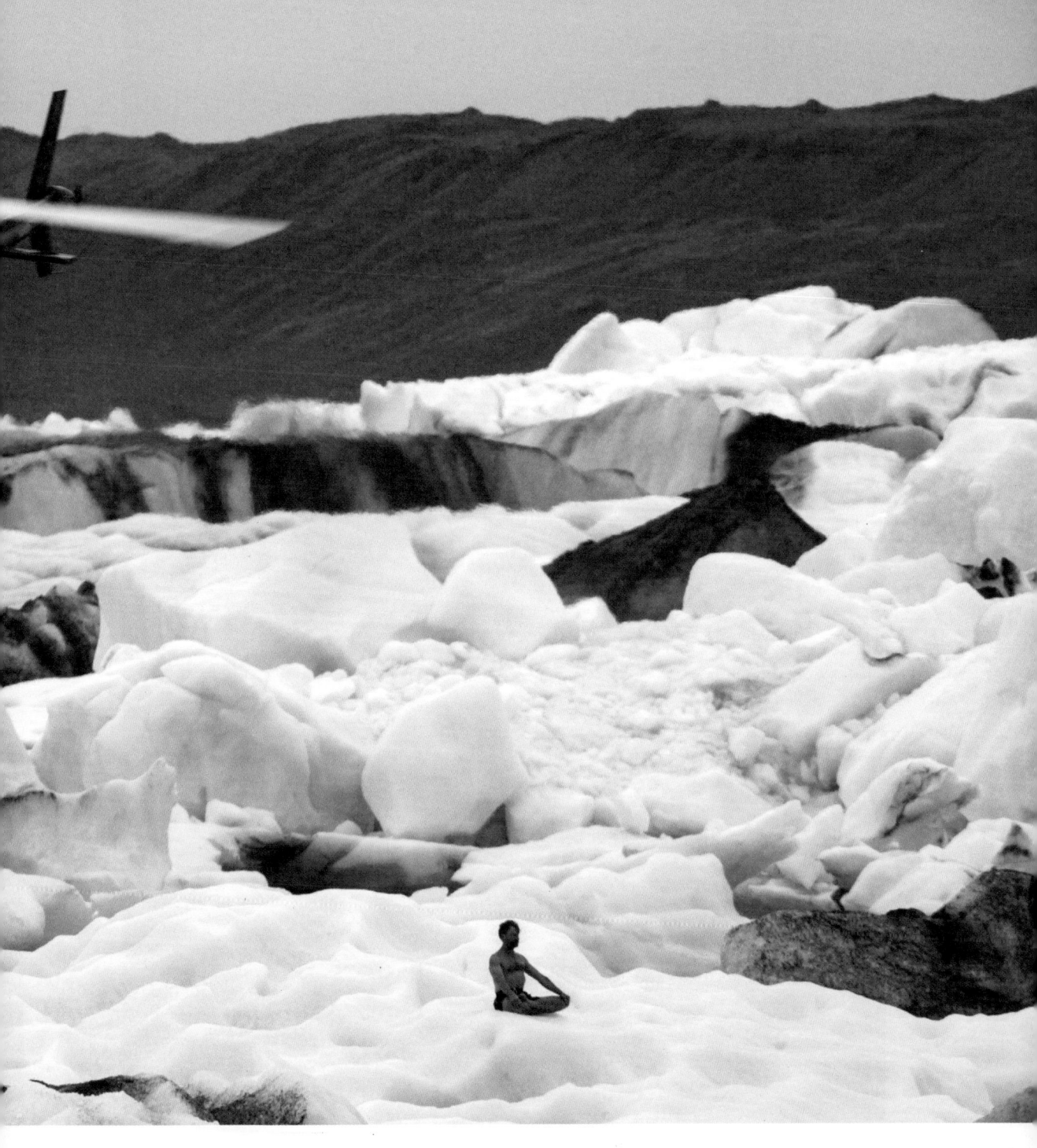

BBC documentary in the making before we had
drones. Technology advances. Our spirits, too?

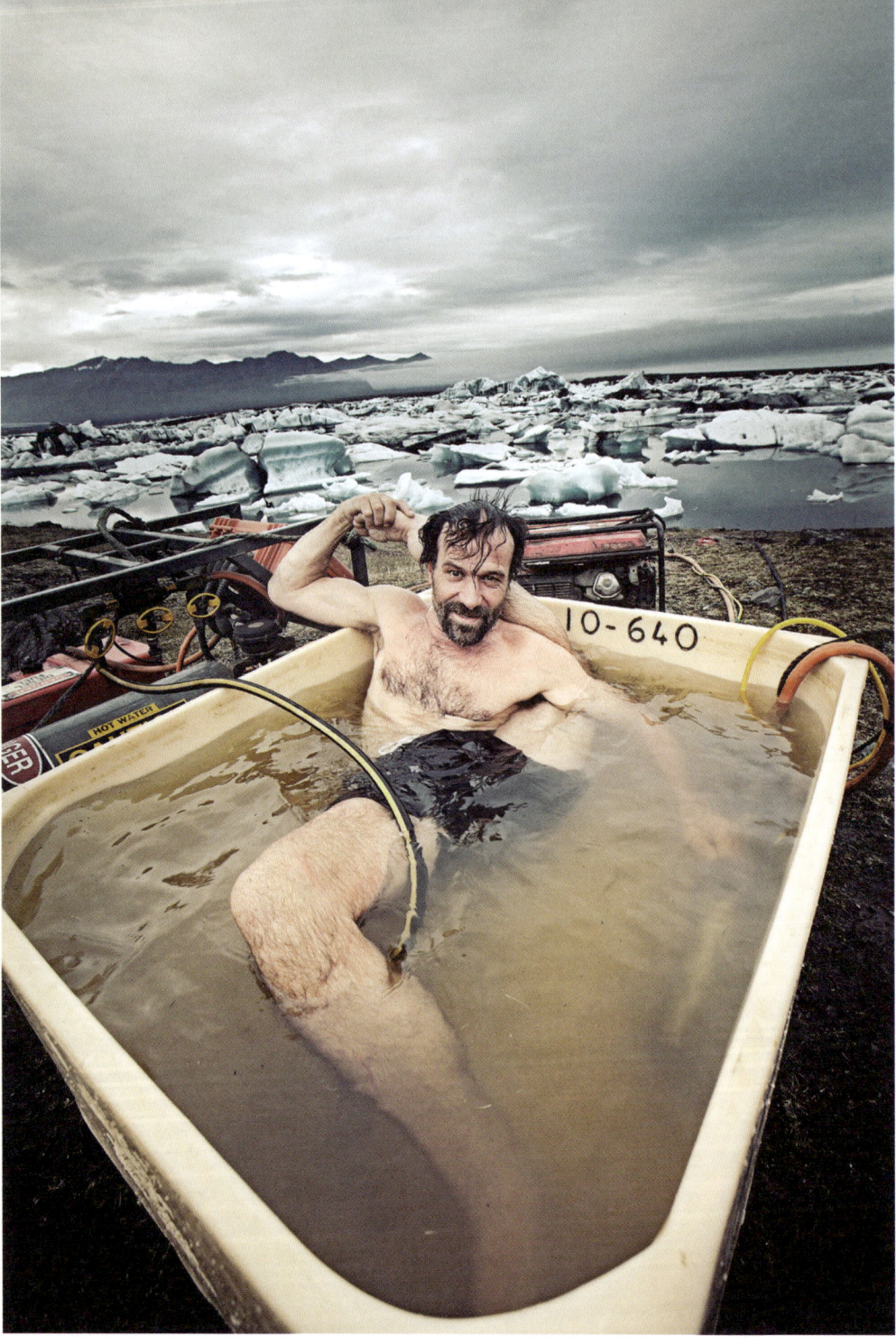

Locking myself up in a warm bath after cold swimming.
Part of the "from the top" scene after scene. Fun, too.

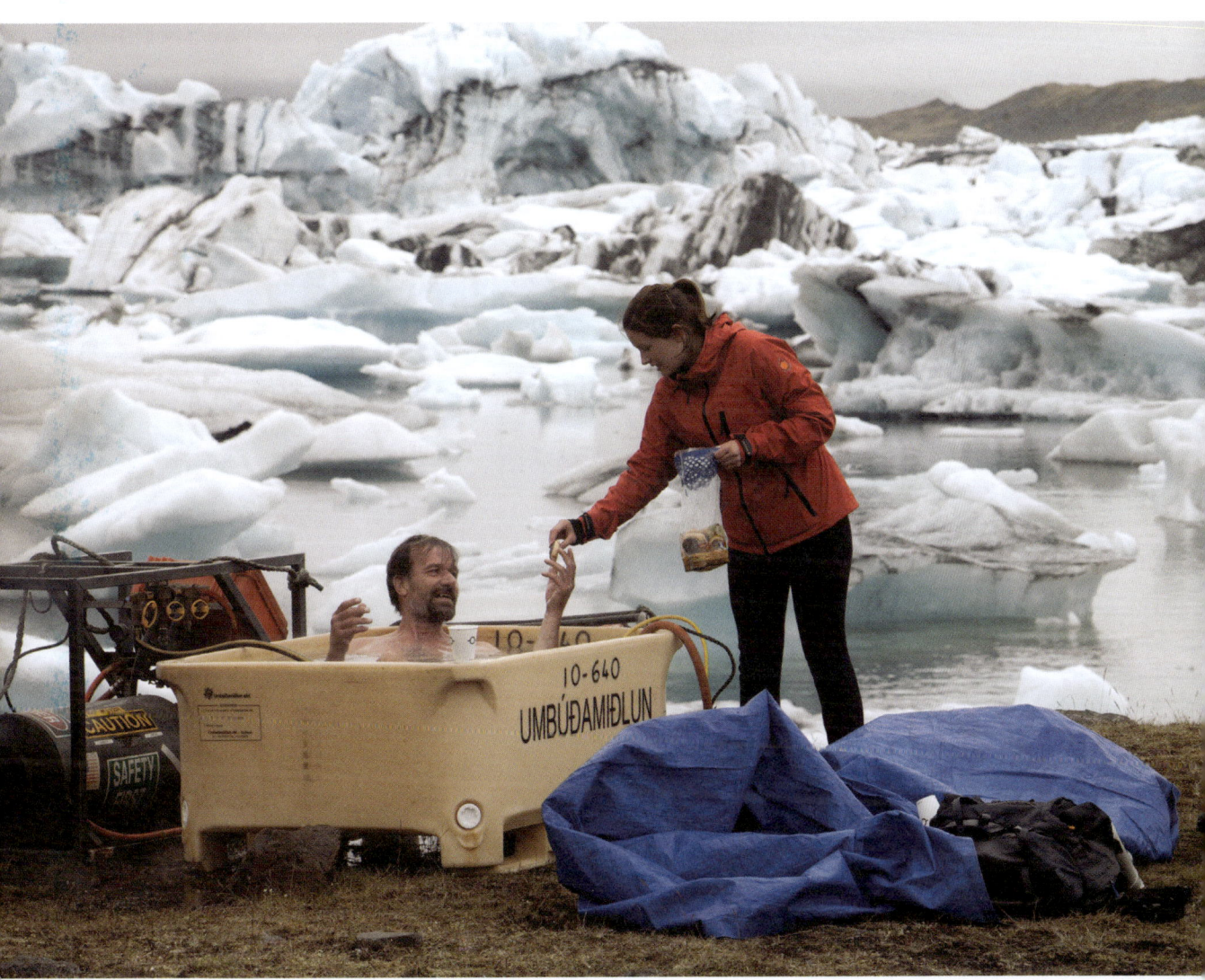

What a setting. Getting coffee while being in a hot tub. After thirty years of training alone, suddenly I am being treated like a VIP.

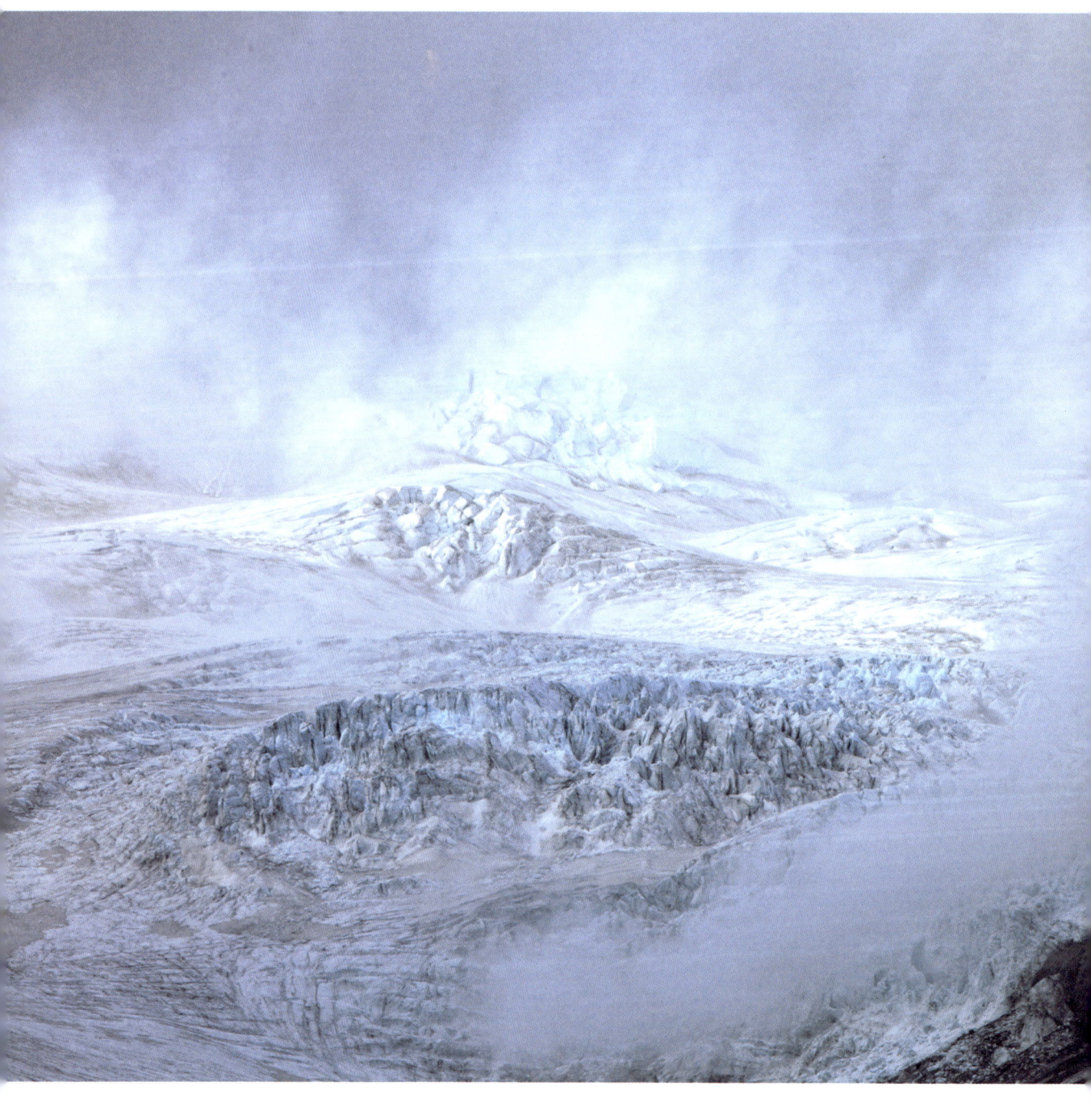

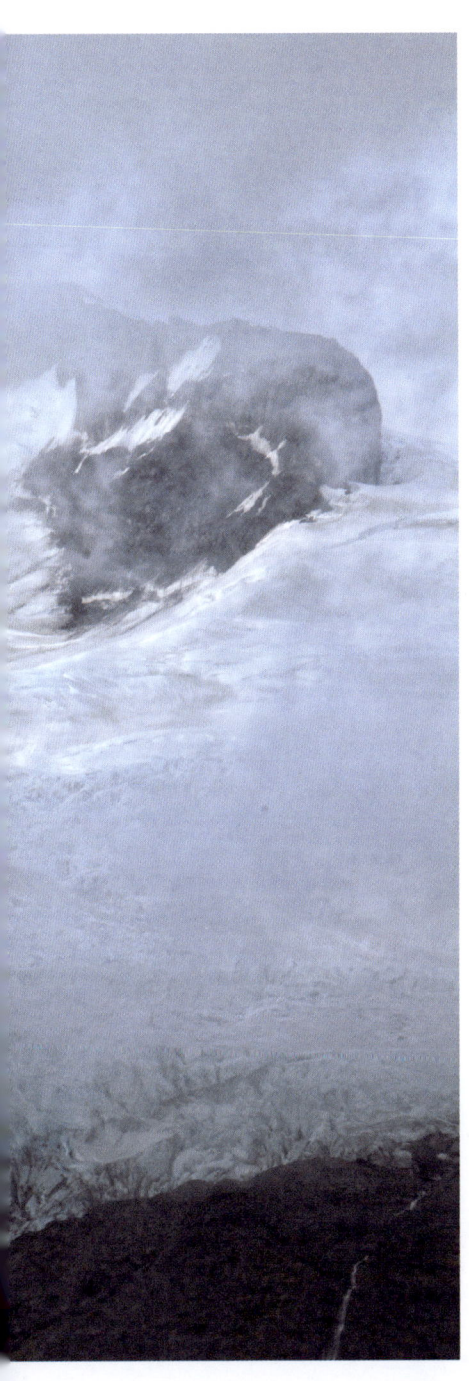

The icy white, the mists, the silence
Speaks more than thousands of words.
You can hear whispers
when you stand still enough.

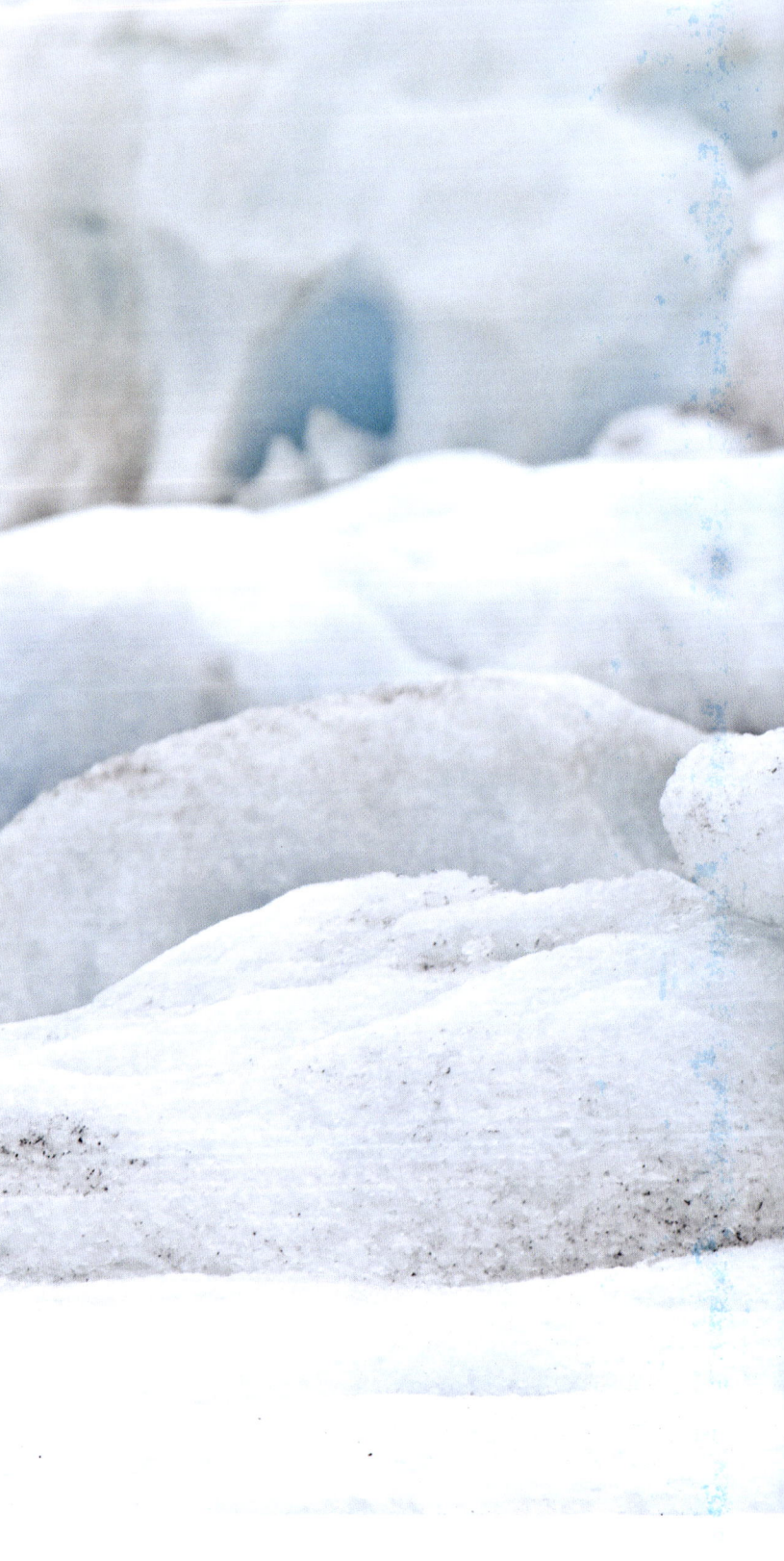

From the top in the
cold freeze!
It looks like the body is doing
nothing, yet internally, you boil.

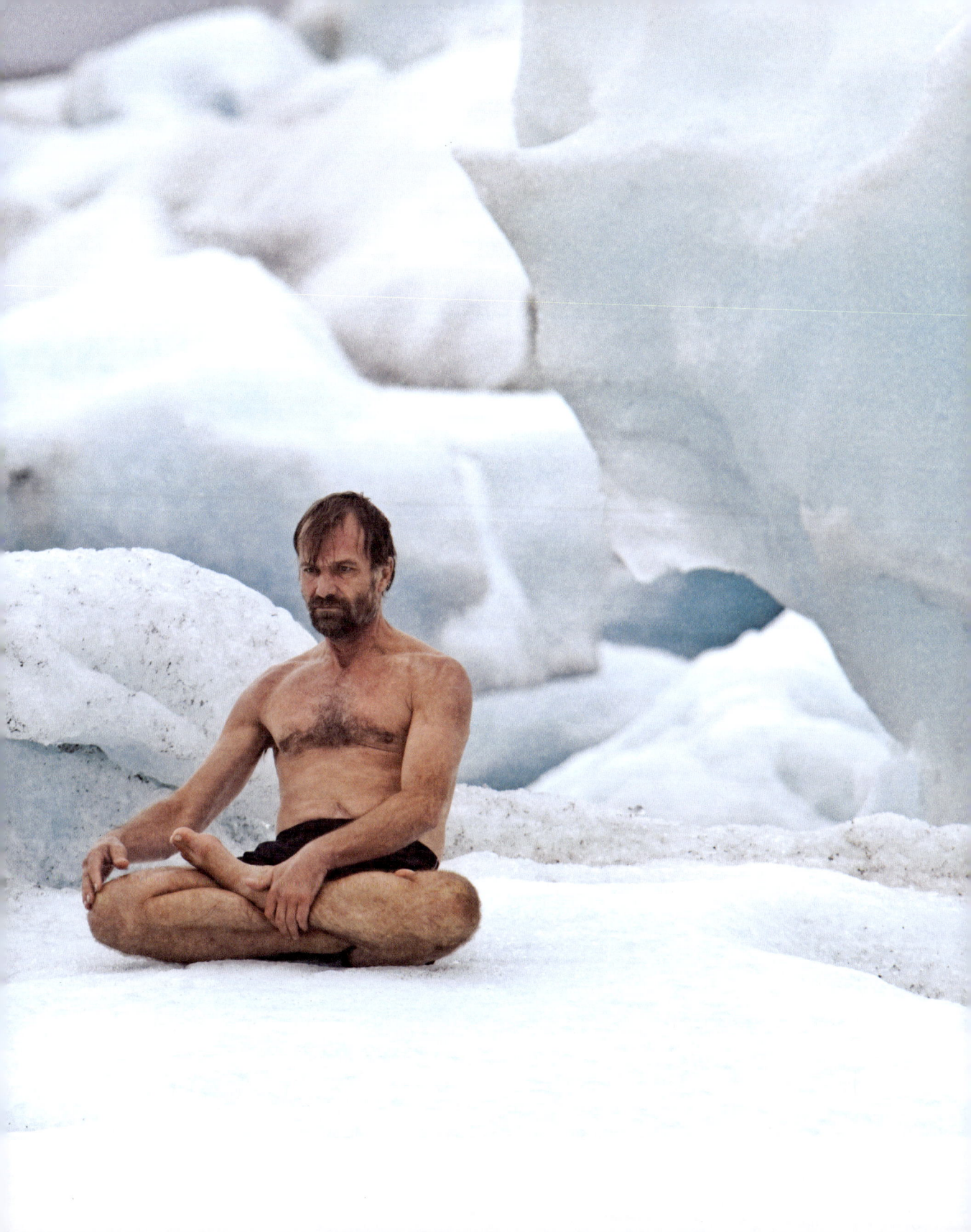

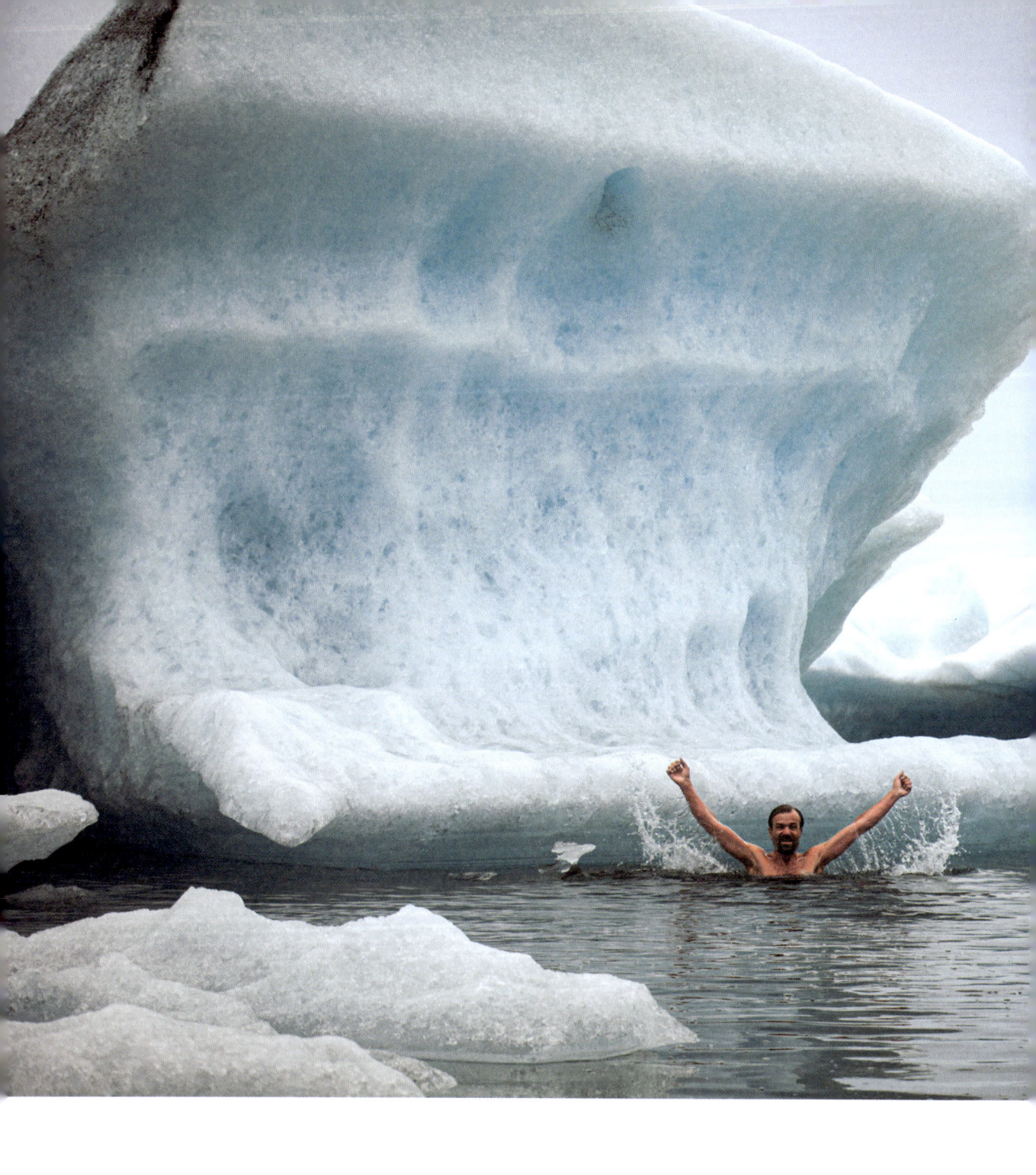

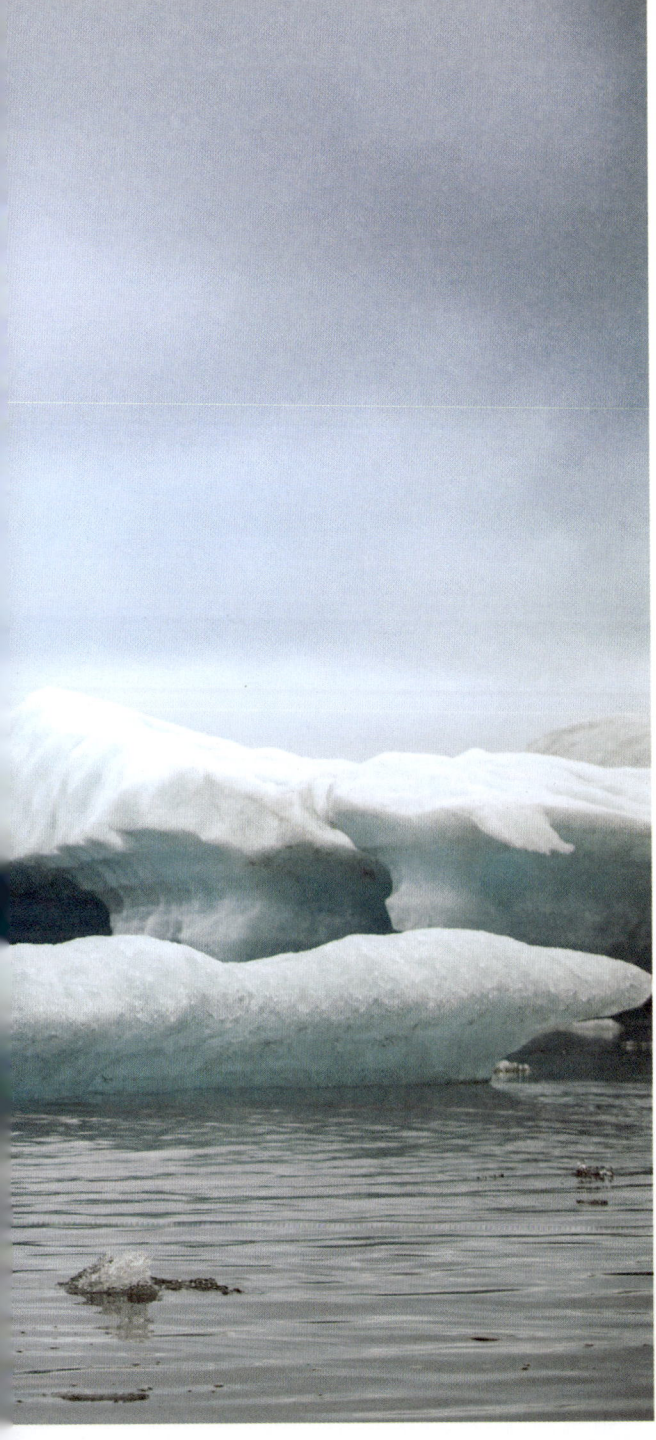

Great memories and a good shot.
It was hard to raise my body out
of the water and then spread
my arms up in the air. Victory.

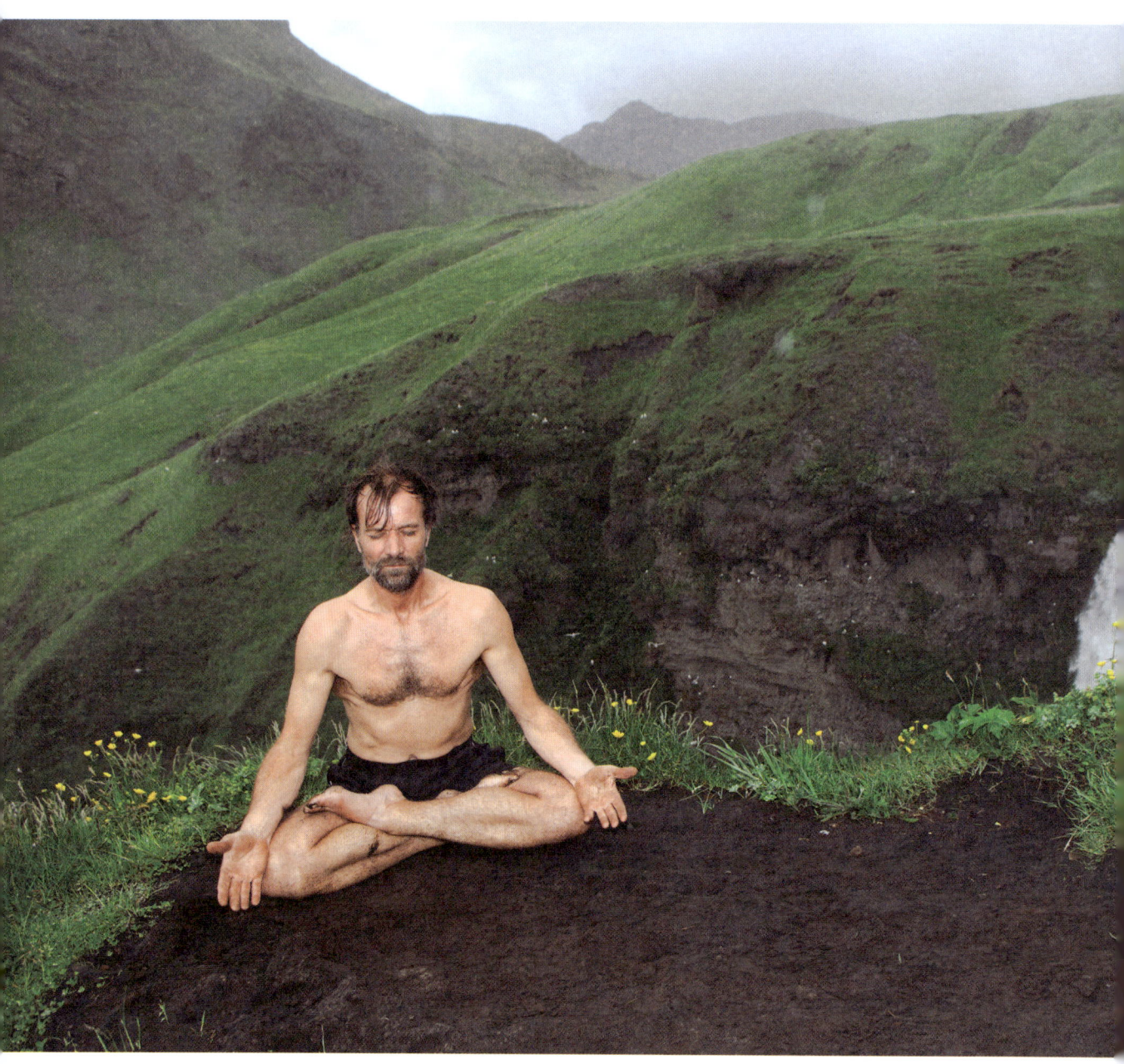

Iceland is volcanic. Black soil. Very fertile.

A deep breath goes deeper than the deepest meditation.

Breathe and be.

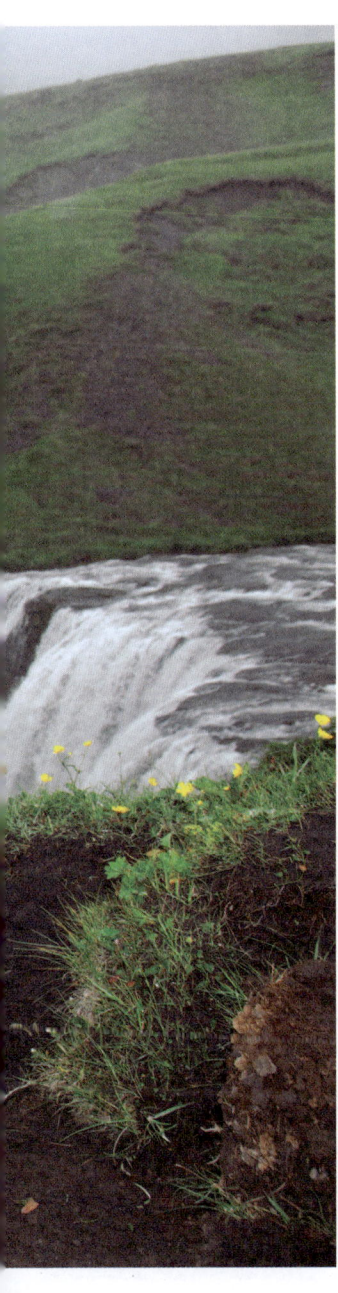

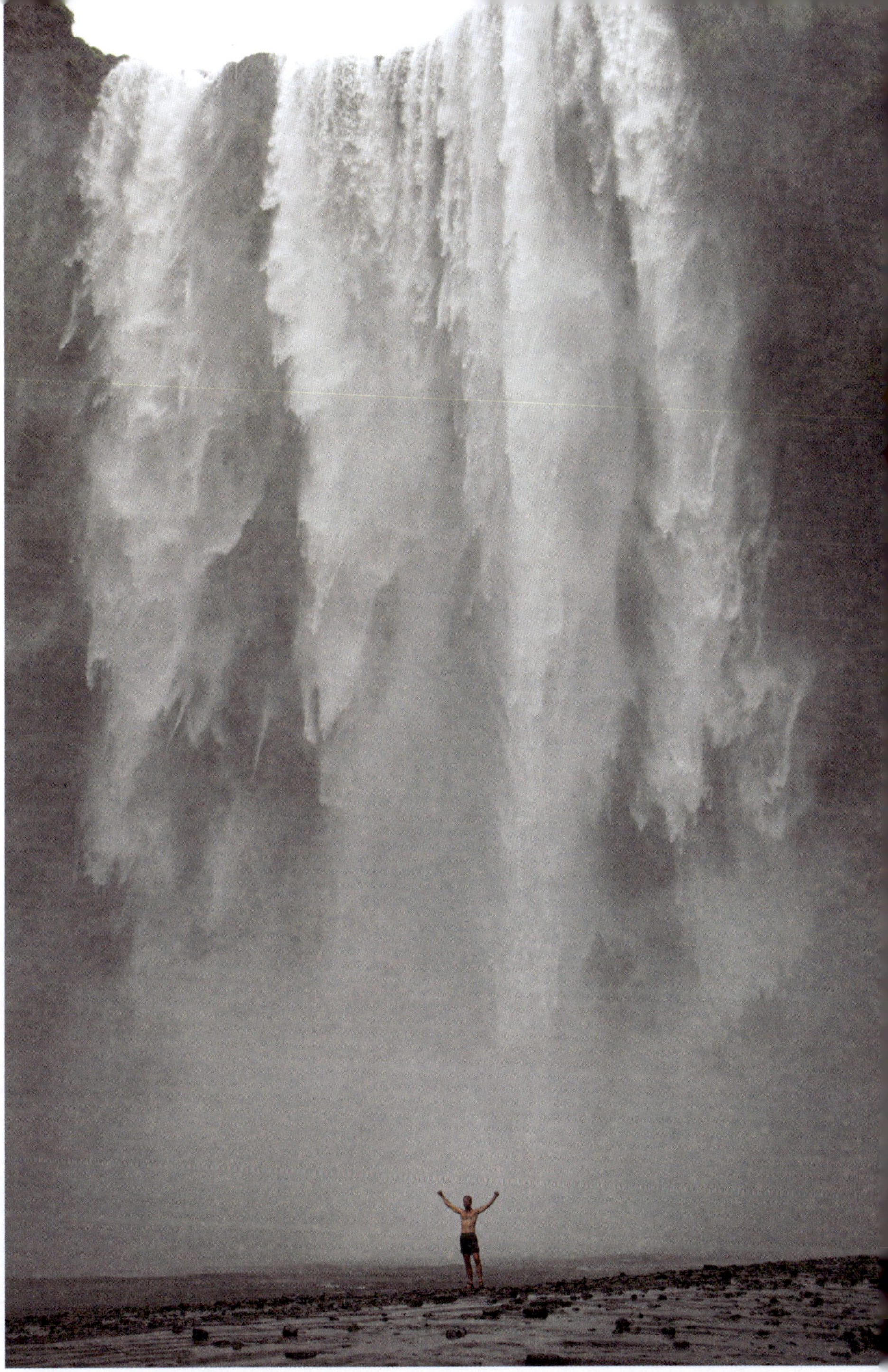

Iceland cascade.

Stay humble and be great, humbly.

In the end we only begin to understand.

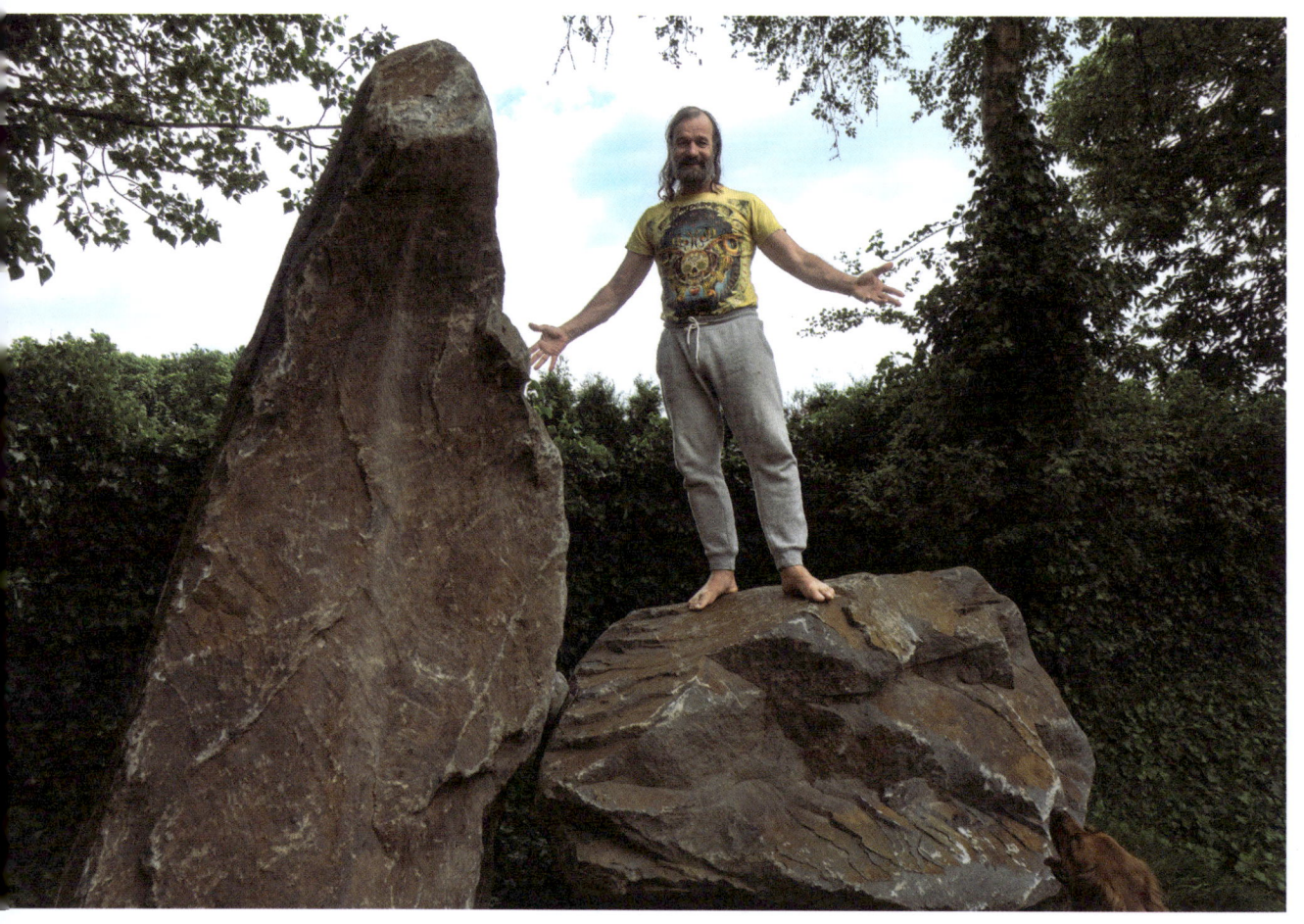

Stroe, Netherlands, at the Wim Hof Method
center, loving the rocks. The one on the left is
our guardian of the center, looking like Mary.

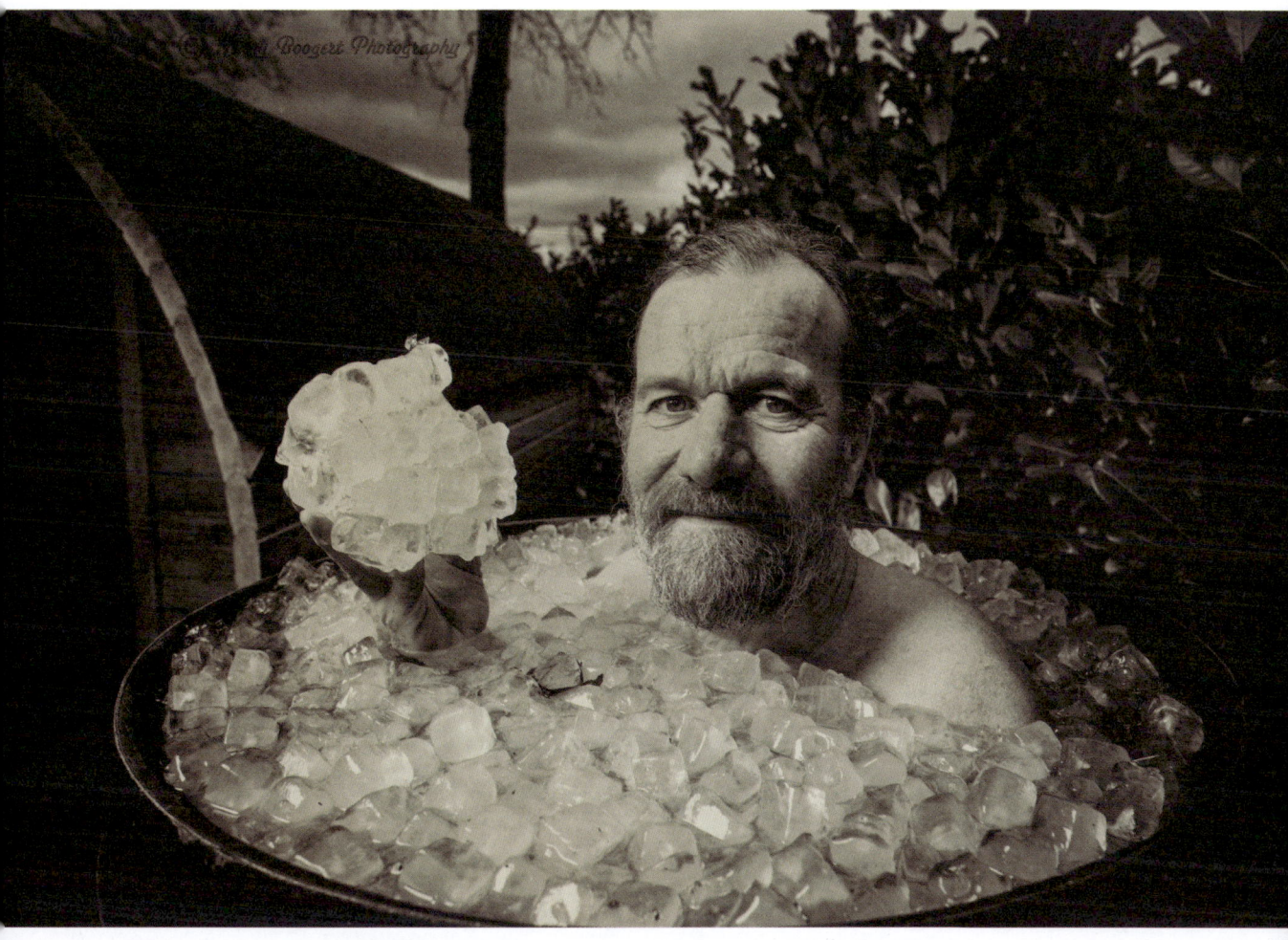

I'm still doing the same discipline
as always, but now the whole
world is joining me. I love it!

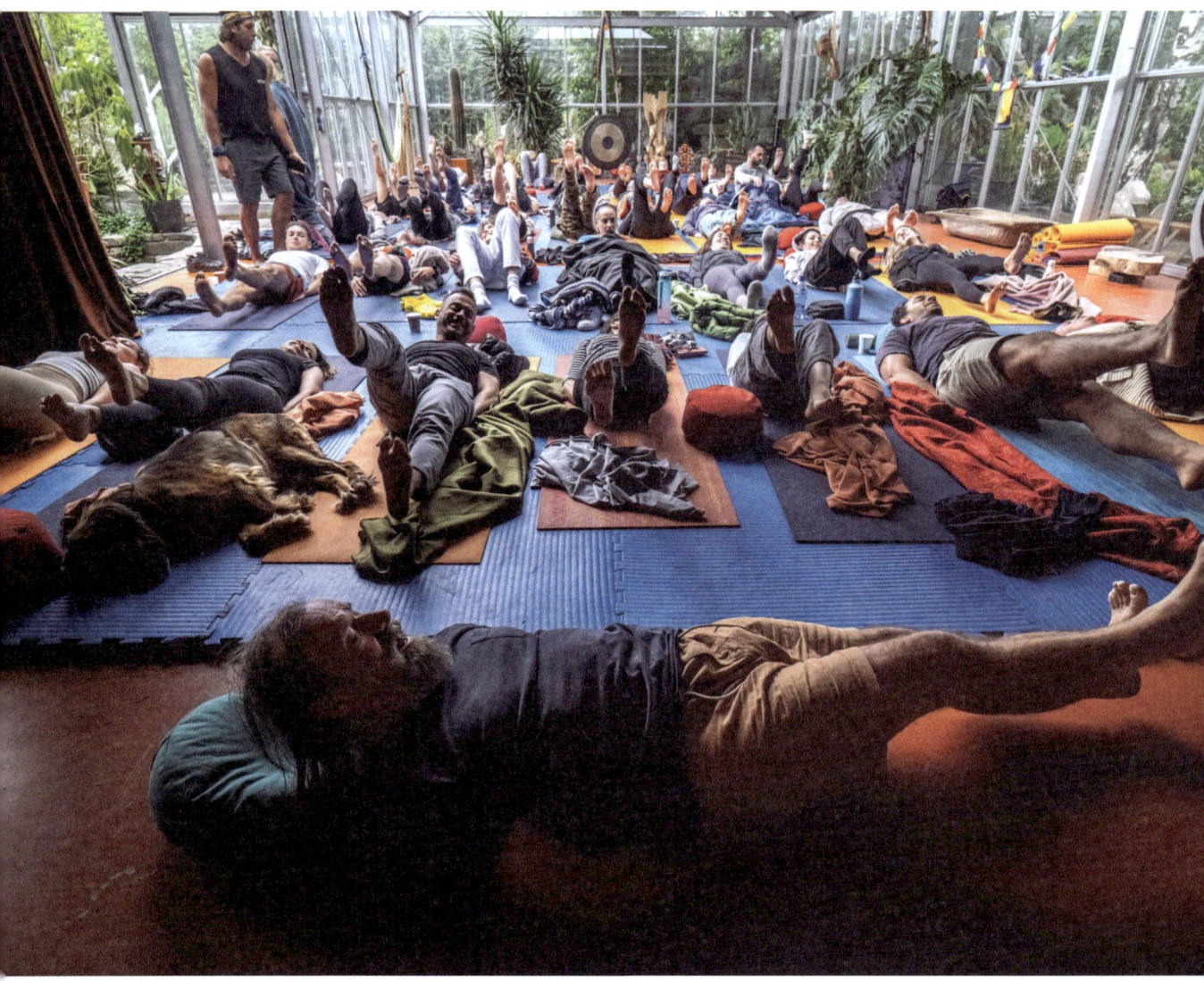

Scissor kicks for five minutes. Bang! Learning to
stay in the moment and not in the pain.

Thus connecting with the periaqueductal gray hemisphere,
deep in our brain where opioids and cannabinoids are
activated. We can have much better control over that!

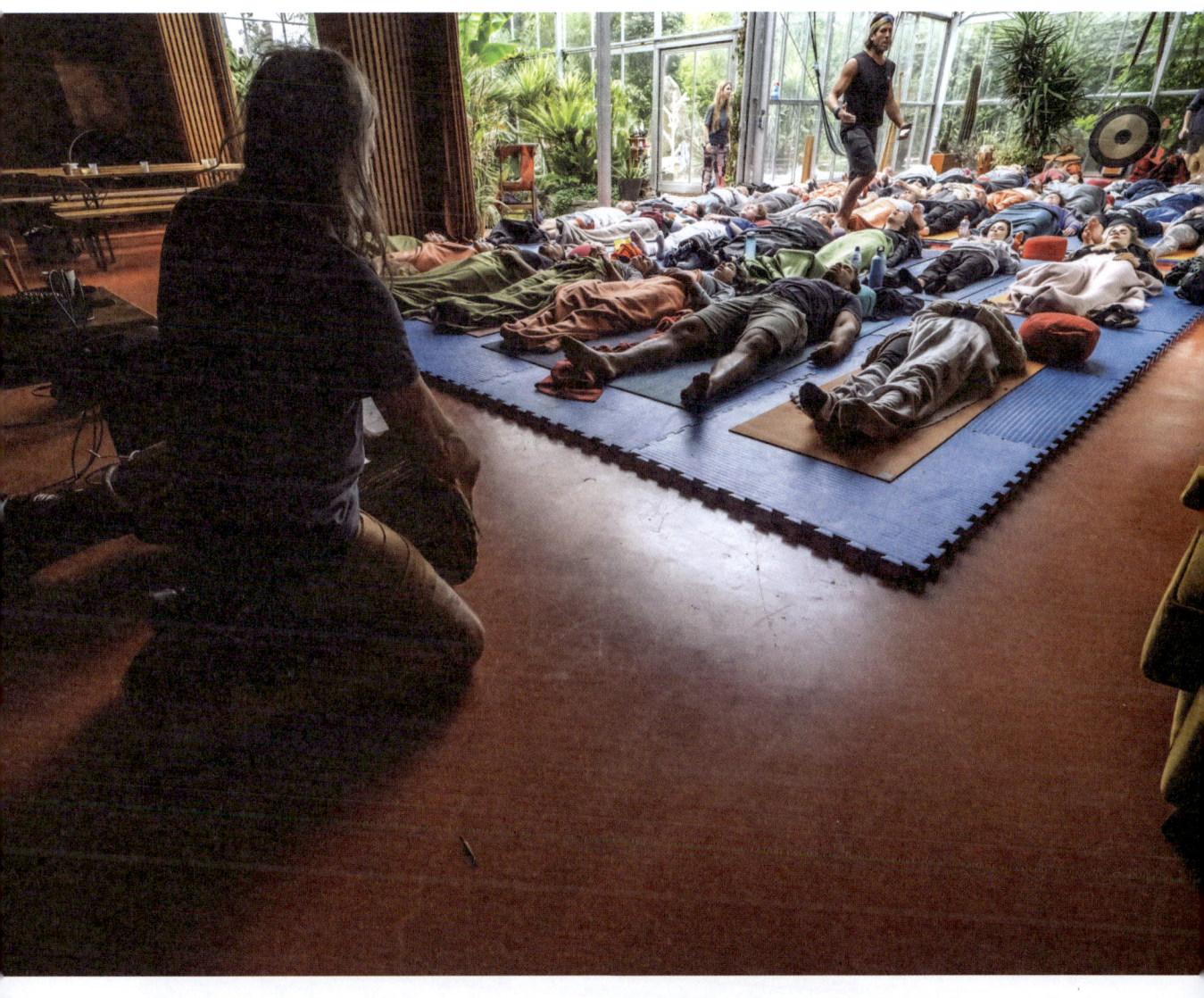

Breathing exercises through our conditioned mind and
body bring us into the absolute depth of our being.

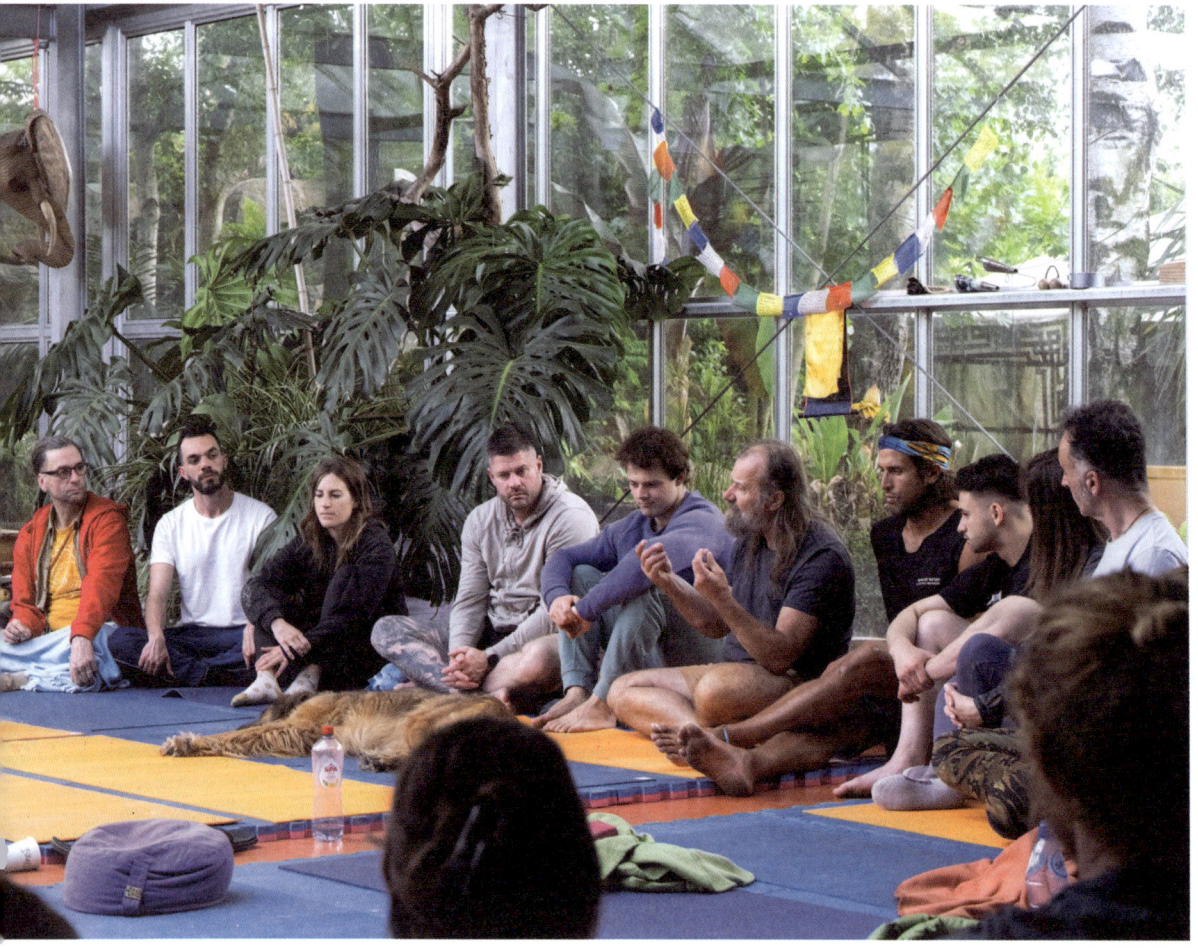

Sharing is caring from the heart.

It is so interesting to hear people opening from the heart instead of the mind. From confidence instead of protocol, about emotions instead of thoughts.

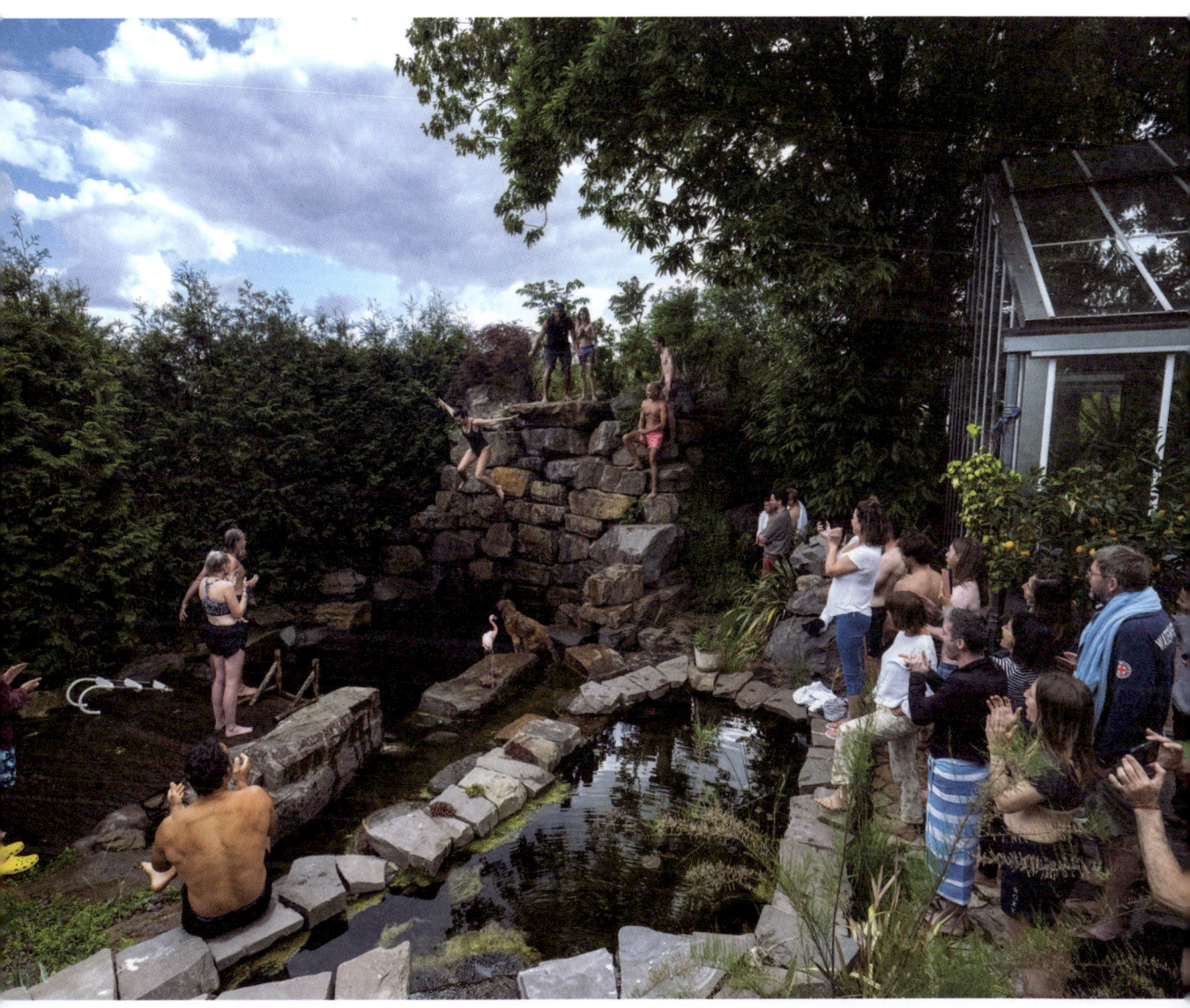

My backyard has become a garden where we play,
challenge, and meet Soul to Soul. Like a family.

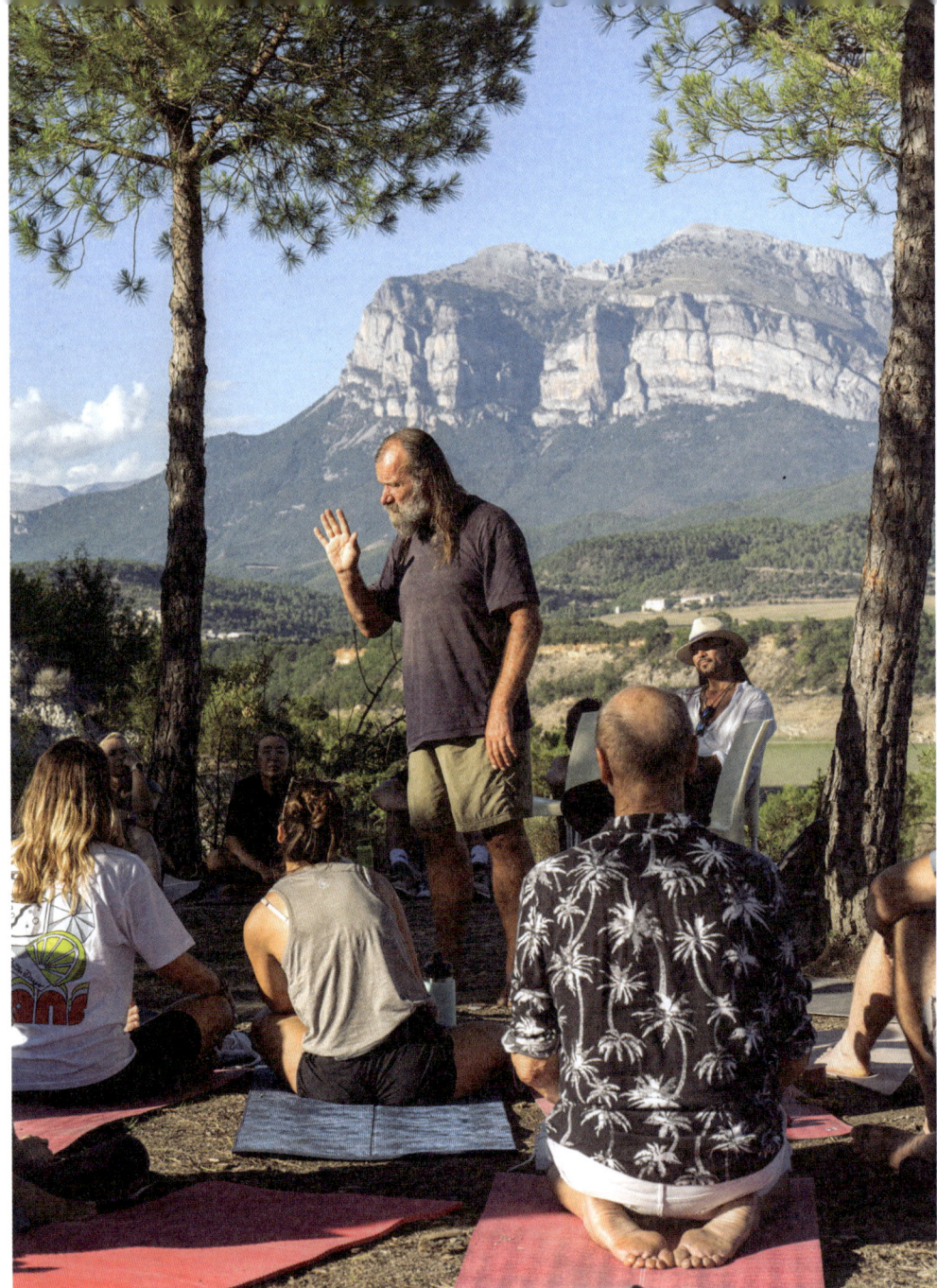

Full circle, back in Spain. The same region. Echoes of the past.

We have our morning speech, intention, breathing, how
to change our brain patterns and find depth.

In the background, the mountain-like rock is
La Peña Montañesa (2,260 meters).

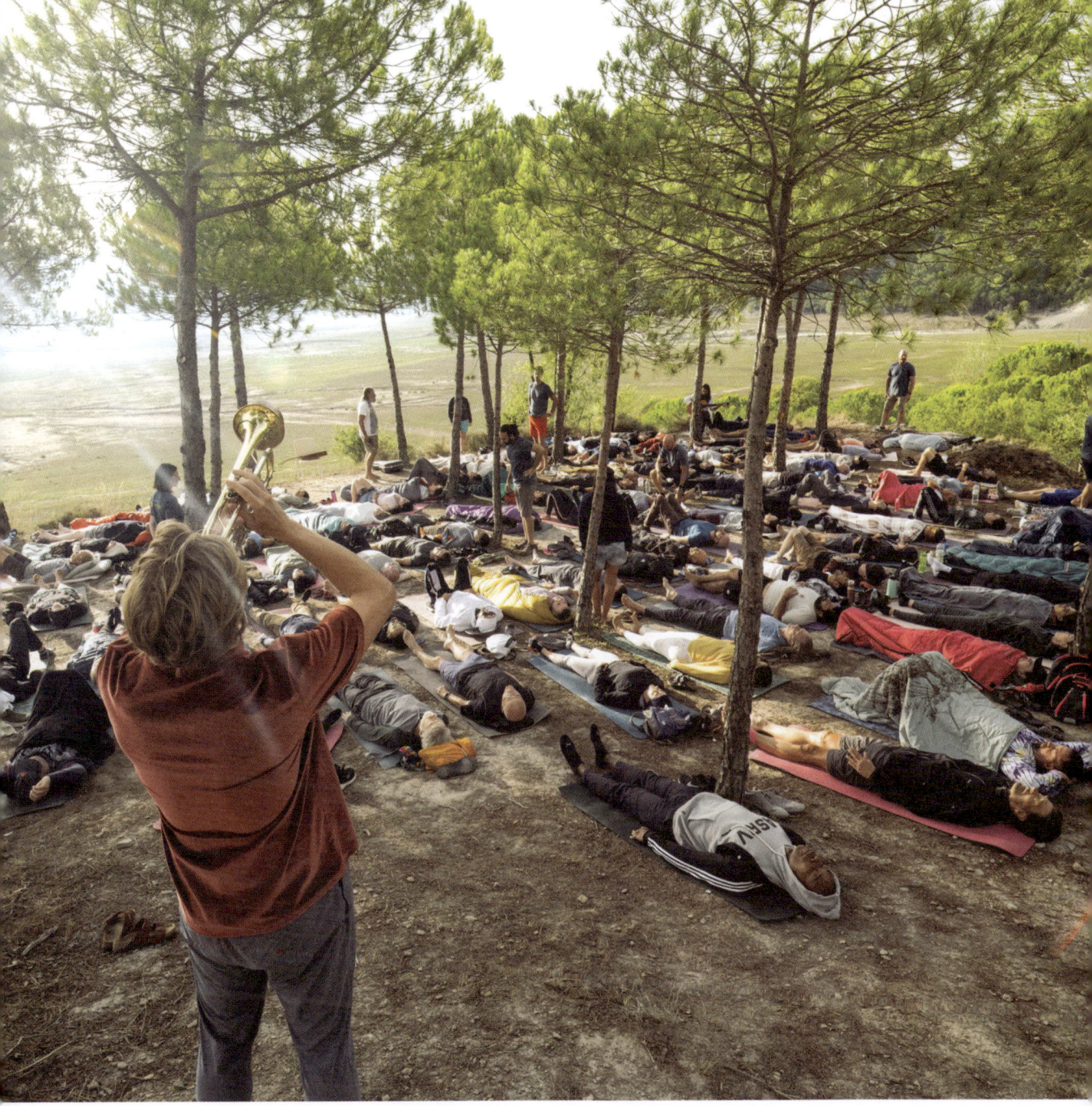

Live music and breathing past conditioned body and
mind. Into the depths, into the now, the clarity of it all.
Morning session in Morillo de Tou, Spanish Pyrenees.

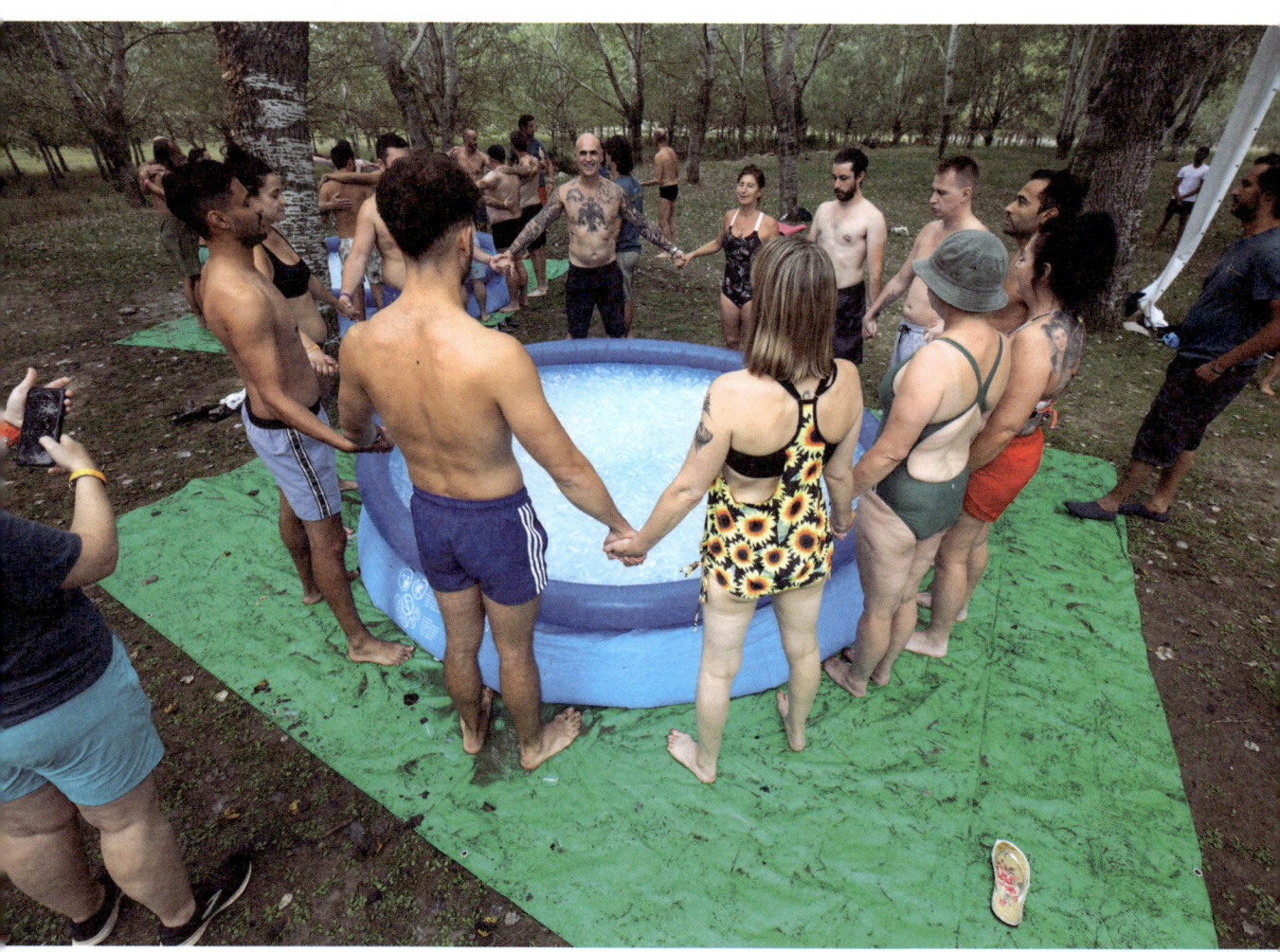

The cold unites past our individualistic
mind; no ego, but we go.

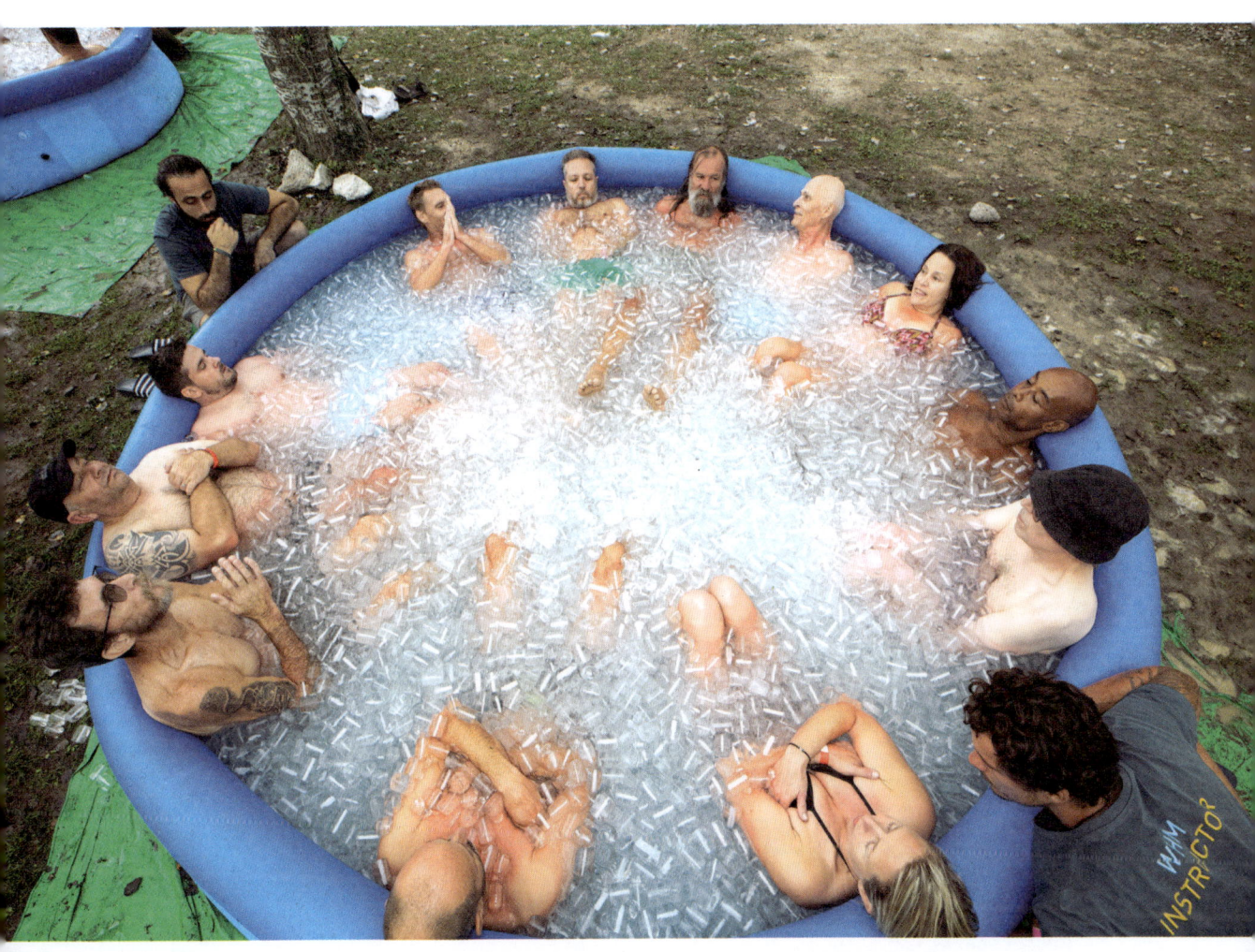

Let the body do what the body is able to do!

Deep meditation is naturally there, so you
can let go. We can automatically connect
neurologically with the deep brain.

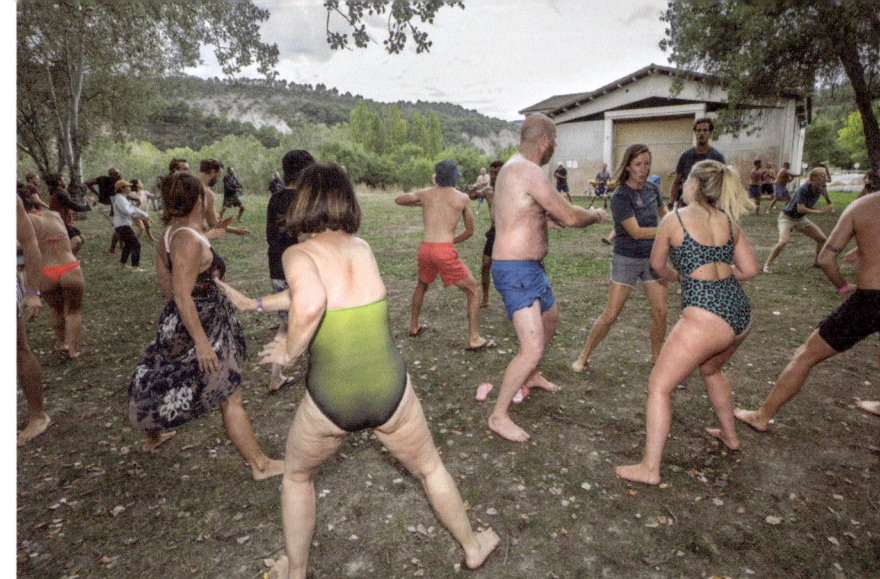

Horse stance after an ice bath of at least ten minutes. It helps bring back the blood flow in a natural way. The sense of accomplishment is amazing, as if you have gone from survival to valuing life as it is. Wonderful.

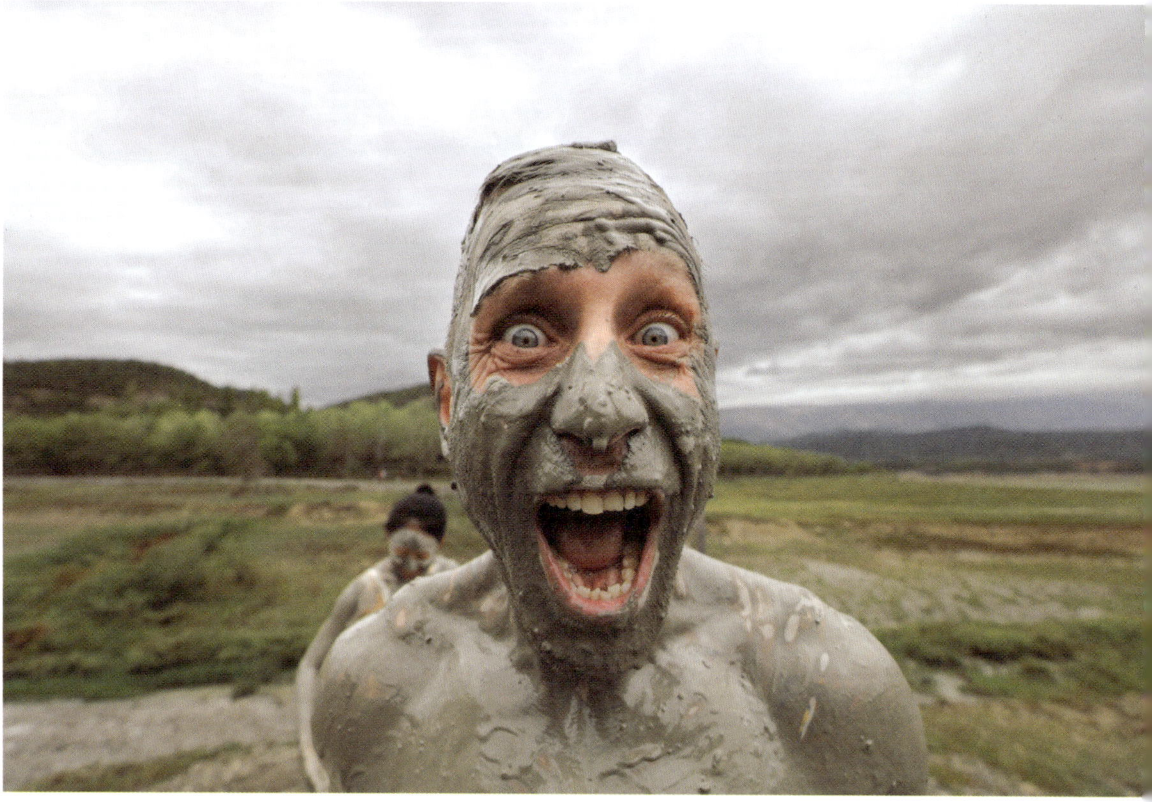

The mud bath is a part of the summer travels. One of my favorites. Great cleanser. We feel great after doing it.

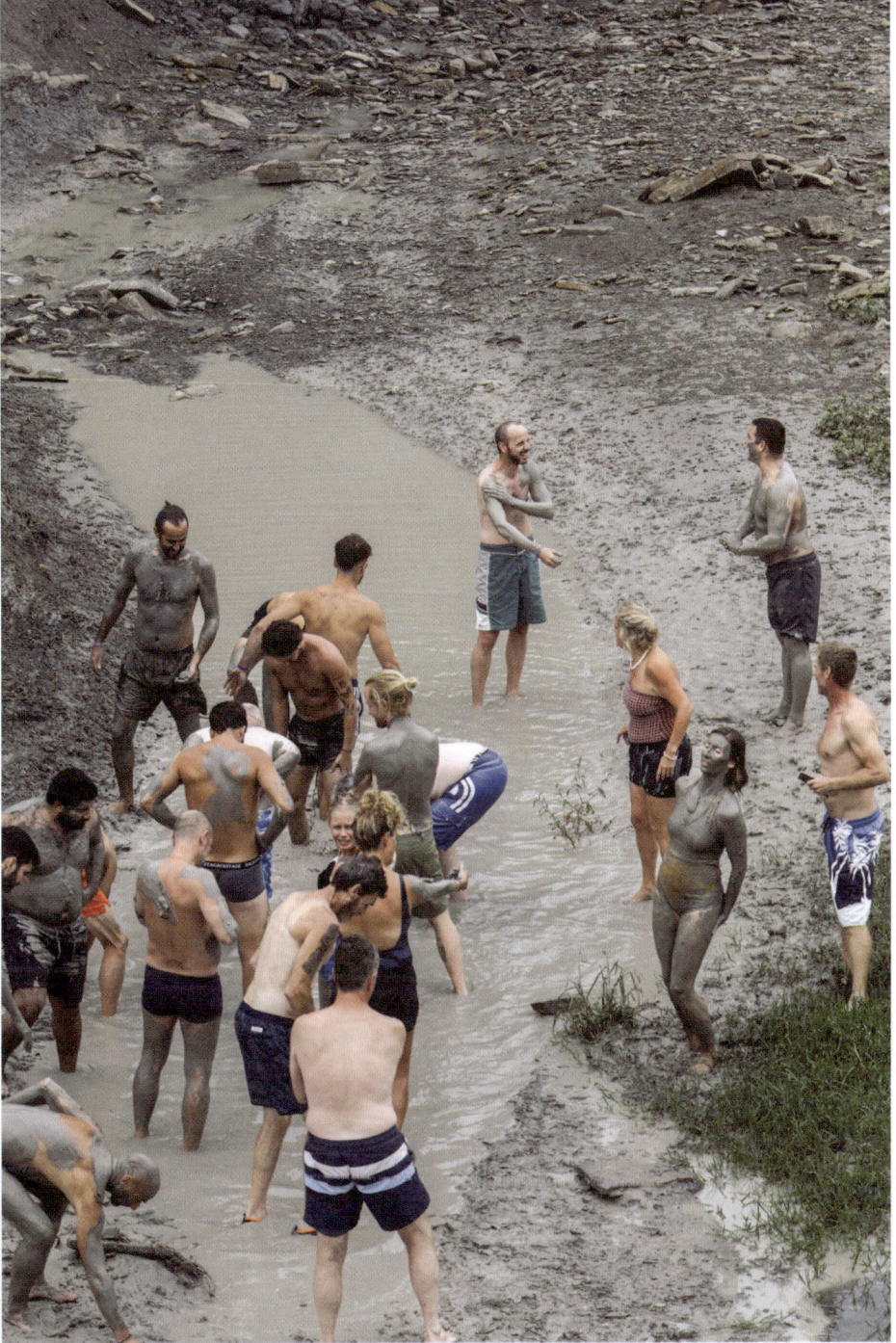

It's fun to dirty yourself with clay. Inhibitions go. We are getting dirty, or cleansed. What a joy it is to go with so many people, sharing fun and the pleasure of the earth while being in a state of heightened awareness. Disentangling thought patterns creates space and energy flow, while having superb fun. You can't fool people with stories; it has to be real. Feeling is understanding.

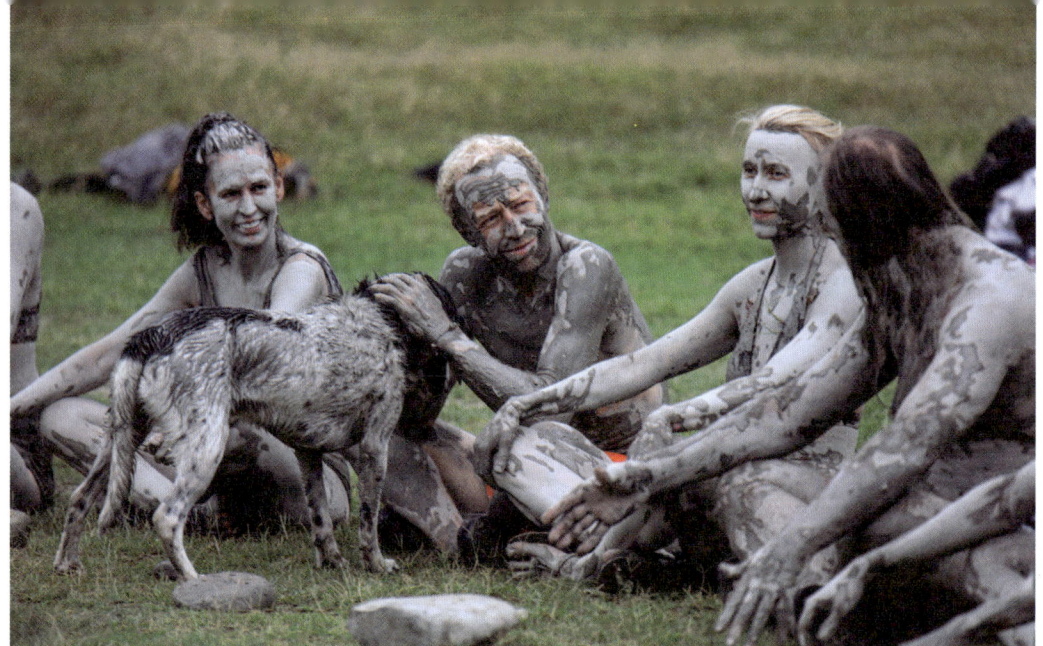

All the same color; the earth's
soil shows no politics.

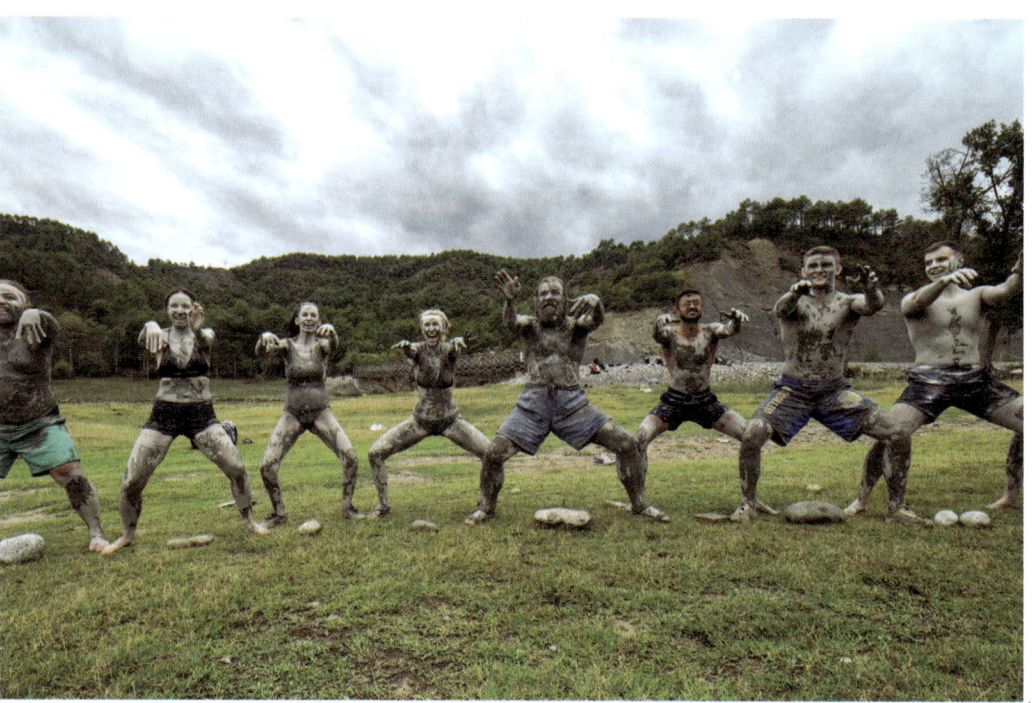

Horse stance ten minutes strong. Ice bath
fifteen minutes strong. Love strong.

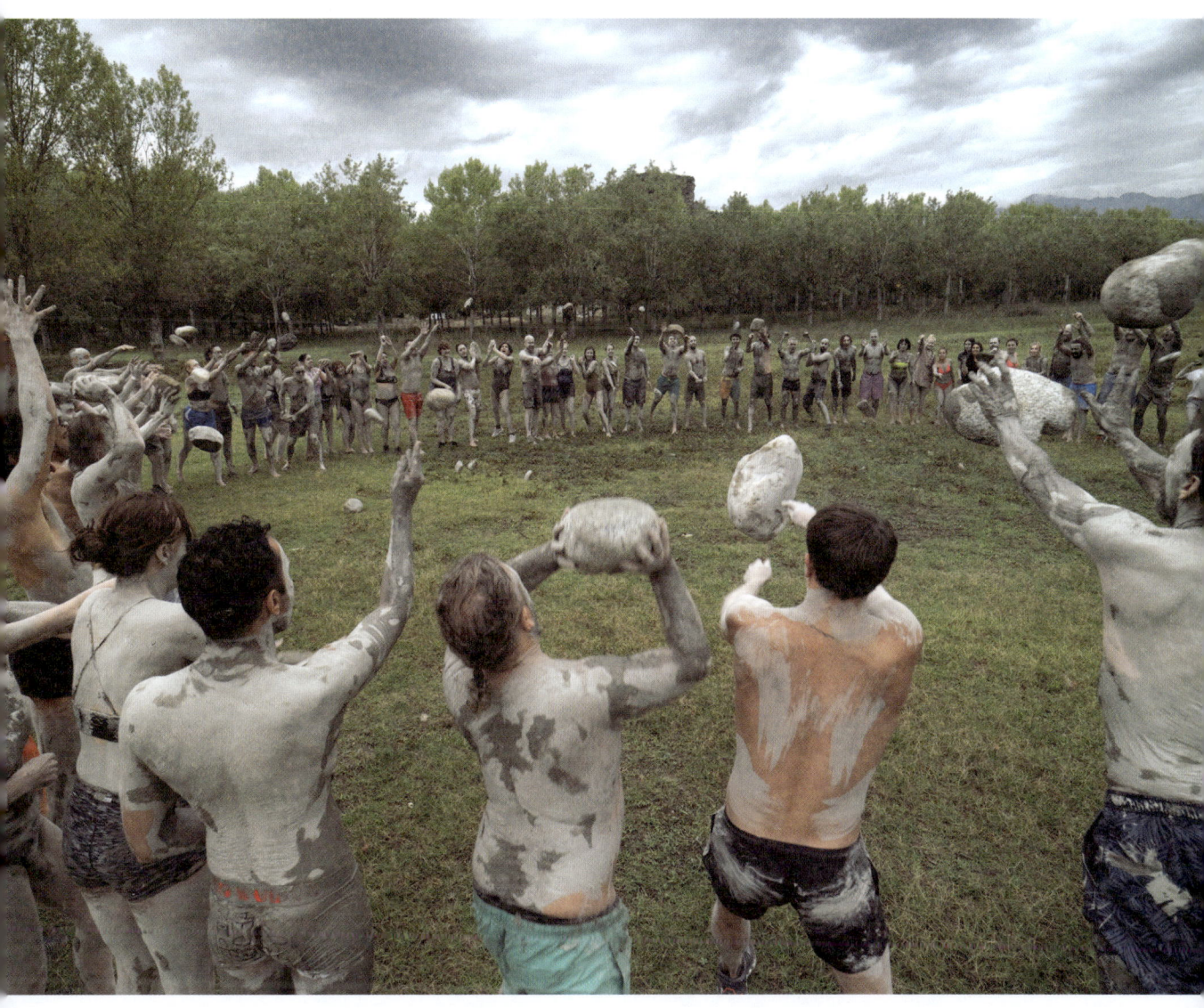

Stone Age. The rocks are loaded with
our willful intent to be thrown out. Go!

FROM THEART

When we see, infinity
The Soul, love, being free
When we feel that and be consciously there
Is when the sun starts shining through, simply

Aware

War is over, inner and out, the conflict gone, like

An overblown cloud

suppression, depression, all of the past

You are in the moment, bottomless depth

Take it all in, expand into the breath

Becoming as great as the heart can be

At your disposal sent out your psyche, free

There is no better way than you heart

Cut the tied up mind, be holy not just a part

As the puzzled mind stays behind

Because of the speed of light, being kind

You will spark for what is all good

Healing each other the way we should

Where you and I come together

Where we understand it's gravity

Being is light as a feather.

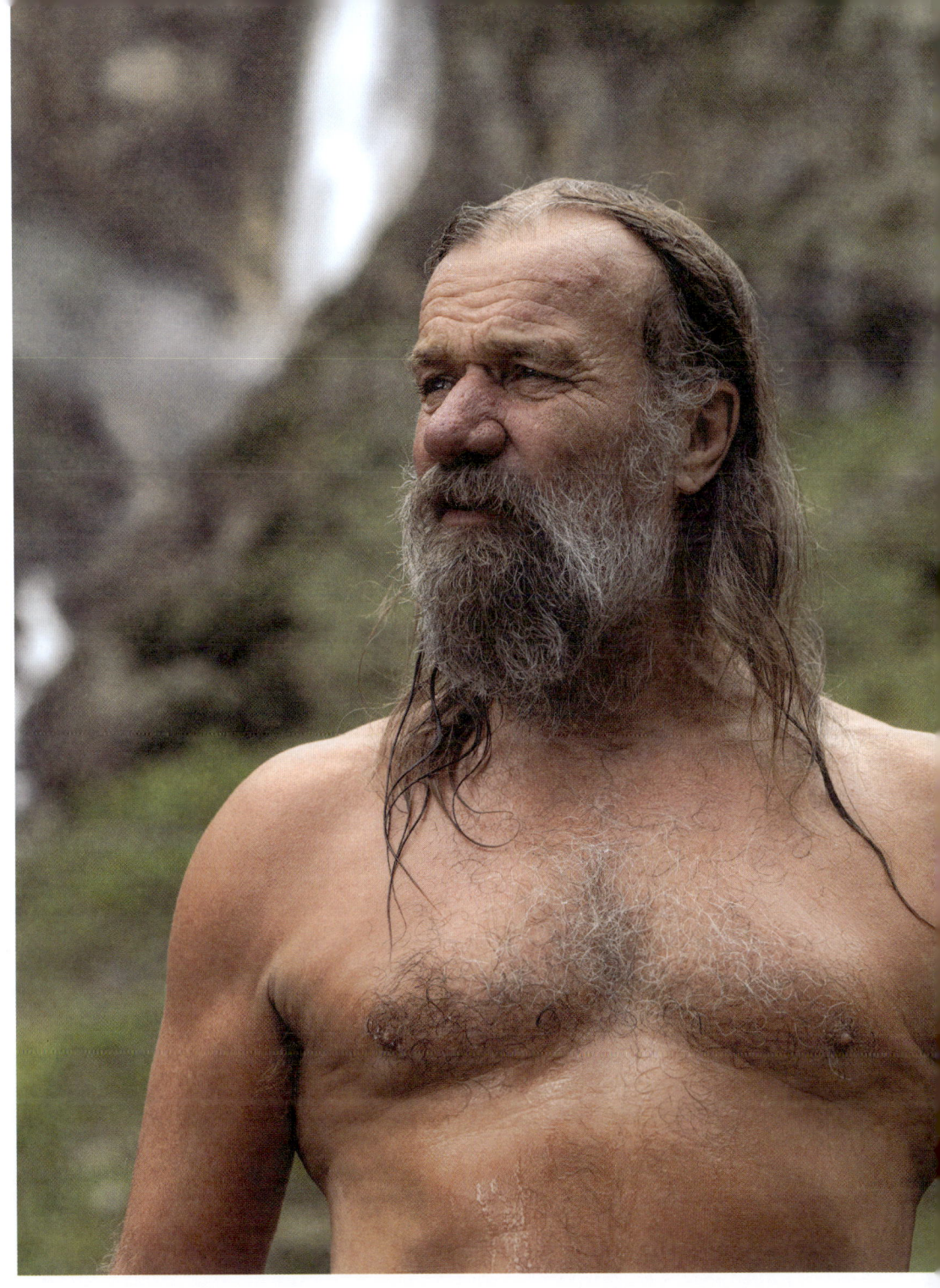

Feeling the power of it all, reflecting it back into nature.
Make the Soul be the predominant presence in life.

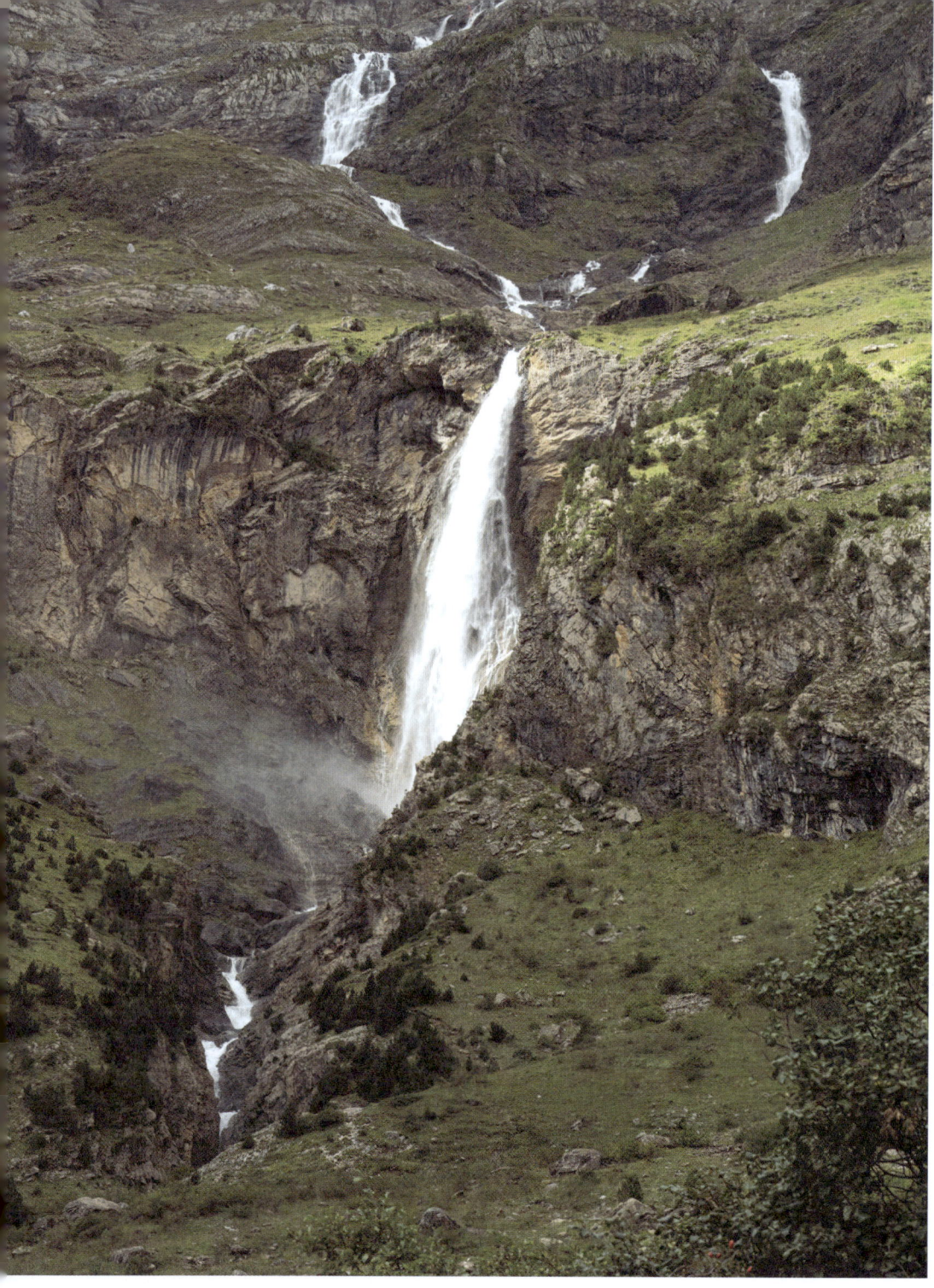

Nature has it. Had it. And is simply the best.
Pineta Valley in the Pyrenees. Let's go!

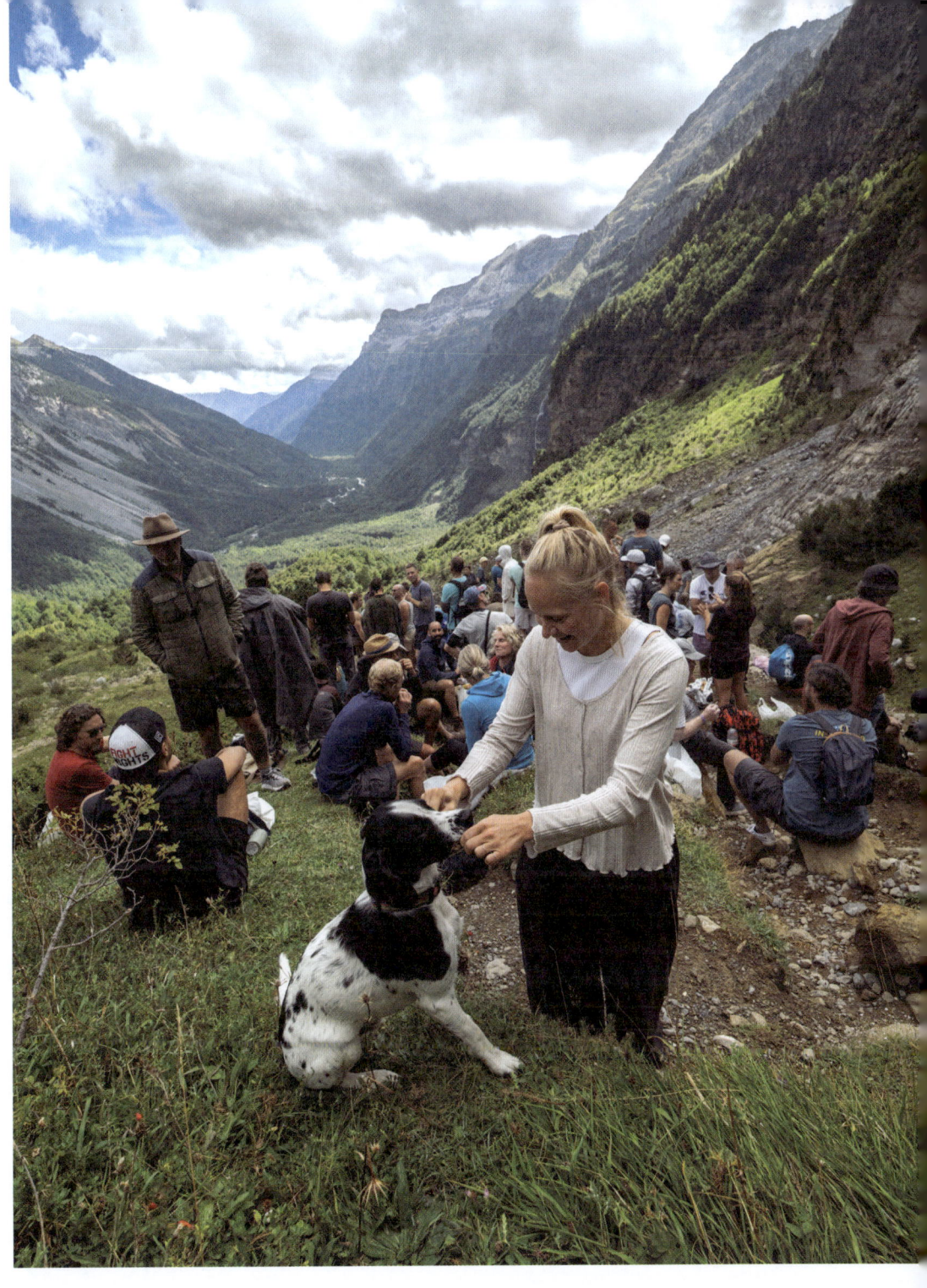

As a family together. So lucky to do
this with so many. Love, love, love.

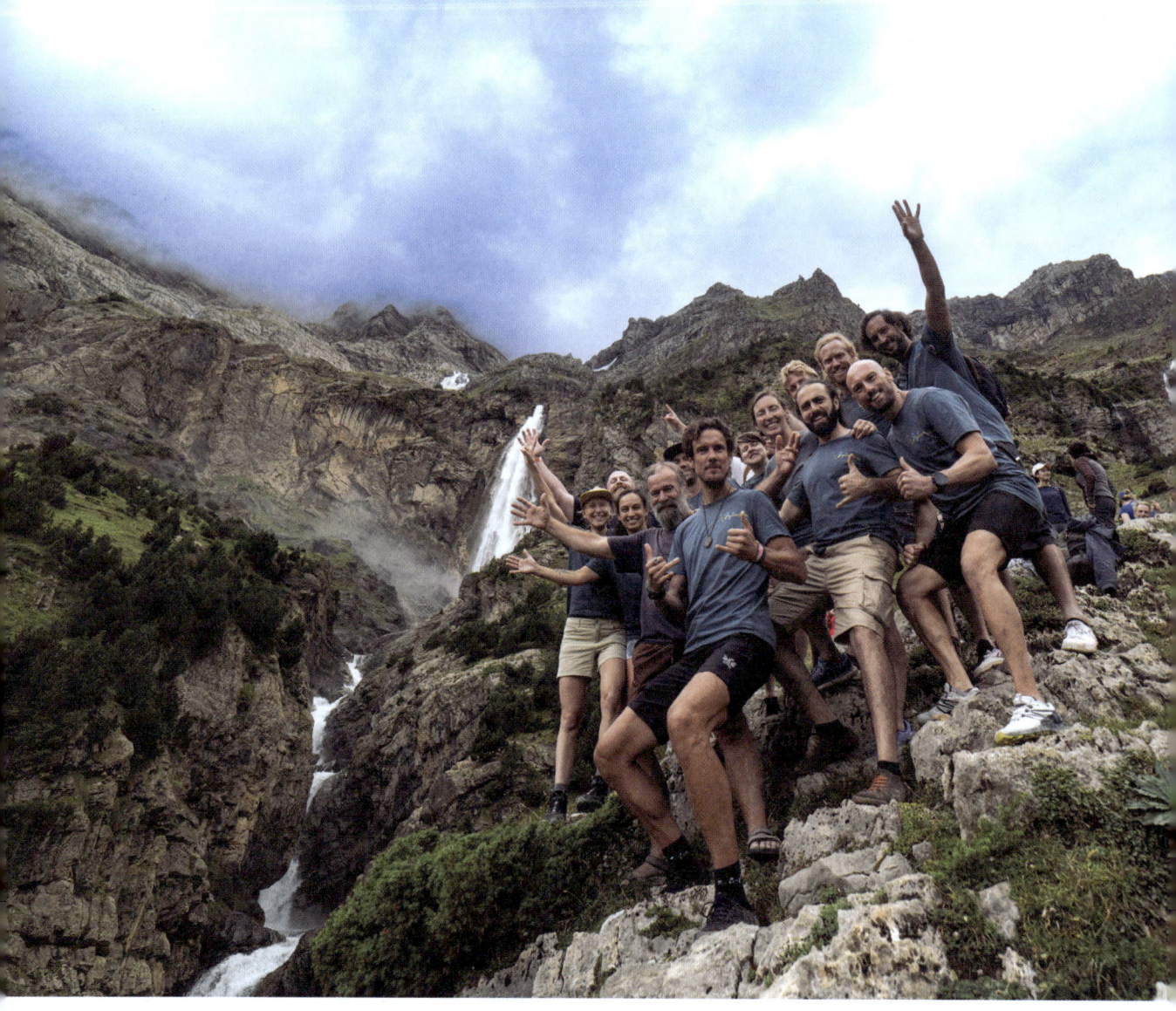

Wim Hof Method Instructors—my team!
A wall of love that can make all change
for the good. So grateful for it all.

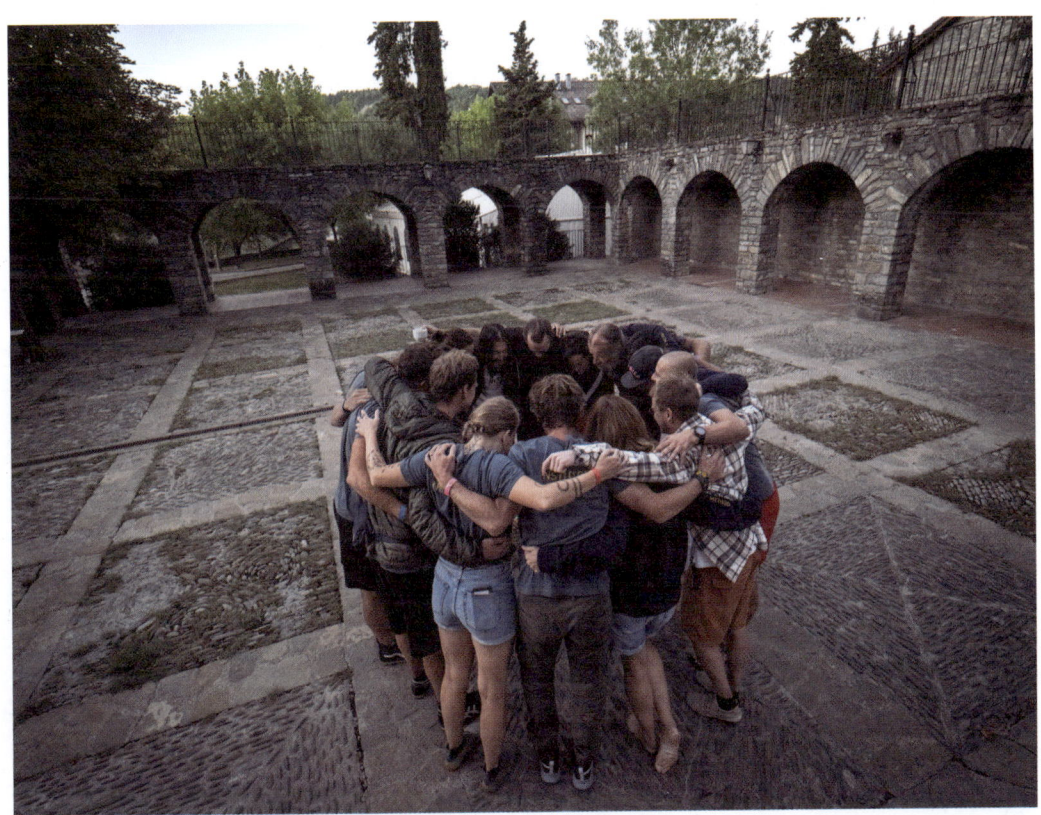

Coming together and sealing
unity through intention.

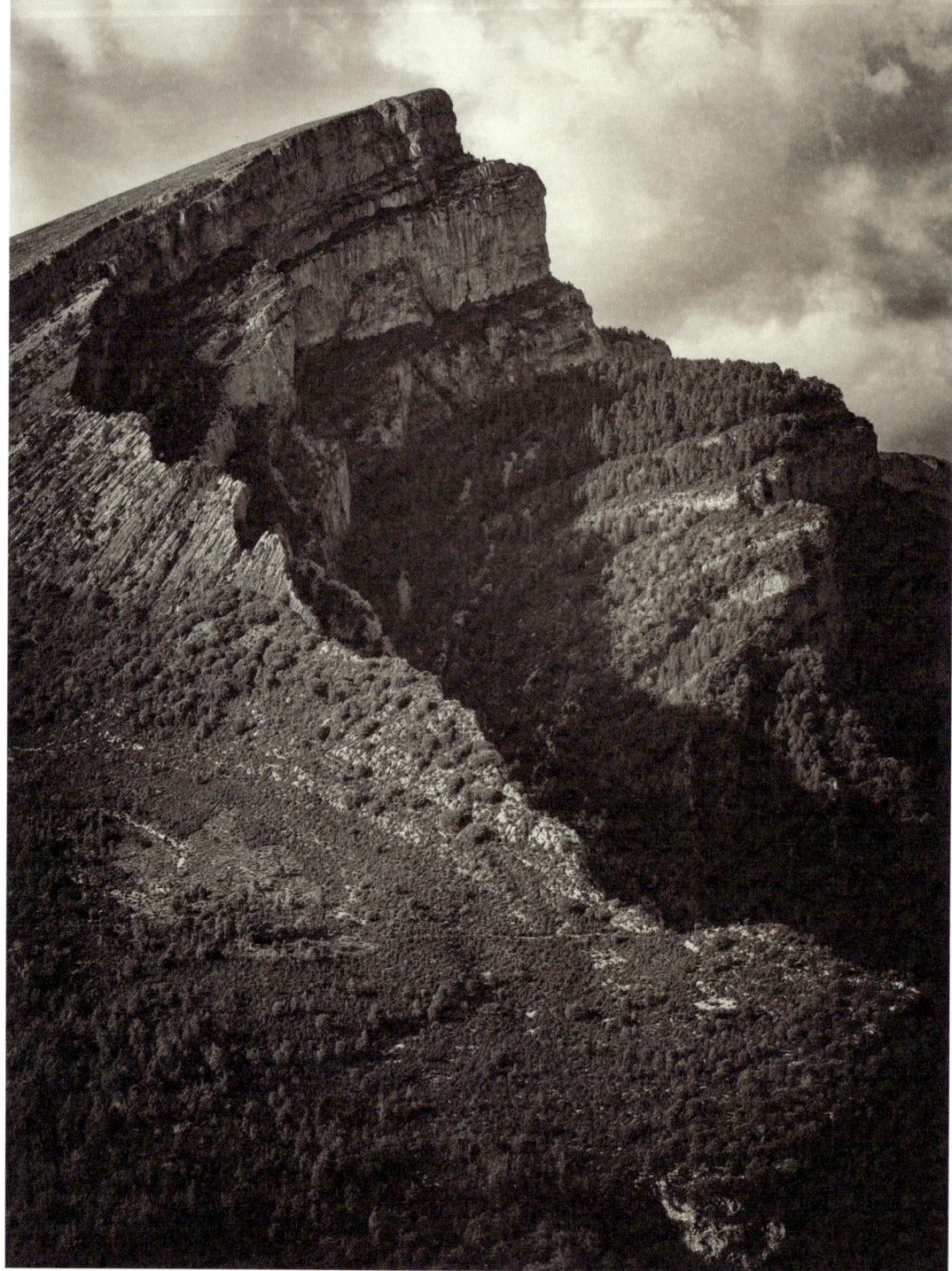

Mountains. Here the tectonic shifting through the geo
collision millions of years ago. The Pyrenees. You can
see the layers that were at the bottom of the sea. Let
your layers shine. We are all pieces of nature.

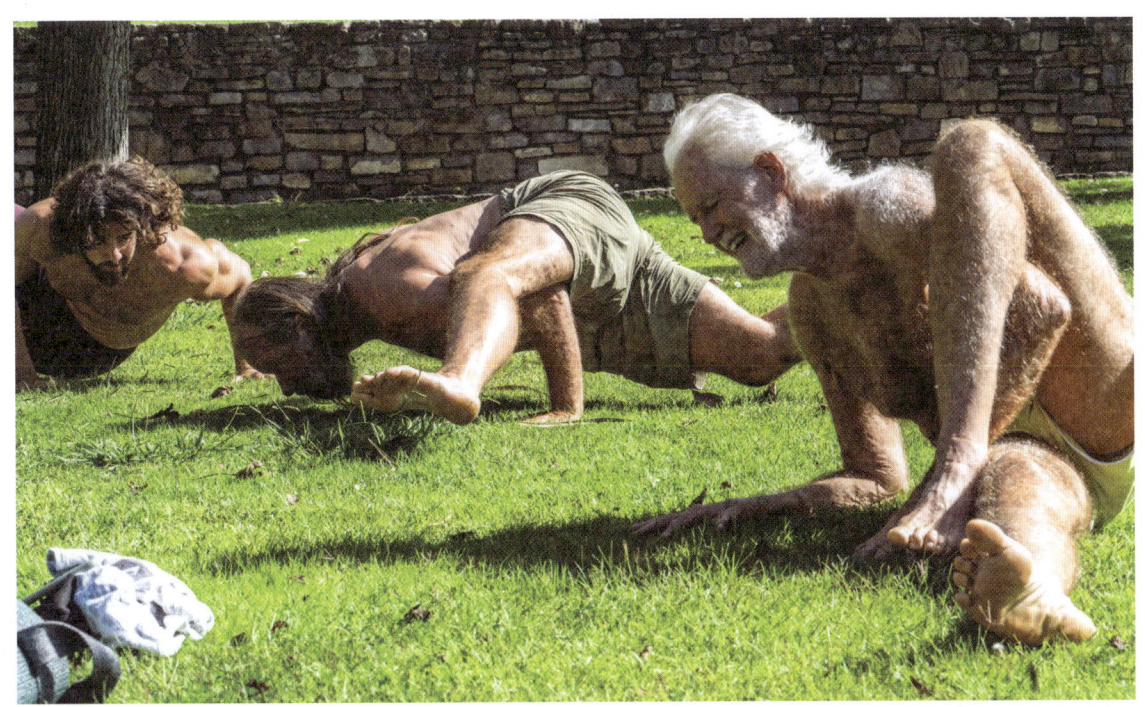

Still doing it after so many years. And
always great to do it together.

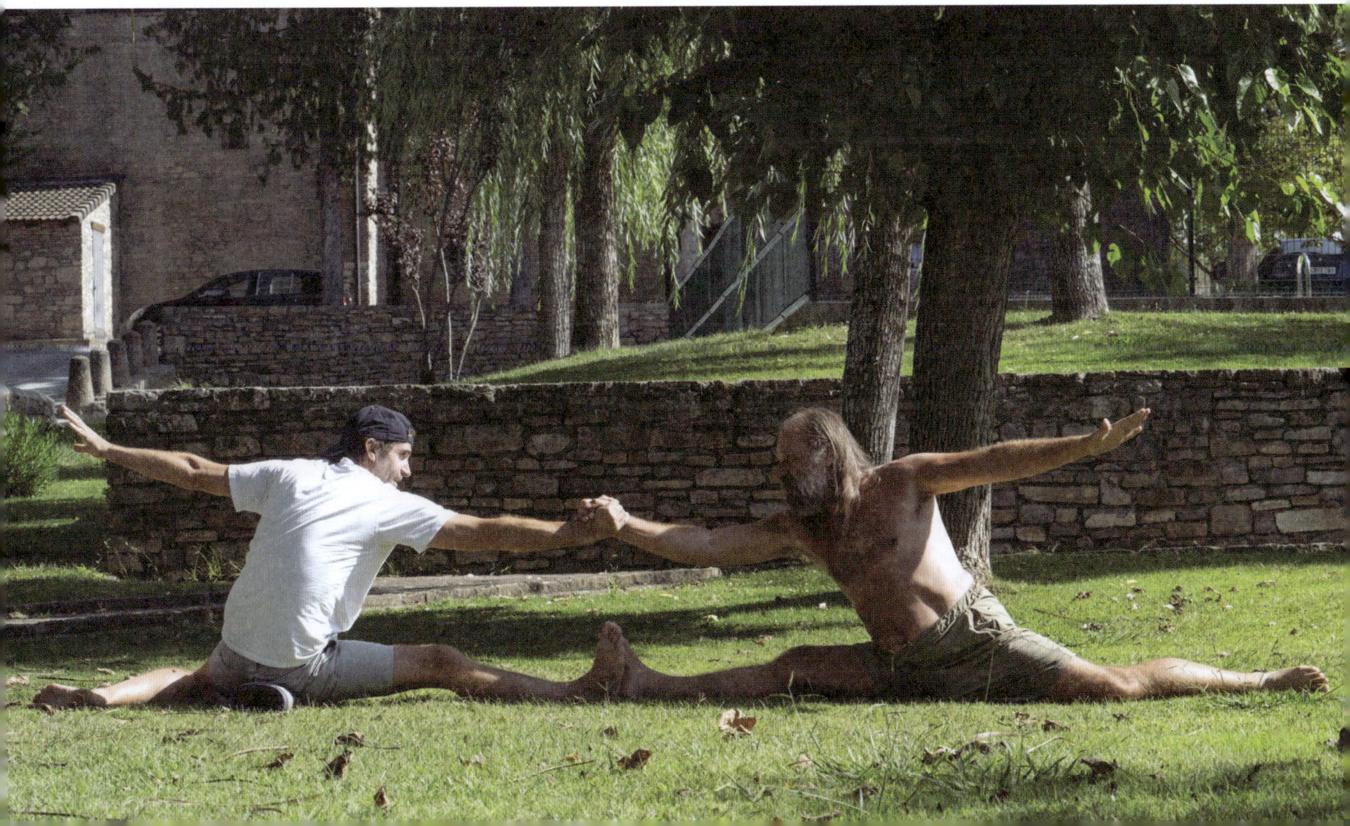

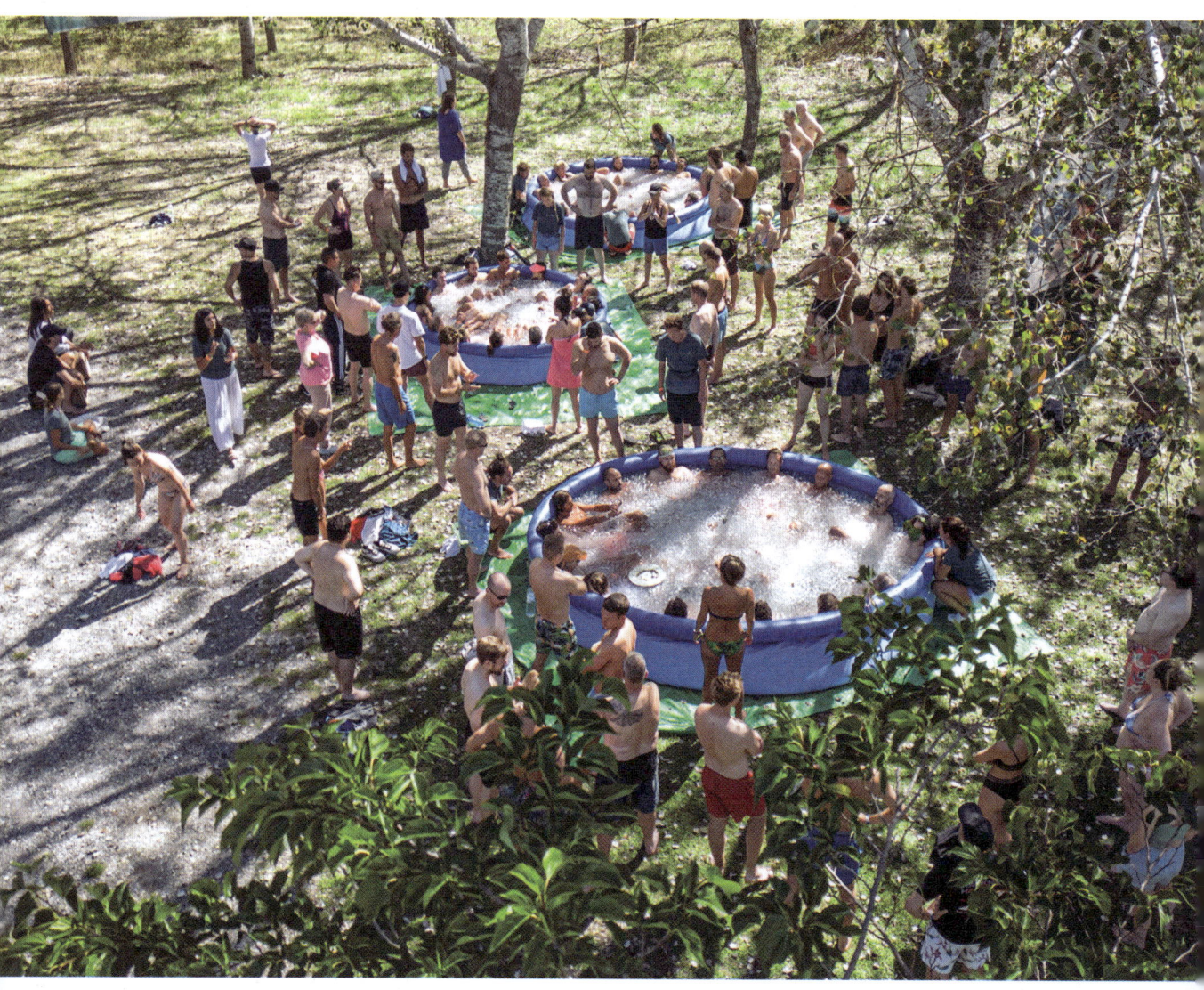

Ice baths as an almost ritualistic session.
Holy it is, or at least wholesome. No. Holy.

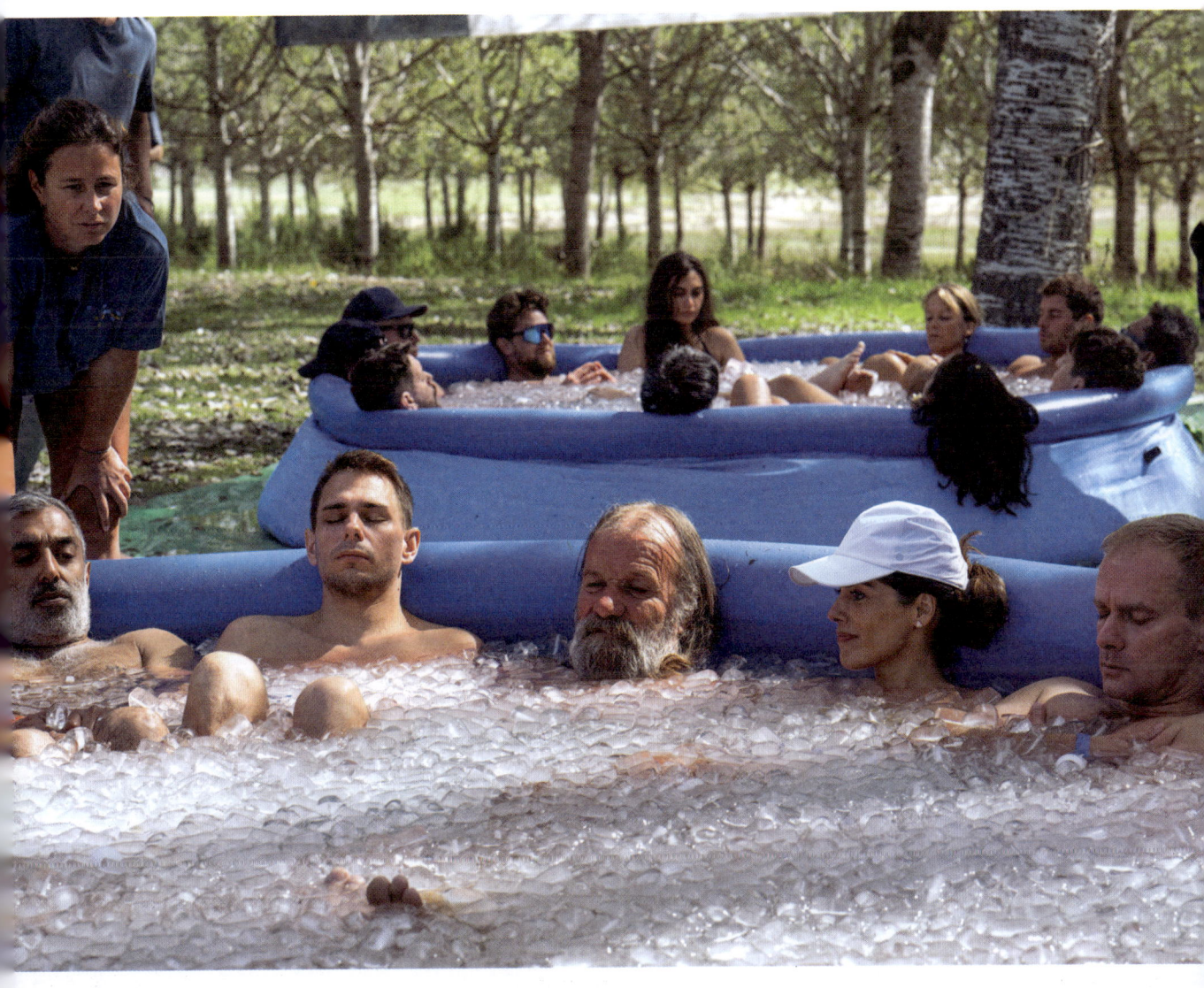

I join like everyone else. It's great to
share the energy. I love the community
all doing it. Real and strong.

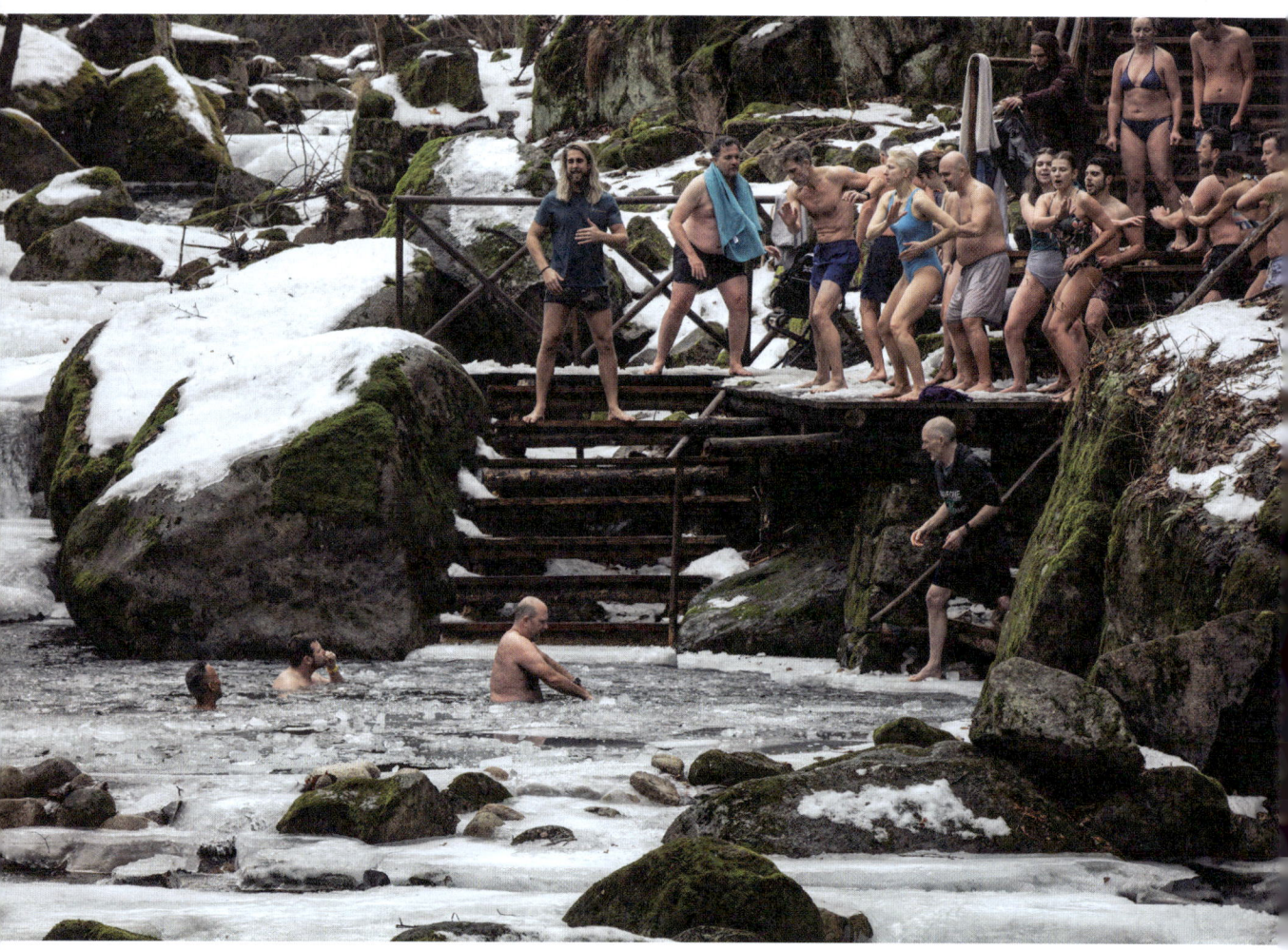

Heading down to the icy water, still seeing division and
tension, yet when you overcome that, you go beyond that mind—
you come together in unison. One mind, one body.

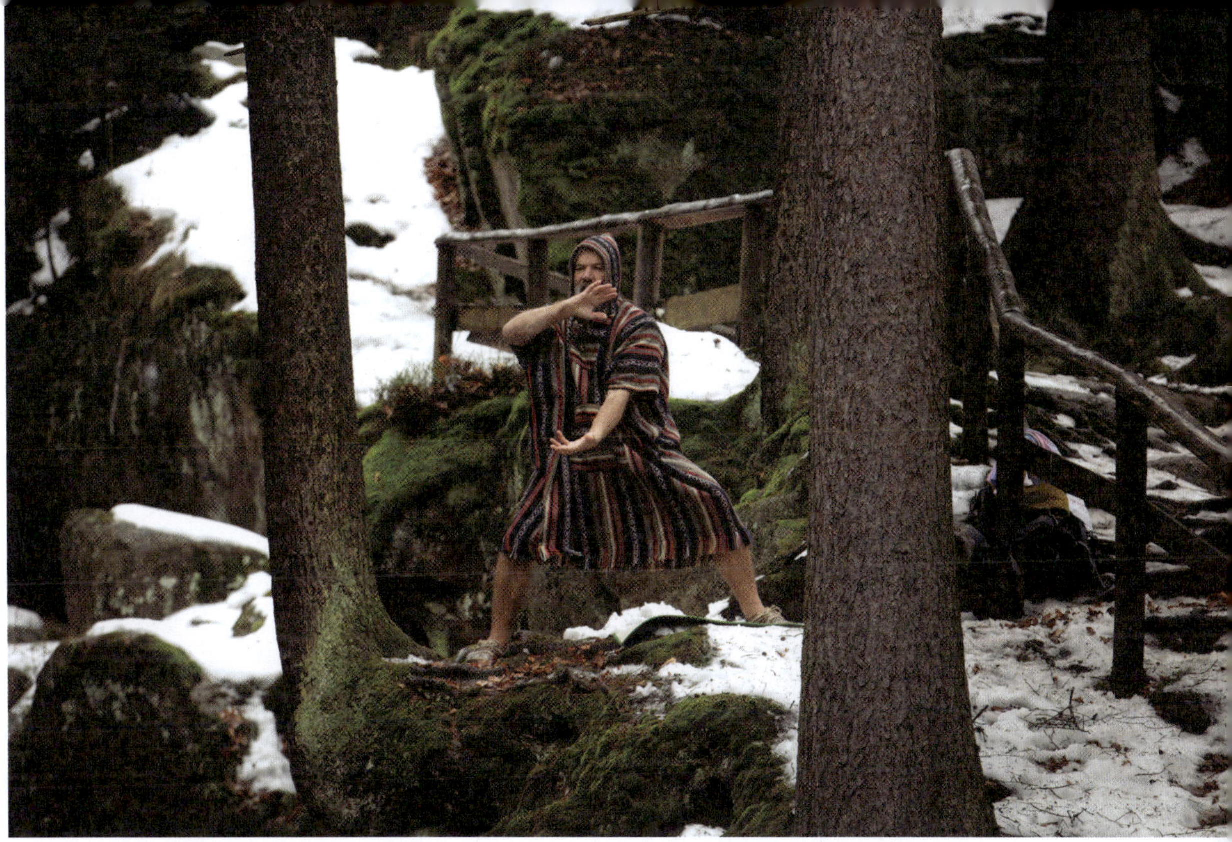

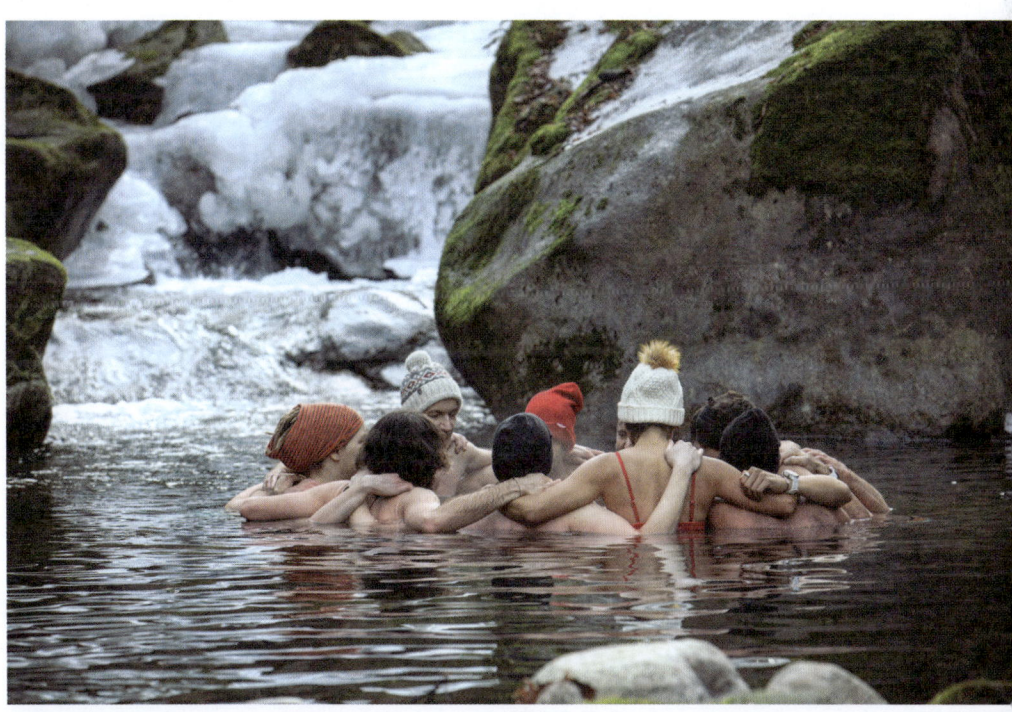

Horse stance at the Wodospad
(waterfall in Polish) in Przesieka.

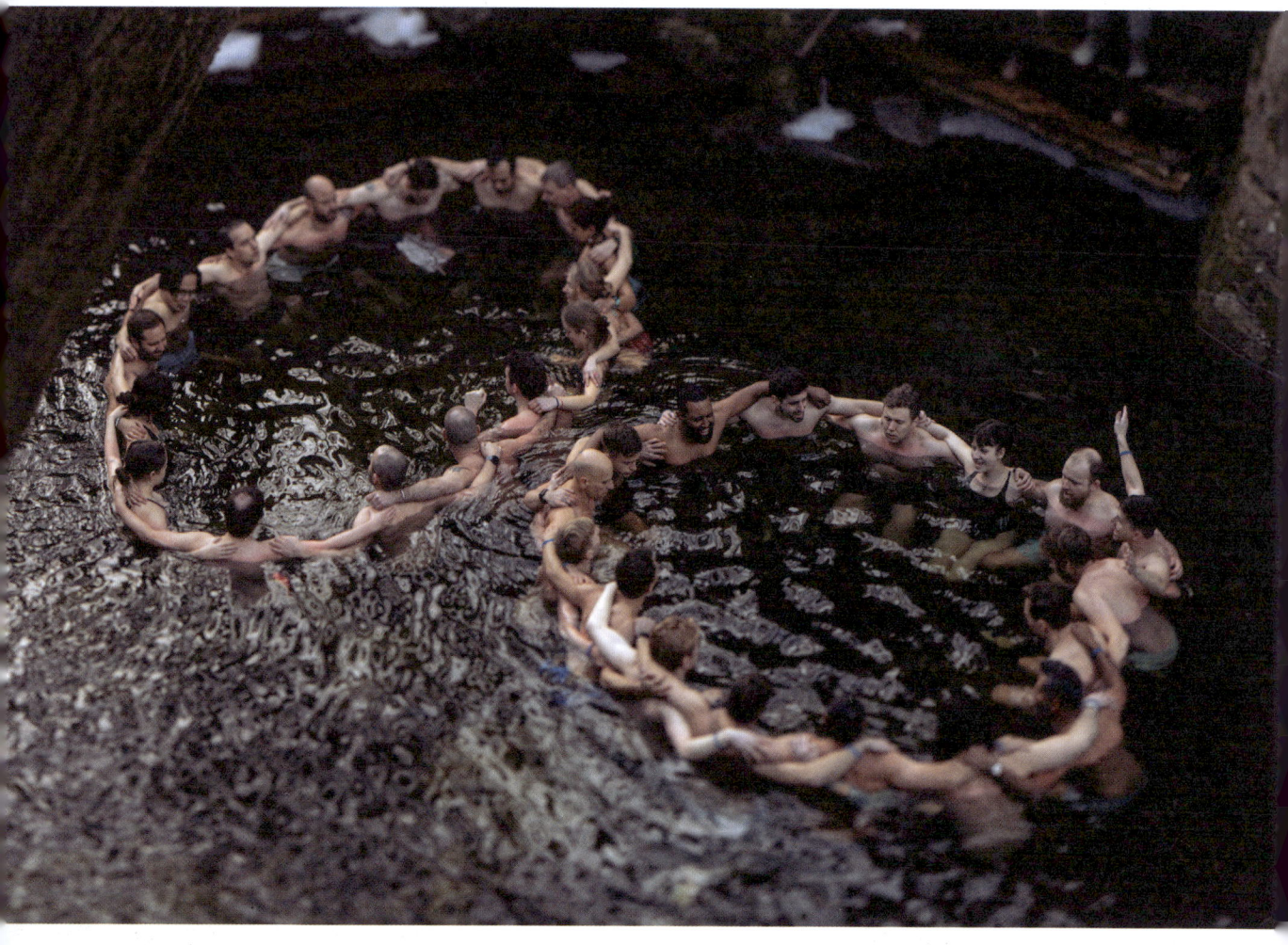

Circles have social power, an energetic connection.
So many people have come together in these
mystical waters. I'm so grateful to you all!

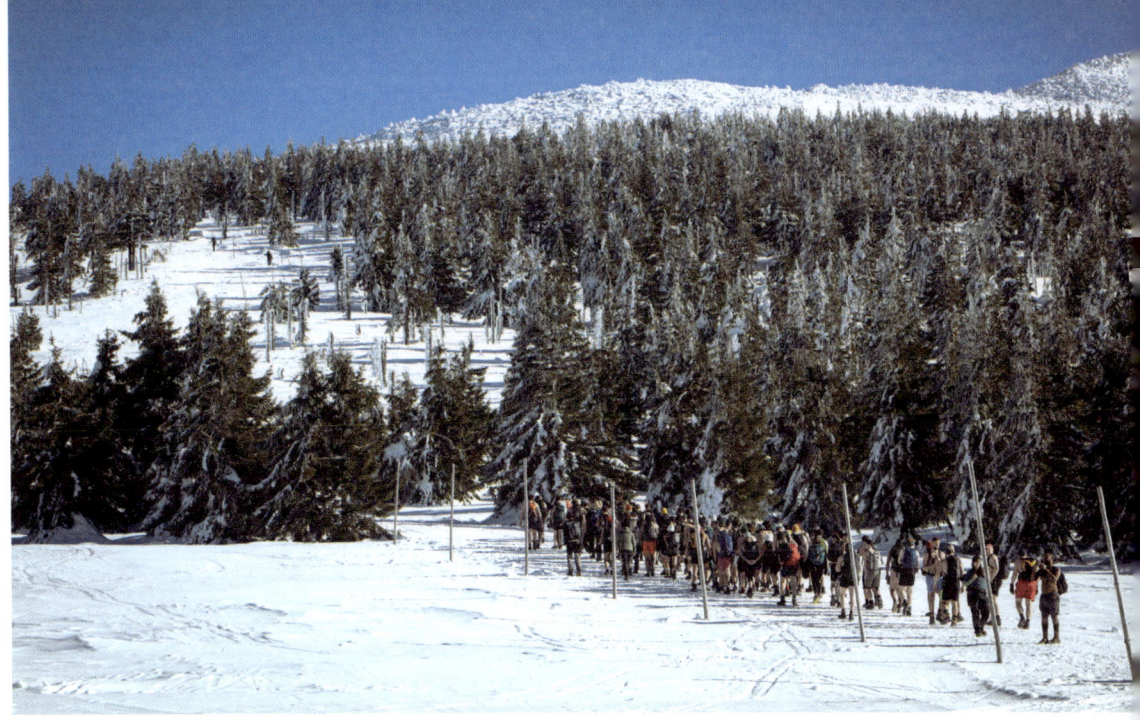

Climbing the mountain, the "holy mountain"—a sacred journey. It is not a competition. To go to the summit or not; it does not matter. The real summit is to get the best out of yourself. You are the leader there.

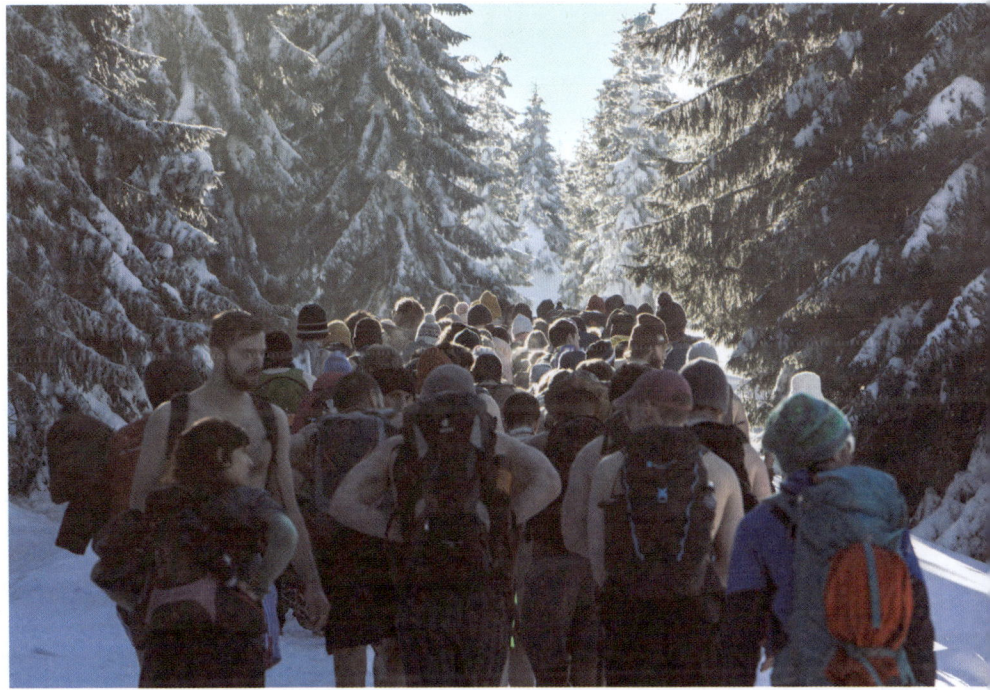

Mammals up mountains, over the world—we are mammals showing the same natural reflexes. Into the elements we go.

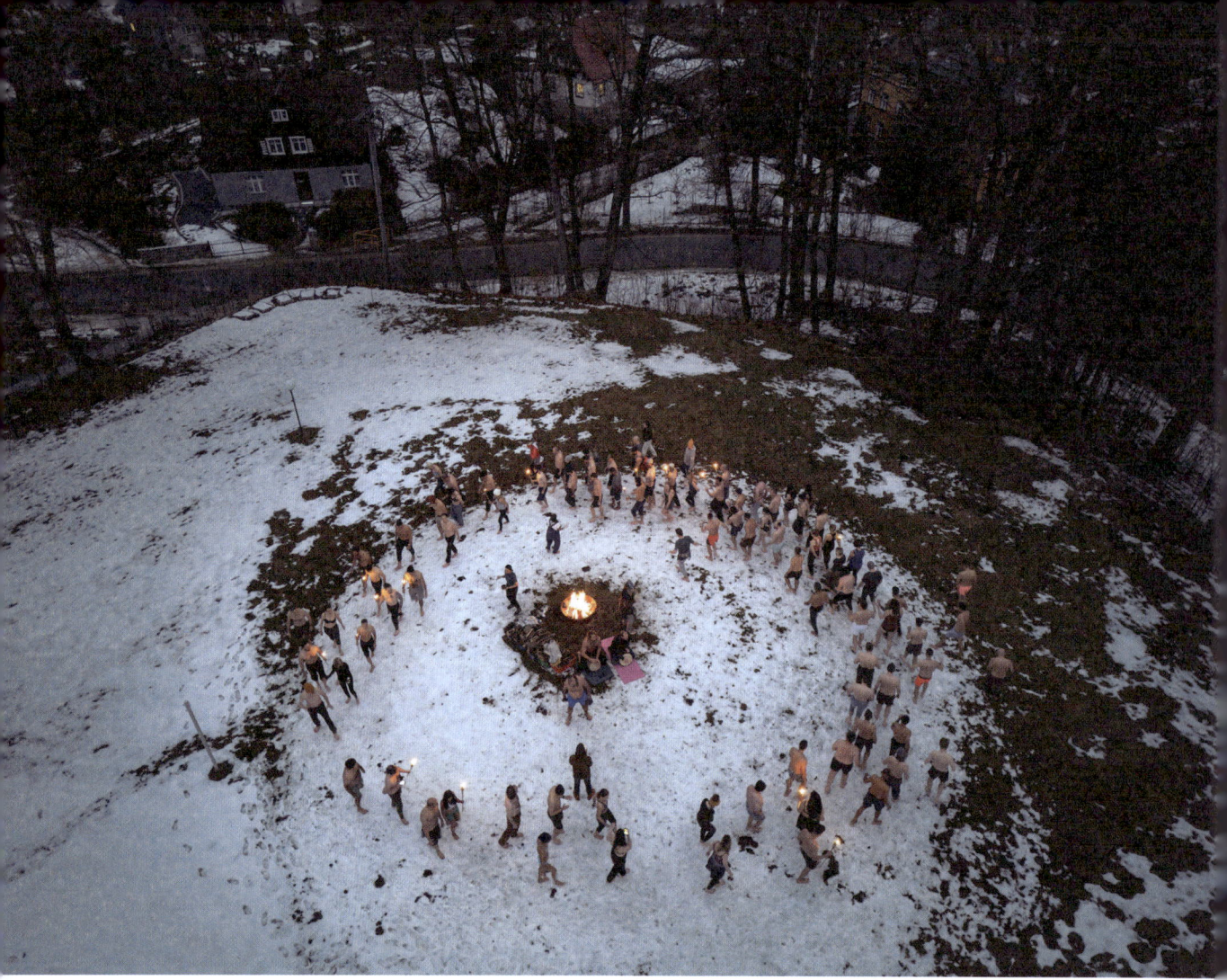

Community you find automatically, naturally, through barefoot exposure in the freezing cold. It seems so simple, but that's all it is. Get out there!

Love and power: is that not our human nature? Through this tribal bath, we remember, literally. We remember with our deeper physiology and tap into the power of social energy that is a big part of our humanity. Share it, together.

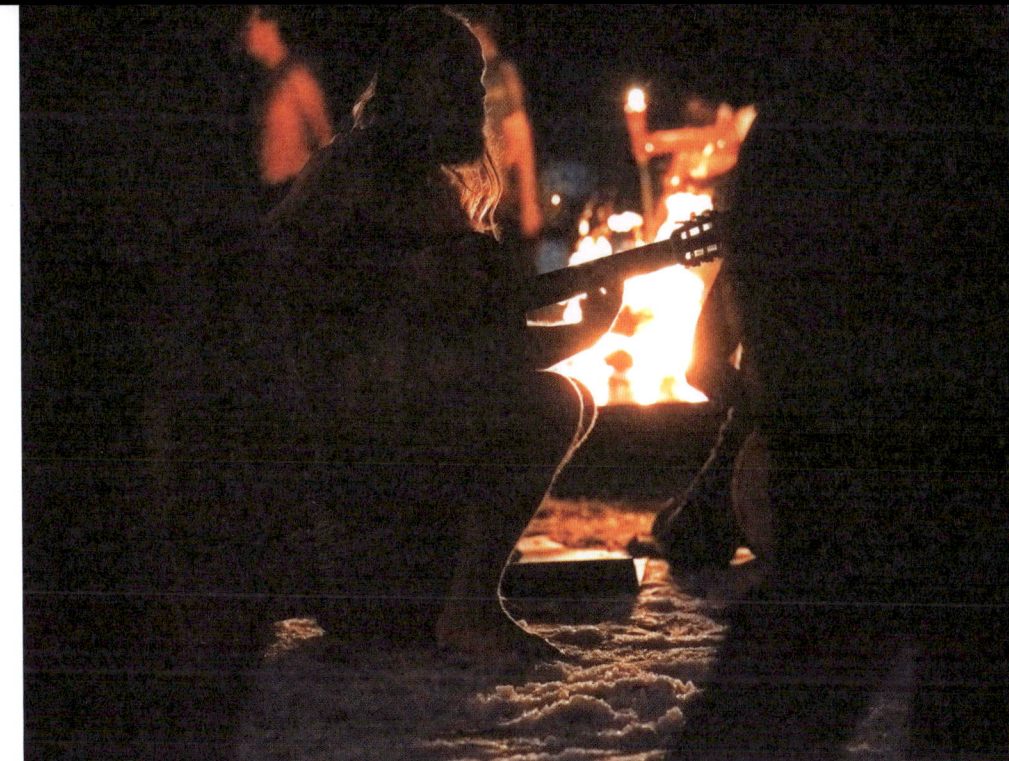

Of course, I join,
making music and
singing. Power
and love songs.
I love the mission,
people, sharing. We
have a good time, a
time for celebration.

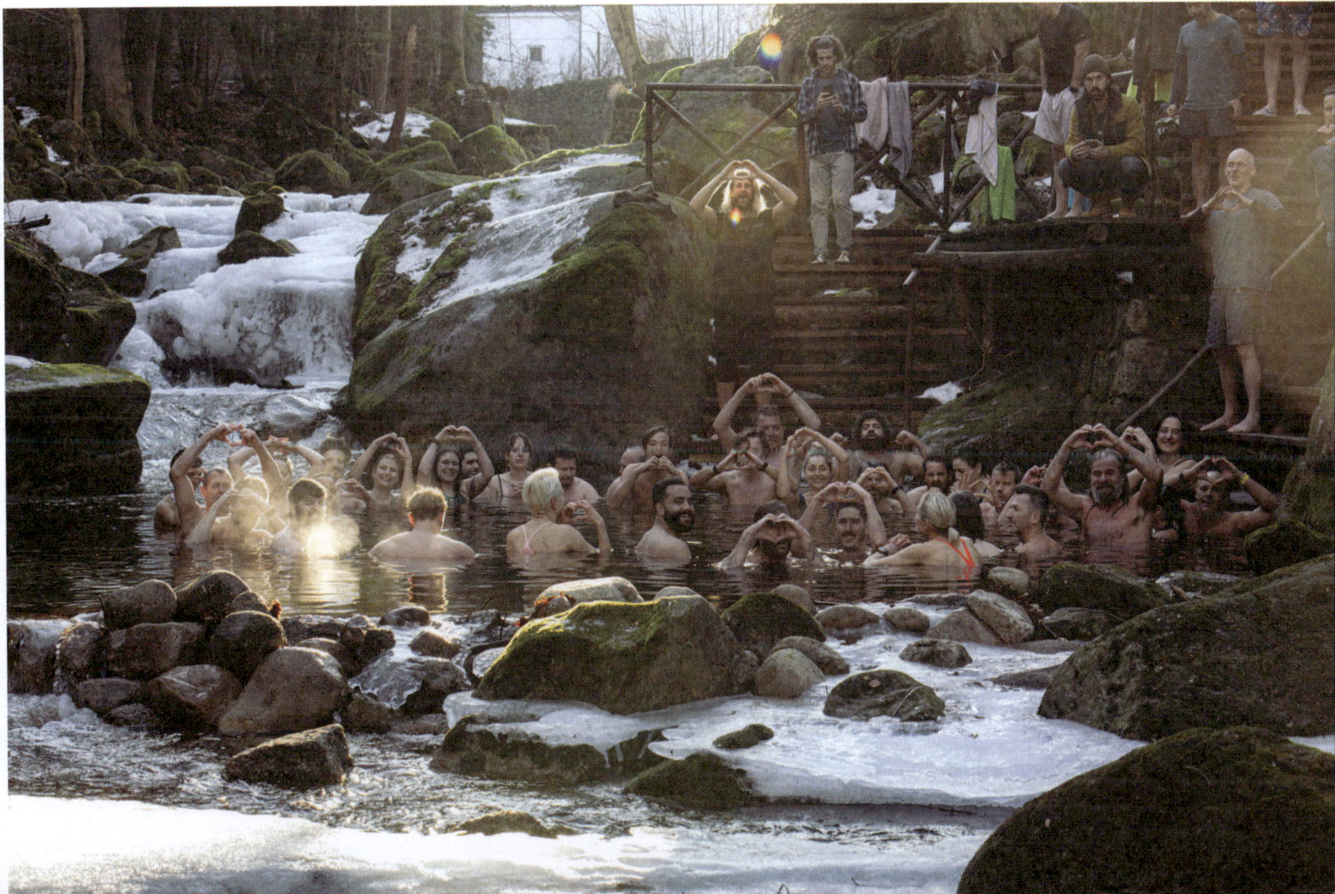

IN THE END, IT IS within the hardship of nature where we find real comfort. Go past your captive mind. Feel your essence. It is with you here and now. Go grab a guitar, go barefoot, dance, laugh, sing! Get back to who you are and what you are. It's just beautiful.

All the love, all the power.

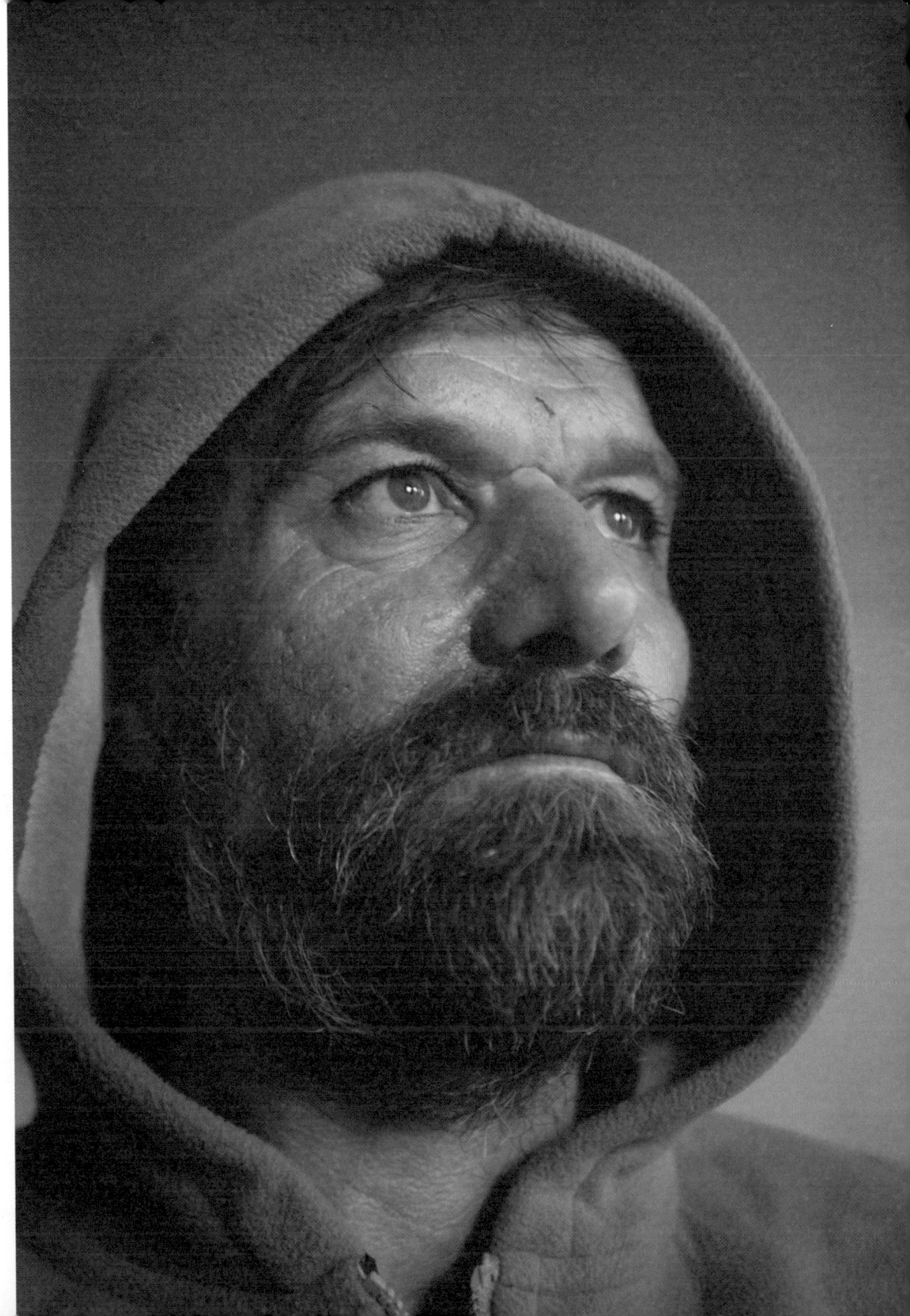

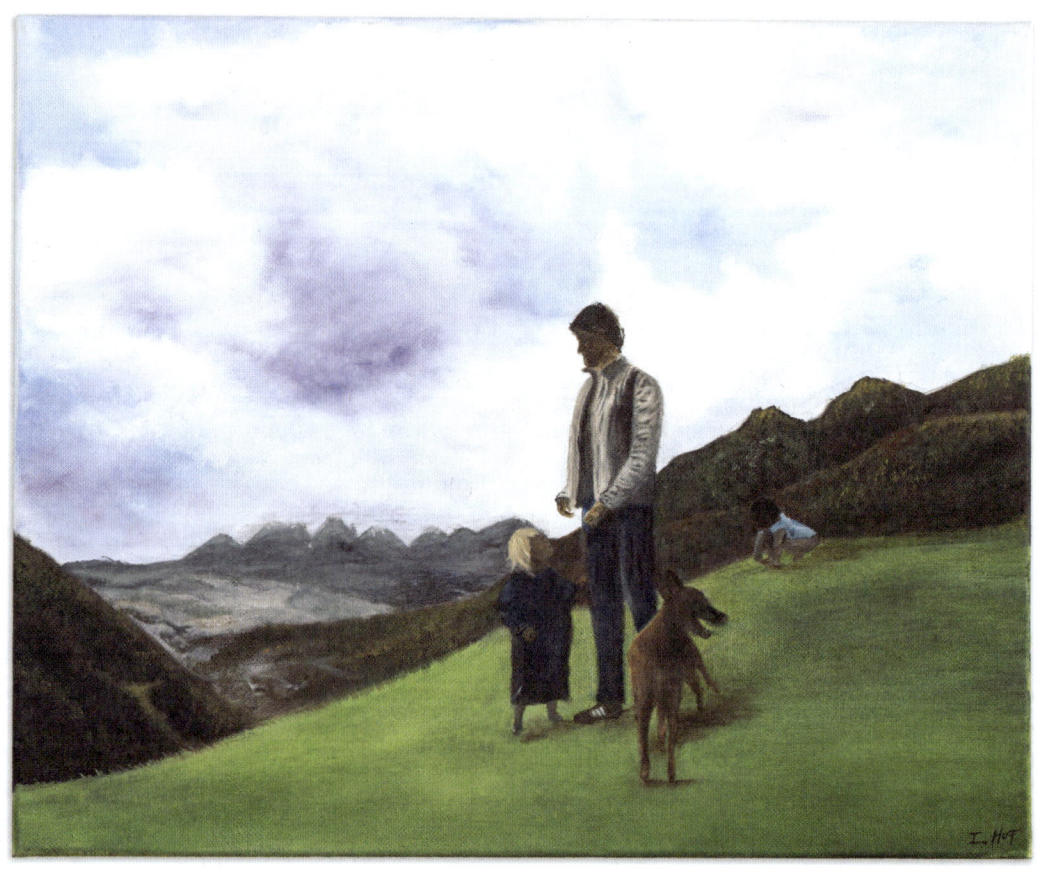

What once was. Painting by Isabelle Hof.

Acknowledgments

Wim Hof

WHAT A JOURNEY IT HAS been! Thank you, Henny, for picking up your camera all those years ago and believing in me when no one else did. This would not be possible without you. Thank you to Jaidree Braddix, Diana Ventimiglia, Tami Simon, and all the team at Sounds True for helping pull this all together with such enthusiasm and heart—and for loving my poems! To my children, who have helped carve out my destiny; still together, changing the world. I love you. To my partner, Erin, who pushes me to get to the core of it all. And to all the beautiful Souls who have become WHM instructors, you are like family to me. Thank you for helping us to change the world. They, along with all the wondrous people I have met over the years in Poland, Spain, the whole world—you fill my heart with gratitude. Pure wonders. I see your faces as I write this. You have all enriched my life and allowed my Soul to mirror. That is something we are gifted: pure experience. I have lost many people in my life, but I have also had the chance to share so much love with so many. I thank you all for that, for believing, for coming together. This is only the beginning!

Special respect to the ones who are flying above, beautiful Souls on their next adventures.

Salvatore, beautiful Olaya, and Javier. Shine on.

XX

Henny Boogert

I FEEL VERY GRATEFUL THAT, after many years of planning and preparation, this book could finally be published.

First, I would like to thank Wim for his patience while I was photographing him. He had to repeat various stunts over and over again, either because the camera was not ready, the light was not proper, or the angle had to be adjusted. Also, I am grateful for having the opportunity to visit some places of enormous natural beauty with Wim. Our cooperation has always been fun and reminds me of the youngsters we were when we met back in 1980s Amsterdam.

A big hug goes out to the team, Sounds True, Jaidree, and Erin, who did a fantastic job developing and producing this book.

Finally, I would like to thank Tobias Müller (text editing), Leonard van Vliet (some photo editing), and Bart Kuijpers Wentinck (Camera Nu scanning).

About Wim Hof

WIM HOF, AKA "THE ICEMAN," became known to the world through his extreme feats of endurance and exposure to cold—such as climbing Mount Kilimanjaro wearing only shorts and shoes, running a barefoot half marathon in the arctic circle, and standing in an ice-filled container for more than 112 minutes. Having embraced the majestic force of nature through decades of self-exploration leading to groundbreaking scientific studies, Wim has created a simple, effective way to stimulate deep physiological processes: the Wim Hof Method is a natural path to foundational health. Now practiced by millions, it has become a global health movement with ongoing university research worldwide.

Wim is a "man on a mission" to help humanity reshape our understanding of what the mind and body are truly capable of. Happiness, strength, and health for all. And it is only just the beginning . . .

About Henny Boogert

HENNY BOOGERT (1962) FIRST GOT into photography at age 16. His first camera was a Pentax ME Super. In 1983, he started his professional specialization at Gerrit Rietveld Academy Amsterdam, where he studied photography for two years. Originally fascinated by documentary photography, he has explored a broad range of other genres since—from apparel and food to nature, sports, reportage, and corporate.

Henny's work is typified by a process in which action and dynamics play essential roles. In many of his photographs we see people moving, not in a glamorous way, but with an emphasis on the purity of their actions, emotions, and facial expressions. His most outstanding project so far, entitled *Images Connect*, took him around the globe for several years capturing students in their rooms.

Henny always appreciates new challenges coming his way. Among the steady elements of his photography is the cooperation with Wim Hof, The Ice Man, which still continues after forty years.

About Sounds True

SOUNDS TRUE WAS FOUNDED IN 1985 by Tami Simon with a clear mission: to disseminate spiritual wisdom. Since starting out as a project with one woman and her tape recorder, we have grown into a multimedia publishing company with a catalog of more than 3,000 titles by some of the leading teachers and visionaries of our time, and an ever-expanding family of beloved customers from across the world.

In more than three decades of evolution, Sounds True has maintained our focus on our overriding purpose and mission: to wake up the world. We offer books, audio programs, online learning experiences, and in-person events to support your personal growth and awakening, and to unlock our greatest human capacities to love and serve.

At SoundsTrue.com you'll find a wealth of resources to enrich your journey, including our weekly *Insights at the Edge* podcast, free downloads, and information about our nonprofit Sounds True Foundation, where we strive to remove financial barriers to the materials we publish through scholarships and donations worldwide.

To learn more, please visit SoundsTrue.com/freegifts or call us toll-free at 800.333.9185.

Together, we can wake up the world.

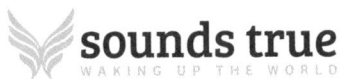